The Physics of
Radiation Therapy

The Physics of Radiation Therapy

FAIZ M. KHAN, Ph.D.

Professor
Department of Therapeutic Radiology
University of Minnesota Medical School
Director
Radiation Physics Section, University Hospitals
Minneapolis, Minnesota

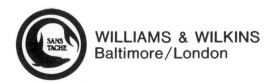
WILLIAMS & WILKINS
Baltimore/London

Editor: George Stamathis
Associate Editor: Jonathan W. Pine, Jr.
Copy Editor: Linda Jadlos
Design: Bert Smith
Production: Anne G. Seitz

Made in the United States of America

Library of Congress Cataloging in Publication Data

Main entry under title:
  Khan, Faiz M.
  The physics of radiation therapy.

  Includes index.
  1. Radiotherapy. 2. Medical physics. I. Title. [DNLM: 1. Radiation. 2. Radiotherapy. 3. Health physics. WN 100 K45p]
RM849.K43 1984   615.8'42'0153   84-5126 ISBN 0-683-04501-6

Composed and printed at the
Waverly Press, Inc.

*To my wife and friend Kathy
and daughters
Sarah, Yasmine and Rachel*

Preface

Most textbooks on radiological physics present a broad field which includes physics of radiation therapy, diagnosis, and nuclear medicine. The emphasis is on the basic physical principles which form a common foundation for these areas. Consequently, the topics of practical interest are discussed only sparingly or completely left out. The need is felt for a book solely dedicated to radiation therapy physics with emphasis on the practical details.

This book is written primarily with the needs of residents and clinical physicists in mind. Therefore, greater emphasis is given to the practice of physics in the clinic. For the residents, the book provides both basic radiation physics and physical aspects of treatment planning, using photon beams, electron beams, and brachytherapy sources. For the clinical physicist, additionally, current information is provided on dosimetry.

Except for some sections in the book dealing with the theory of absorbed dose measurements, the book should also appeal to the radiotherapy technologists. Of particular interest to them are the sections on treatment techniques, patient setups, and dosimetric calculations.

Since the book is designed for a mixed audience, a careful balance had to be maintained between theory and practical details. A conscious effort was made to make the subject palatable to those not formally trained in physics (*e.g.* residents and technicians) without diminishing the value of the book to the physicist. This object was hopefully achieved by a careful selection of the topics, simplification of the mathematical formalisms, and ample references to the relevant literature.

In developing this text, I have been greatly helped by my physics colleagues, Drs. Jeff Williamson, Chris Deibel, Barry Werner, Ed Cytacki, Bruce Gerbi, and Subhash Sharma. I wish to thank them for reviewing the text in its various stages of development. My great appreciation goes to Sandi Kuitunen who typed the manuscript and provided the needed organization for this lengthy project. I am also thankful to Kathy Mitchell and Lynne Olson who prepared most of the illustrations for the book.

Finally, I greatly value my association with Dr. Seymour Levitt, the chairman of this department, from whom I got much of the clinical philosophy I needed as a physicist.

FAIZ M. KHAN

Contents

CONTENTS

Check out some of these

CHAPTER 1

Structure of Matter

1.1 THE ATOM

All matter is composed of individual entities called elements. Each element is distinguishable from the others by the physical and chemical properties of its basic component—the atom. Originally thought to be the "smallest" and "indivisible" particle of matter, the atom is now known to have a substructure and can be "divided" into smaller components. Each atom consists of a small central core, the nucleus, where most of the atomic mass is located and a surrounding "cloud" of electrons moving in orbits around the nucleus. Whereas the radius of the atom (radius of the electronic orbits) is about 10^{-10} m, the nucleus has a much smaller radius, namely, about 10^{-14} m. Thus, for a particle of size comparable to nuclear dimensions, it will be quite possible to penetrate several atoms of matter before a collision happens. As will be pointed out in the chapters ahead, it is important to keep track of those particles that have not interacted with the atoms (the primary beam) and those that have suffered collisions (the scattered beam).

1.2 THE NUCLEUS

The properties of atoms are derived from the constitution of their nuclei and the number and the organization of the orbital electrons.

The nucleus contains two kinds of fundamental particles, protons and neutrons. Whereas protons are positively charged, neutrons have no charge. Since the electron has a negative *unit charge* (1.60×10^{-19} coulombs) and the proton has a positive unit charge, the number of protons in the nucleus is equal to the number of electrons outside the nucleus, thus making the atom electrically neutral.

An atom is completely specified by the formula $_{Z}^{A}X$, where X is the chemical symbol for the element, A is the *mass number*, defined as the number of nucleons (neutrons and protons in the nucleus), and Z is the *atomic number*, denoting the number of protons in the nucleus (or the number of electrons outside the nucleus). An atom represented in such a manner is also called a *nuclide*. For example, $_{1}^{1}H$ and $_{2}^{4}He$ represent atoms or nuclei or nuclides of hydrogen and helium, respectively.

On the basis of different proportions of neutrons and protons in the nuclei, atoms have been classified into the following categories: *isotopes*, atoms having nuclei with the same number of protons but different number of neutrons; *isotones*, having the same number of neutrons but different number of protons; *isobars*, with the same number of nucleons but different number of protons; and *isomers*, containing the same number of protons as well as neutrons. The last category, namely isomers, represents identical atoms except that they differ in their nuclear energy states. For example, $^{131m}_{54}$Xe (m stands for metastable state) is an isomer of $^{131}_{54}$Xe.

It has been observed that certain combinations of neutrons and protons result more in stable (nonradioactive) nuclides than others. For instance, stable elements in the low atomic number range have an almost equal number of neutrons, N, and protons, Z. However, as Z increases beyond about 20, the neutron to proton ratio for stable nuclei becomes greater than 1 and keeps on increasing with Z. This is evident in Fig. 1.1 which shows a plot of the ratios of neutrons to protons in stable nuclei.

Nuclear stability has also been analyzed in terms of even and odd number of neutrons and protons. Of about 300 different stable isotopes, more than half have even numbers of protons and neutrons, and are known as even-even nuclei. This suggests that nuclei gain stability when neutrons and protons are mutually paired. On the other hand, only four stable nuclei exist which have both odd Z and odd N, namely $^{2}_{1}$H, $^{6}_{3}$Li, $^{10}_{5}$B, and $^{14}_{7}$N. About 20% of the stable nuclei have even Z and odd N and about the same proportion have odd Z and even N.

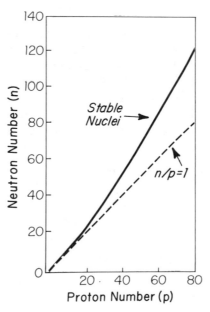

Figure 1.1.   A plot of neutrons *vs.* protons in stable nuclei.

1.3 ATOMIC MASS AND ENERGY UNITS

Masses of atoms and atomic particles are conveniently given in terms of atomic mass unit (amu). An amu is defined as $1/12$ of the mass of a $^{12}_{6}C$ nucleus, a carbon isotope. Thus, the nucleus of $^{12}_{6}C$ is arbitrarily assigned the mass equal to 12 amu. In basic units of mass,

$$1 \text{ amu} = 1.66 \times 10^{-27} \text{ kg}$$

The mass of an atom expressed in terms of amu is known as *atomic mass* or *atomic weight*. Another useful term is *gram atomic weight* which is defined as the mass in grams numerically equal to the atomic weight. According to Avogadro's hypothesis, every gram atomic weight of a substance contains the same number of atoms. The number, referred to as *Avogadro's number, N_A*, has been measured by many investigators and its currently accepted value is 6.0228×10^{23} atoms per gram atomic weight.

From the above definitions, one can calculate other quantities of interest such as the number of atoms per gram, grams per atom, and electrons per gram. Considering helium as an example, its atomic weight, A_W, is equal to 4.0026.

Therefore,

$$\text{Number atoms/g} = \frac{N_A}{A_W} = 1.505 \times 10^{23}$$

$$\text{Grams/atom} = \frac{A_W}{N_A} = 6.646 \times 10^{-24}$$

$$\text{Number electrons/g} = \frac{N_A \cdot Z}{A_W} = 3.009 \times 10^{23}$$

The masses of atomic particles, according to the atomic mass unit, are electron = 0.000548 amu, proton = 1.00727 amu, and neutron = 1.00866 amu.

Since the mass of an electron is much smaller than that of a proton or neutron and since protons and neutrons have nearly the same mass, equal to approximately 1 amu, all the atomic masses in units of amu are very nearly equal to the mass number. However, it is important to point out that the mass of an atom is not exactly equal to the sum of the masses of constituent particles. The reason for this is that, when the nucleus is formed, a certain mass is destroyed and converted into energy which acts as a "glue" to keep the nucleons together. This mass difference is called the *mass defect*. Looking at it from a different perspective, an amount of energy equal to the mass defect must be supplied to separate the nucleus into individual nucleons. Therefore, this energy is also called the *binding energy of the nucleus.*

The basic unit of energy is the joule and is equal to the work done when a force of 1 newton acts through a distance of 1 m. The newton, in turn, is a unit of force given by the product of mass (1 kg) and acceleration (1 m/sec^2). However, a more convenient energy unit in atomic and nuclear physics is the electron volt (eV), defined as the kinetic energy acquired by an electron in passing through a potential difference of 1 V. It can be shown that the work done in this case is given by the product of potential difference and the charge on the electron. Therefore, we have:

$$1 \text{ eV} = 1 \text{ V} \times 1.607 \times 10^{-19} \text{ coulombs} = 1.602 \times 10^{-19} \text{ J}$$

Multiples of this unit are:

$$1 \text{ keV} = 1000 \text{ eV}$$

$$1 \text{ million eV (MeV)} = 10^6 \text{ eV}$$

According to the Einstein's *principle of equivalence of mass and energy*, a mass m is equivalent to energy E and the relationship is given by

$$E = mc^2 \tag{1.1}$$

where c is the velocity of light (3×10^8 m/sec). For example, a mass of 1 kg, if converted to energy, is equivalent to

$$E = 1 \text{ kg} \times (3 \times 10^8 \text{ m/sec})^2$$

$$= 9 \times 10^{16} \text{ J} = 5.62 \times 10^{29} \text{ MeV}$$

The mass of an electron at rest is sometimes expressed in terms of its energy equivalent, E_0. Since its mass is 9.1×10^{-31} kg, we have from Equation 1.1:

$$E_0 = 0.511 \text{ MeV}$$

Another useful conversion is that of amu to energy. It can be shown that:

$$1 \text{ amu} = 931 \text{ MeV}$$

1.4 DISTRIBUTION OF ORBITAL ELECTRONS

According to the model proposed by Niels Bohr in 1913, the electrons revolve around the nucleus in specific orbits and are prevented from leaving the atom by the centripetal force of attraction between the positively charged nucleus and the negatively charged electron.

On the basis of classical physics, an accelerating or revolving electron must radiate energy. This would result in a continuous decrease of the radius of the orbit with the electron eventually spiraling into the nucleus. However, the data on the emission or absorption of radiation by elements reveal that the change of energy is not continuous but discrete. To explain the observed line spectrum of hydrogen, Bohr theorized that the sharp lines of the spectrum represented electron jumps from one orbit down to another with the emission of light of a particular frequency or a quantum of energy. He proposed two fundamental postulates: 1) electrons can exist only in those orbits for which

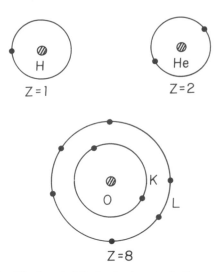

Figure 1.2. Electron orbits for hydrogen, helium, and oxygen.

the angular momentum of the electron is an integral multiple of $h/2\pi$, where h is the Planck's constant (6.62×10^{-34} J-sec); 2) no energy is gained or lost while the electron remains in any one of the permissible orbits.

The arrangement of electrons outside the nucleus is governed by the rules of quantum mechanics and the Pauli exclusion principle (not discussed here). Although the actual configuration of electrons is rather complex and dynamic, one may simplify the concept by assigning electrons to specific orbits. The innermost orbit or shell is called the K shell. The next shells are L, M, N, and O. The maximum number of electrons in an orbit is given by $2n^2$, where n is the orbit number. For example, a maximum of 2 electrons can exist in the first orbit, 8 in the second, and 18 in the third. Figure 1.2 shows the electron orbits of hydrogen, helium, and oxygen atoms.

Electron orbits can also be considered as energy levels. The energy in this case is the potential energy of the electrons. With the opposite sign it may also be called as the *binding energy* of the electron.

1.5 ATOMIC ENERGY LEVELS

It is customary to represent the energy levels of the orbital electrons by what is known as the *energy level diagram* (Fig. 1.3). The binding energies of the electrons in various shells depend on the magnitude of Coulomb force of attraction between the nucleus and the orbital electrons. Thus, the binding energies for the higher Z atoms are greater because of the greater nuclear charge. In the case of tungsten ($Z = 74$), the electrons in the K, L, and M shells have binding energies of about 69,500, 11,000, and 2,500 eV, respectively. The so-called valence electrons, which are responsible for chemical reactions and bonds between atoms as well as the emission of optical radiation spectra, normally occupy the outer shells. If energy is imparted to one of these valence

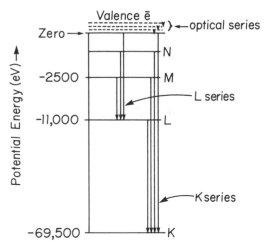

Figure 1.3. A simplified energy level diagram of the tungsten atom (not to scale). Only few possible transitions are shown for illustration. Zero of the energy scale is arbitrarily set at the position of the valence electrons when the atom is in the unexcited state.

electrons to raise it to a higher energy (higher potential energy but lower binding energy) orbit, this will create a state of atomic instability. The electron will fall back to its normal position with the emission of energy in the form of optical radiation. The energy of the emitted radiation will be equal to the energy difference of the orbits between which the transition took place.

If the transition involved inner orbits, such as K, L, and M shells where the electrons are more tightly bound (because of larger coulomb forces), the absorption or emission of energy will involve higher energy radiation. Also, if sufficient energy is imparted to an inner orbit electron so that it is completely ejected from the atom, the vacancy or the hole created in that shell will be almost instantaneously filled by an electron from a higher level orbit, resulting in the emission of radiation. This is the mechanism for the production of *characteristic x-rays*.

1.6 NUCLEAR FORCES

As discussed earlier, the nucleus contains neutrons which have no charge and protons with positive charge. But how are these particles held together, in spite of the fact that electrostatic repulsive forces exist between particles of similar charge? Earlier, in Section 1.3, the terms mass defect and binding energy of the nucleus were mentioned. It was then suggested that the energy required to keep the nucleons together is provided by the mass defect. However, the nature of the forces involved in keeping the integrity of the nucleus is quite complex and will be discussed here only briefly.

The only forces in nature are the following: nuclear, electrostatic, magnetic, and gravitational. Of these, the magnetic and gravitational forces involved in the nucleus are very weak. The electrostatic force is quite strong but it is repulsive and tends to disrupt the nucleus. A force much larger than the electrostatic force is the *nuclear force* that accounts of the binding energy of nuclei.

The nuclear force is a *short range force* which comes into play when the distance between the nucleons becomes smaller than the nuclear diameter ($\sim 10^{-14}$ m). If we assume that a nucleon has zero potential energy when it is an infinite distance apart from the nucleus, then as it approaches close enough to the nucleus to be within the range of nuclear forces, it will experience strong attraction and will "fall" into the *potential well* (Fig. 1.4a). This potential well is formed as a result of the mass defect and provides the nuclear binding energy. It acts as a *potential barrier* against any nucleon escaping the nucleus.

In the case of a positively charged particle approaching the nucleus, there will be a potential barrier due to the coulomb forces of repulsion, preventing the particle from approaching the nucleus. If, however, the particle is able to get close enough to the nucleus so as to be within the range of the nuclear forces, the repulsive forces will be overcome and the particle will be able to enter the nucleus. Figure 1.4b illustrates the potential barrier against a charged particle such as an α particle (traveling $^4_2$He nucleus) approaching a $^{238}_{92}$U nucleus. Conversely, the barrier serves to prevent an α particle escaping from the nucleus. Although it appears, according to the classical ideas, that an α particle would require a minimum energy equal to the *height of the potential barrier* (30 MeV) in order to penetrate the $^{238}_{92}$U nucleus or escape from it, the

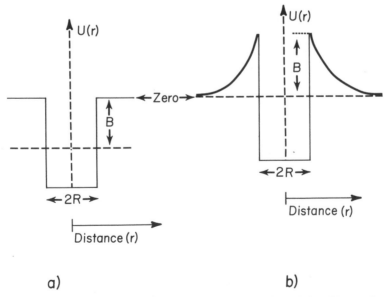

a)   b)

Figure 1.4. Energy level diagram of a particle in a nucleus: a) particle with no charge; b) particle with positive charge; $U(r)$ is the potential energy as a function of distance r from the center of the nucleus. B is the barrier height; R is the nuclear radius.

data show that the barrier can be crossed with much lower energies. This has been explained by a complex mathematical theory known as wave mechanics, in which particles are considered to be associated with de Broglie waves.

1.7 NUCLEAR ENERGY LEVELS

The shell model of the nucleus assumes that the nucleons are arranged in shells representing discrete energy states of the nucleus similar to the atomic energy levels. If energy is imparted to the nucleus, it may be raised to an excited state, and when it returns to a lower energy state, it will give off energy equal to the energy difference of the two states. Sometimes the energy is radiated in steps, corresponding to the intermediate energy states, before the nucleus settles down to the stable or ground state.

Figure 1.5 shows an energy level diagram with a decay scheme for a cobalt-60 ($^{60}_{27}$Co) nucleus which has been made radioactive in a reactor by bombarding stable $^{59}_{27}$Co atoms with neutrons. The excited $^{60}_{27}$Co nucleus first emits a particle, known as β^- particle and then, in two successive jumps, emits packets of energy, known as photons. The emission of a β^- particle is the result of a nuclear transformation in which one of the neutrons in the nucleus disintegrates into a proton, an electron, and a neutrino. The electron and neutrino are emitted instantaneously and share the released energy with the recoiling nucleus. The process of β decay will be discussed in the next chapter.

1.8 PARTICLE RADIATION

The term radiation applies to the emission and propagation of energy through space or a material medium. By particle radiation we mean energy propagated by traveling corpuscles that have a definite rest mass and within limits have a definite momentum and defined position at any instant. However, the distinction between particle radiation and electromagnetic waves, both of which represent modes of energy travel, became less sharp when, in 1925, de

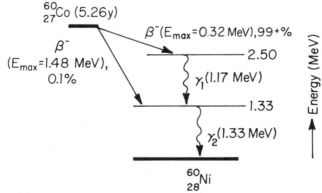

Figure 1.5.   Energy level diagram for the decay of $^{60}_{27}$Co nucleus.

Table 1.1.
Elementary particles*

Particle	Symbol	Charge	Mass
Electron	e^-, β^-	-1	0.000548 amu
Positron	e^+, β^+	$+1$	0.000548 amu
Proton	$p, {}^1_1H^+$	$+1$	1.00727 amu
Neutron	$n, {}^1_0n$	0	1.00866 amu
Neutrino	ν	0	$<1/2000\ m_0$†
Mesons	Π^+, Π^-	$+1, -1$	$273\ m_0$
	Π°	0	$264\ m_0$
	μ^+, μ^-	$+1, -1$	$207\ m_0$
	K^+, K^-	$+1, -1$	$967\ m_0$
	K°	0	$973\ m_0$

* This is only a partial list. Many other elementary particles besides the common ones listed above have been discovered.
† (m_0 = rest mass of an electron).

Broglie introduced a hypothesis concerning the dual nature of matter. He theorized that not only do photons (electromagnetic waves) sometimes appear to behave like particles (exhibit momentum), but material particles such as electrons, protons, and atoms have some type of wave motion associated with them (show refraction and other wave-like properties).

Besides protons, neutrons, and electrons discussed earlier, many other atomic and subatomic particles have been discovered. These particles can travel with high speeds, depending on their kinetic energy, but never attain exactly the speed of light in a vacuum. Also, they interact with matter and produce varying degrees of energy transfer to the medium.

The so-called *elementary particles* have either zero or unit charge (equal to that of an electron). All other particles have charges that are whole multiples of the electronic charge. Some elementary particles of interest in radiological physics are listed in Table 1.1. Their properties and clinical applications will be discussed later in this book.

1.9 ELECTROMAGNETIC RADIATION

A. Wave Model

Electromagnetic radiation constitutes the mode of energy propagation for such phenomena as light waves, heat waves, radio waves, microwaves, untraviolet rays, x-rays, and γ rays. These radiations are called "electromagnetic" because they were first described, by Maxwell, in terms of oscillating electric and magnetic fields. As illustrated in Fig. 1.6 an electromagnetic wave can be represented by the spatial variations in the intensities of an electric field (E) and a magnetic field (H), the fields being at right angles to each other at any given instant. Energy is propagated with the speed of light (3×10^8 m/sec in vacuum) in the Z direction. The relationship between wavelength λ, frequency

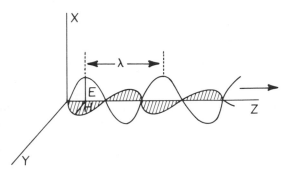

Figure 1.6. Graph showing electromagnetic wave at a given instant of time. E and H are respectively the peak amplitudes of electric and magnetic fields. The two fields are perpendicular to each other.

ν, and velocity of propagation c is given by

$$c = \nu\lambda \qquad (1.2)$$

In the above equation, c should be expressed in meters/sec, λ in meters, and ν in cycles/sec or hertz.

Figure 1.7 shows a spectrum of electromagnetic radiations with wavelengths ranging anywhere from 10^7 (radio waves) to 10^{-13} m (ultrahigh energy x-rays). Since wavelength and frequency are inversely related, the frequency spectrum corresponding to the above range will be 3×10^1–3×10^{21} cycles/sec. It is interesting to note that only a very small portion of the electromagnetic spectrum constitutes visible light bands. The wavelengths of the wave to which the human eye responds range from 4×10^{-7} (blue light) to 7×10^{-7} m (red).

The wave nature of the electromagnetic radiation can be demonstrated by experiments involving phenomena such as interference and diffraction of light. Similar effects have been observed with x-rays using crystals which possess interatomic spacing comparable to the x-ray wavelengths. However, as the wavelength becomes very small or the frequency becomes very large, the dominant behavior of electromagnetic radiations can only be explained by considering their particle or quantum nature.

B. Quantum Model

In order to explain the results of certain experiments involving interaction of radiation with matter, such as the photoelectric effect and the Compton scattering, one has to consider electromagnetic radiations as particles rather than waves. The amount of energy carried by such a packet of energy, or photon, is given by:

$$E = h\nu \qquad (1.3)$$

where E is the energy (joules) carried by the photon, h is the Planck's constant $(6.62 \times 10^{-34}$ J-sec), and ν is the frequency (cycles/sec). By combining equations

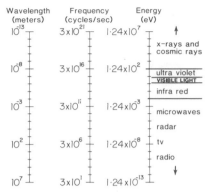

Figure 1.7. The electromagnetic spectrum. Ranges are approximate.

1.2 and 1.3, we have

$$E = \frac{hc}{\lambda} \tag{1.4}$$

If E is to be expressed in electron volts (eV) and λ in meters (m), then, since $1 \text{ eV} = 1.602 \times 10^{-19}$ J,

$$E = \frac{1.24 \times 10^{-6}}{\lambda} \tag{1.5}$$

The above equations indicate that as the wavelength becomes shorter or the frequency becomes larger, the energy of the photon becomes greater. This is also seen in Fig. 1.7.

CHAPTER 2

Nuclear Transformations

2.1 RADIOACTIVITY

Radioactivity, first discovered by Henri Becquerel in 1896, is a phenomenon in which radiation is given off by the nuclei of the elements. This radiation can be in the form of particles or electromagnetic radiation or both.

Figure 2.1 illustrates a method in which radiation emitted by radium can be separated by a magnetic field. Since α particles (helium nuclei) are positively charged, and β^- particles (electrons) are negatively charged, they are deflected in opposite directions. The difference in the radii of curvature indicates that the α particles are much heavier than β particles. On the other hand, γ rays, which are similar to x-rays except for their nuclear origin, have no charge and, therefore are unaffected by the magnetic field.

It was mentioned in the first chapter (Section 1.6) that there is a potential barrier preventing particles from entering or escaping the nucleus. Although, the particles inside the nucleus possess kinetic energy, this energy, in a stable nucleus, is not sufficient for any of the particles to penetrate the nuclear barrier. However, a radioactive nucleus has excess energy which is constantly redistributed among the nucleons by mutual collisions. As a matter of probability, one of the particles may gain enough energy to escape from the nucleus, thus enabling the nucleus to achieve a state of lower energy. Also, the emission of a particle may still leave the nucleus in an excited state. In that case, the nucleus will continue stepping down to the lower energy states by emitting particles or γ rays until the stable or the ground state has been achieved.

2.2 DECAY CONSTANT

The process of radioactive *decay* or *disintegration* is a statistical phenomenon. Whereas, it is not possible to know when a particular atom will disintegrate, one can accurately predict, in a large collection of atoms, the proportion that will disintegrate in a given time. The mathematics of radioactive decay is based on a simple fact that the number of atoms disintegrating per unit time, $\Delta N/\Delta t$, is proportional to the number of radioactive atoms, N, present. Symbolically,

$$\frac{\Delta N}{\Delta t} \propto N \quad \text{or} \quad \frac{\Delta N}{\Delta t} = -\lambda N \tag{2.1}$$

where λ is a constant of proportionality called the *decay constant*. The minus sign indicates that the number of the radioactive atoms decreases with time.

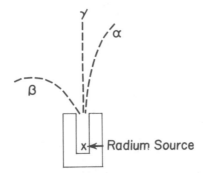

Figure 2.1. Diagrammatic representation of the separation of three types of radiation emitted by radium under the influence of magnetic field (applied perpendicular to the plane of the paper).

If ΔN and Δt are so small that they can be replaced by their corresponding differentials, dN and dt, then Equation 2.1 becomes a differential equation. The solution of this equation yields the following equation:

$$N = N_0 e^{-\lambda t} \tag{2.2}$$

where N_0 is the initial number of radioactive atoms and e is the number denoting the base of the natural logarithm ($e = 2.718$). Equation 2.2 is the well known exponential equation for radioative decay.

2.3 ACTIVITY

The rate of decay is referred to as the *activity* of a radioactive material. If $\Delta N/\Delta t$ in Equation 2.1 is replaced by A, the symbol for activity, then

$$A = - \lambda N \tag{2.3}$$

Similarly, Equation 2.2 can be expressed in terms of activity:

$$A = A_0 e^{-\lambda t} \tag{2.4}$$

where A is the activity remaining at time t and A_0 is the original activity equal to λN_0.

The unit of activity is the curie (Ci), defined as:

$$1 \text{ Ci} = 3.7 \times 10^{10} \text{ distintegrations/sec (dps)}[1]$$

Fractions of this unit are:

$$1 \text{ mCi} = 10^{-3} \text{ Ci} = 3.7 \times 10^7 \text{ dps}$$

$$1 \text{ } \mu\text{Ci} = 10^{-6} \text{ Ci} = 3.7 \times 10^4 \text{ dps}$$

$$1 \text{ nCi} = 10^{-9} \text{ Ci} = 3.7 \times 10^1 \text{ dps}$$

---

[1] This definition is based on the rate of decay of 1 g of radium which was originally measured to be 3.7×10^{10} dps. Although the recent measurements have established the decay rate as 3.61×10^{10} dps/g of radium, the original definition of curie remains unchanged.

$$1 \text{ pCi} = 10^{-12} \text{ Ci} = 3.7 \times 10^{-2} \text{ dps}$$

Recently, another unit of activity, the becquerel (Bq), has been proposed. The becquerel is a smaller but more basic unit than the curie and is defined as:

$$1 \text{ Bq} = 1 \text{ dps} = 2.70 \times 10^{-11} \text{ Ci}$$

2.4 THE HALF-LIFE AND THE MEAN LIFE

The term *half-life*, $T_{1/2}$, of a radioactive substance is defined as the time required for either the activity or the number of radioactive atoms to decay to half the initial value. By substituting $N/N_0 = \frac{1}{2}$ in Equation 2.2 or $A/A_0 = \frac{1}{2}$ in Equation 2.4, at $t = T_{1/2}$, we have

$$\frac{1}{2} = e^{-\lambda \cdot T1/2} \quad \text{or} \quad T_{1/2} = \frac{\ln 2}{\lambda}$$

where ln 2 is the natural logarithm of 2 having a value of 0.693. Therefore,

$$T_{1/2} = \frac{0.693}{\lambda} \tag{2.5}$$

Figure 2.2a illustrates the exponential decay of a radioactive sample as a function of time, expressed in units of half-life. It can be seen that after one half-life, the activity is $\frac{1}{2}$ the initial value, after two half-lives, it is $\frac{1}{4}$ and so on. Thus, after n half-lives, the activity will be reduced to $\frac{1}{2}^n$ of the initial value.

Although an exponential function can be plotted on a linear graph (Fig. 2.2a), it is better plotted on a semilog paper, since it yields a straight line, as demonstrated in Fig. 2.2b. This general curve applies to any radioactive material and can be used to determine the fractional activity remaining if the elapsed time is expressed as a fraction of half-life.

The *mean* or *average life* is the average lifetime for the decay of radioative atoms. Although, in theory, it will take an infinite amount of time for all the atoms to decay, the concept of average life, T_a, can be understood in terms of an imaginary source which decays at a constant rate equal to the initial activity and produces the same total number of disintegrations as the given source decaying exponentially from time $t = 0$ to $t = \infty$. Since the initial activity = λN_0 (from Equation 2.3) and the total number of disintegrations must be equal to N_0, we have:

$$T_a \lambda N_0 = N_0 \quad \text{or} \quad T_a = \frac{1}{\lambda} \tag{2.6}$$

Comparing Equations 2.5 and 2.6, we obtain the following relationship between half-life and average life.

$$T_a = 1.44 \ T_{1/2} \tag{2.7}$$

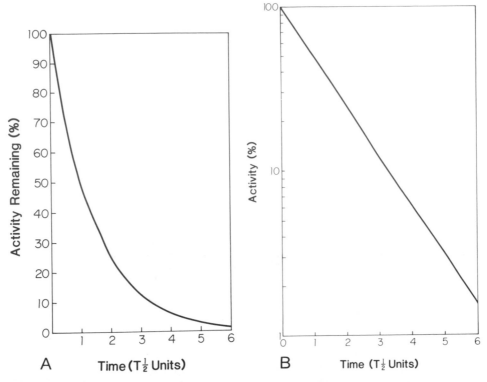

Figure 2.2. General decay curve. Activity as a percentage of initial activity plotted against time in units of half-life. A, plot on linear graph; B, plot on semilogarithmic graph.

Example 1

(a) Calculate the number of atoms in 1 g of ^{226}Ra.

(b) What is the activity of 1 g of ^{226}Ra (half-life = 1622 years)?

(a) In Section 1.3, we showed that:

$$\text{Number of atoms/g} = \frac{N_A}{A_W}$$

where N_A = Avogadro's number = 6.02×10^{23} atoms per gram atomic weight and A_W is the atomic weight. Also, we stated in the same section that A_W is very nearly equal to the mass number. Therefore, for ^{226}Ra

$$\text{Number of atoms/g} = \frac{6.02 \times 10^{23}}{226} = 2.66 \times 10^{21}$$

(b) Activity = λN (Equation 2.3, ignoring the minus sign). Since $N = 2.66 \times 10^{21}$ atoms/g (example above) and

$$\lambda = \frac{0.693}{T_{1/2}}$$

$$= \frac{0.693}{(1622 \text{ years}) \times (3.15 \times 10^7 \text{ sec/year})}$$

$$= 1.356 \times 10^{-11}/\text{sec}$$

Therefore,

$$\text{Activity} = 2.66 \times 10^{21} \times 1.356 \times 10^{-11} \text{ dps/g}$$

$$= 3.61 \times 10^{10} \text{ dps/g}$$

$$= 0.975 \text{ Ci/g}$$

The activity per unit mass of a radionuclide is termed the *specific activity*. As shown in the above example, the specific activity of radium is slightly less than 1 *Ci/g*, although the curie was originally defined as the decay rate of 1 g of radium. The reason for this discrepancy, as mentioned before, is the current revision of the actual decay rate of radium without modification of the original definition of the curie.

High specific activity of certain radionuclides can be advantageous for a number of applications. For example, the use of elements as tracers in studying biochemical processes requires that the mass of the incorporated element should be so small that it does not interfere with the normal metabolism and yet it should exhibit measurable activity. Another example is the use of radioisotopes as teletherapy sources. One reason why cobalt-60 is preferable to cesium-137, in spite of its lower half-life (5.26 years for ^{60}Co *vs.* 30.0 years for ^{137}Cs) is its much higher specific activity. The interested reader may verify this fact by actual calculations! (It should be assumed in these calculations that the specific activities are for pure forms of the nuclides.)

Example 2

(a) Calculate the decay constant for cobalt-60 ($T_{1/2} = 5.26$ years) in units of month^{-1}.

(b) What will be the activity of a 5000-Ci ^{60}Co source after 4 years?

(a) From Equations 2.5, we have

$$\lambda = \frac{0.693}{T_{1/2}}$$

since $T_{1/2} = 5.26$ years $= 63.12$ months. Therefore,

$$\lambda = \frac{0.693}{63.12} = 1.0979 \times 10^{-2} \text{ month}^{-1}$$

(b) $t = 4$ years $= 48$ months. From Equations 2.4, we have

$$A = A_0 e^{-\lambda t}$$
$$= 5000 \times e^{-1.0979\times10^{-2}\times48}$$
$$= 2952 \; Ci$$

Alternatively:

$$t = 4 \text{ years} = \frac{4}{5.26} \; T_{1/2} = 0.760 \; T_{1/2}$$

Therefore,

$$A = 5000 \times \frac{1}{2^{0.760}} = 2952 \; Ci$$

Alternatively: reading the fractional activity from the universal decay curve given in Fig. 2.2, at time $= 0.76 \; T_{1/2}$ and then multiplying it with the initial activity, we get the desired answer.

Example 3

When will 5 mCi of ^{131}I $(T_{1/2} = 8.05$ days) and 2 mCi of ^{32}P $(T_{1/2} = 14.3$ days) have equal activities? for ^{131}I:

$$A_0 = 5 \text{ mCi}$$

and

$$\lambda = \frac{0.693}{8.05} = 8.609 \times 10^{-2} \; \text{day}^{-1}$$

For ^{32}P:

$$A_0 = 2 \text{ mCi}$$

and

$$\lambda = \frac{0.693}{14.3} = 4.846 \times 10^{-2} \; \text{day}^{-1}$$

Suppose the activities of the two nuclides are equal after t days. Then, from Equation 2.4,

$$5 \times e^{-8.609 \times 10^{-2} \times t} = 2 \times e^{-4.846 \times 10^{-2} \times t}$$

Taking the natural log of both sides,

$$\ln 5 - 8.609 \times 10^{-2} \times t = \ln 2 - 4.846 \times 10^{-2} \times t$$

or $1.609 - 8.609 \times 10^{-2} \times t = 0.693 - 4.846 \times 10^{-2} \times t$

or $t = 23.34$ days

Alternatively: one may plot the activity of each sample as a function of time. The activities of the two samples will be equal at the time when the two curves intersect each other.

2.5 RADIOACTIVE SERIES

There are a total of 103 elements known today. Of these, the first 92 (from $Z = 1$ to $Z = 92$) occur naturally. The others have been produced artificially. In general, the elements with lower Z tend to be stable while the ones with higher Z are radioactive. It appears that as the number of particles inside the nucleus increases, the forces that keep the particles together become less effective and, therefore, the chances of particle emission are increased. This is suggested by the observation that all elements with Z greater than 82 (lead) are radioactive.

All naturally occurring radioactive elements have been grouped into three series: the uranium series, the actinium series, and the thorium series. The uranium series originates with ^{238}U having a half-life of 4.51×10^9 years and goes through a series of transformations involving the emission of α and β particles. γ rays are also produced as a result of some of these transformations. The actinium series starts from ^{235}U with a half-life of 7.13×10^8 years and the thorium series begins with ^{232}Th with half-life of 1.39×10^{10} years. All the series terminate at the stable isotopes of lead with mass numbers 206, 207, and 208, respectively. As an example and because it includes radium as one of its decay products, the uranium series is represented in Fig. 2.3.

2.6 RADIOACTIVE EQUILIBRIUM

Many radioactive nuclides undergo successive transformations in which the original nuclide, called the *parent*, gives rise to a radioactive product nuclide, called the *daughter*. The naturally occurring radioactive series provides examples of such transitions. If the half-life of the parent is longer than that of the daughter, then after a certain period of time, a condition of *equilibrium* will be achieved, that is, the ratio of daughter activity to parent activity will become constant. In addition, the apparent decay rate of the daughter nuclide is then governed by the half-life or disintegration rate of the parent.

Two kinds of radioactive equilibria have been defined, depending upon the half-lives of the parent and the daughter nuclides. If the half-life of the parent is not much longer than that of the daughter, then the type of equilibrium established is called the *transient equilibrium*. On the other hand, if the half-life of the parent is much longer than that of the daughter, then it can give rise to what is known as the *secular equilibrium*.

Figure 2.4 illustrates the transient equilibrium between the parent ^{99}Mo ($T_{1/2} = 67$ h) and the daughter ^{99m}Tc ($T_{1/2} = 6$ h). The secular equilibrium is

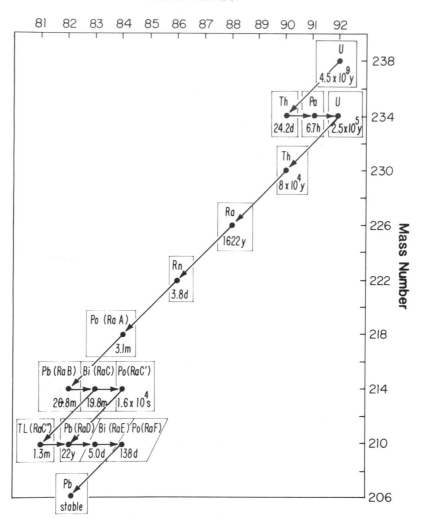

Figure 2.3. The uranium series. Data are from Ref. 1.

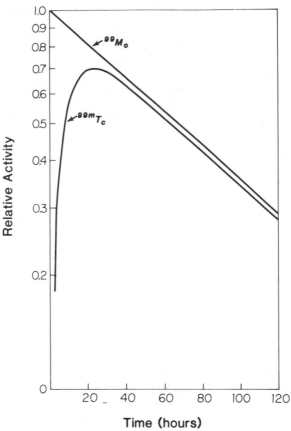

Figure 2.4. Illustration of transient equilibrium by the decay of ^{99}Mo to ^{99m}Tc. It has been assumed that only 88% of the ^{99}Mo atoms decay to ^{99m}Tc.

illustrated in Fig. 2.5 showing the case of ^{222}Rn ($T_{1/2} = 3.8$ days) achieving equilibrium with its parent, ^{226}Ra ($T_{1/2} = 1622$ years).

A general equation can be derived relating the activities of the parent and daughter:

$$A_2 = A_1 \frac{\lambda_2}{\lambda_2 - \lambda_1} (1 - e^{-(\lambda_2 - \lambda_1)t}) \tag{2.8}$$

where A_1 and A_2 are the activities of the parent and the daughter, respectively. λ_1 and λ_2 are the corresponding decay constants. In terms of the half-lives, T_1 and T_2, of the parent and daughter, respectively, the above equation can be rewritten as:

$$A_2 = A_1 \frac{T_1}{T_1 - T_2} (1 - e^{-0.693 \frac{T_1 - T_2}{T_1 T_2} t}) \tag{2.9}$$

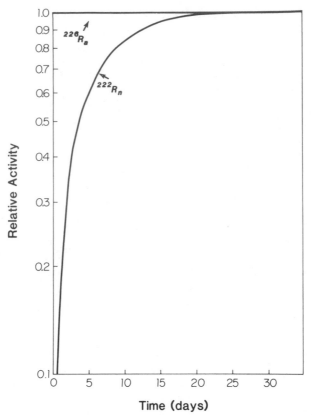

Figure 2.5. Illustration of secular equilibrium by the decay of ^{226}Ra to ^{222}Rn.

Equation 2.9, when plotted, will initially exhibit a growth curve for the daughter before approaching the decay curve of the parent (Figs. 2.4 and 2.5). In the case of a transient equilibrium, the time t to reach the equilibrium value is very large compared to the half-life of the daughter. This makes the exponential term in Equation 2.9 negligibly small. Thus, after the transient equilibrium has been achived, the relative activities of the two nuclides is given by:

$$\frac{A_2}{A_1} = \frac{\lambda_2}{\lambda_2 - \lambda_1} \tag{2.10}$$

or, in terms of half-lives:

$$\frac{A_2}{A_1} = \frac{T_1}{T_1 - T_2} \tag{2.11}$$

A practical example of the transient equilibrium is the ^{99}Mo generator producing ^{99m}Tc for diagnostic procedures. Such a generator is sometimes called "cow" since the daughter product, in this case ^{99m}Tc, is removed or "milked" at regular intervals. Each time the generator is completely milked, the growth of the daughter and the decay of the parent are governed by Equation 2.9. It may be mentioned that not all the ^{99}Mo atoms decay to ^{99m}Tc. Approximately 12% promptly decay to ^{99}Tc without passing through the metastable state of ^{99m}Tc (1). Thus, the activity of ^{99}Mo should be effectively reduced by 12% for the purpose of calculating ^{99m}Tc activity, using any of Equations 2.8–2.11.

Since in the case of a secular equilibrium, the half-life of the parent substance is very long compared with the half-life of the daughter, λ_2 is much greater than λ_1. Therefore, λ_1, can be ignored in Equation 2.8:

$$A_2 = A_1(1 - e^{-\lambda_2 t}) \tag{2.12}$$

The above equation gives the initial build-up of the daughter nuclide, approaching the activity of the parent asymptotically (Fig. 2.5). At the secular equilibrium, after a long time, the product $\lambda_2 t$ becomes large and the exponential term in Equation 2.12 approaches zero. Thus, at secular equilibrium and thereafter:

$$A_2 = A_1 \tag{2.13}$$

or

$$\lambda_2 N_2 = \lambda_1 N_1 \tag{2.14}$$

Radium source in a sealed tube or needle (to keep in the radon gas) is an excellent example of secular equilibrium. After an initial period of time (approximately 1 month), all the daughter products are in equilibrium with the parent and we have the relationship:

$$\lambda_1 N_1 = \lambda_2 N_2 = \lambda_3 N_3 = \dots \tag{2.15}$$

2.7 MODES OF RADIOACTIVE DECAY

A. α Particle Decay

Radioactive nuclides with very high atomic numbers (greater than 82) decay most frequently with the emission of an α particle. It appears that as the number of protons in the nucleus increases beyond 82, the Coulomb forces of repulsion between the protons become large enough to overcome the nuclear forces that bind the nucleons together. Thus, the unstable nucleus emits a particle composed of two protons and two neutrons. This particle, which is in fact a helium nucleus, is called the α particle.

As a result of α decay, the atomic number of the nucleus is reduced by two and the mass number is reduced by four. Thus, a general reaction for α decay can be written as:

$$_Z^A X \rightarrow {}_{Z-2}^{A-4} Y + {}_2^4 \text{He} + Q$$

where Q represents the total energy released in the process and is called the *disintegration energy*. This energy which is equivalent to the difference in mass between the parent nucleus and product nuclei, appears as kinetic energy of the α particle and the kinetic energy of the product nucleus. The equation also shows that the charge is conserved, since the charge on the parent nucleus is Ze (where e is the electronic charge), on the product nucleus it is $(Z - 2)$e and on the α particle it is 2e.

A typical example of α decay is the transformation of radium to radon:

$$_{88}^{226}\text{Ra} \xrightarrow[\text{1622 years}]{T_{1/2}} {}_{86}^{222}\text{Rn} + {}_2^4\text{He} + 4.87 \text{ MeV}$$

Since the momentum of the α particle must be equal to the recoil momentum of the radon nucleus and since the radon nucleus is much heavier than the α particle, it can be shown that the kinetic energy possessed by the radon nucleus is negligibly small (0.09 MeV) and that the disintegration energy appears almost entirely as the kinetic energy of the α particle (4.78 MeV).

It has been found that the α particles emitted by radioactive substances have kinetic energies of about 5 to 10 MeV. From a specific nuclide, they are emitted with discrete energies.

B. β Particle Decay

The process of radioactive decay, which is accompanied by the ejection of a positive or a negative electron from the nucleus, is called the β decay. The negative electron or negatron is denoted by β^- and the positive electron or positron is represented by β^+. Neither of these particles exists as such inside the nucleus but is created at the instant of the decay process. The basic transformations may be written as:

$$_0^1\text{n} \rightarrow {}_1^1\text{p} + {}_{-1}^0\beta + \tilde{\nu} \quad (\beta^- \text{ decay})$$

$$_1^1\text{p} \rightarrow {}_0^1\text{n} + {}_{+1}^0\beta + \nu \quad (\beta^+ \text{ decay})$$

where $_0^1\text{n}$, $_1^1\text{p}$, $\tilde{\nu}$, and ν stand for neutron, proton, antineutrino, and neutrino, respectively. The last two particles, namely antineutrino and neutrino, are identical particles but with opposite spins. They carry no charge and practically no mass.

B.1. NEGATRON EMISSION

The radionuclides with an excessive number of neutrons or a high neutron to proton (n/p) ratio lie above the region of stability (see Fig. 1.1). These nuclei tend to reduce the n/p ratio in order to achieve stability. This is accomplished by emitting a negative electron. The direct emission of neutron, in order to reduce the n/p ratio, is rather uncommon and occurs with some nuclei produced as a result of fission reactions.

The general equation for the negatron or β^- decay is written as:

$$_Z^A X \rightarrow \,_{Z+1}^{A} Y + \,_{-1}^{0}\beta + \tilde{\nu} + Q$$

where Q is the disintegration energy for the process. This energy is provided by the difference in mass between the initial nucleus $_Z^A X$ and the sum of the masses of the product nucleus $_{Z+1}^{A} Y$ and the particles emitted.

The energy Q is shared between the emitted particles (including γ rays if emitted by the daughter nucleus) and the recoil nucleus. As discussed in Section 2.7, the kinetic energy possessed by the recoil nucleus is negligible because of its much greater mass compared to the emitted particles. Thus, the entire disintegration energy is carried by the emitted particles. If there was only one kind of particle involved, all the particles emitted in such a disintegration would have the same energy equal to Q, thus yielding a sharp line spectrum. However, the observed spectrum in the β decay is continuous, which suggests that there is more than one particle emitted in this process. For these reasons, Wolfgang Pauli (1931) introduced the hypothesis that a second particle, later known as the neutrino,[2] accompanied each β particle emitted and shared the available energy.

The experimental data show that the β particles are emitted with all energies ranging from zero to the maximum energy characteristic of the β transition.

Figure 2.6 shows the distribution of energy among the β particles of ^{32}P. The overall transition is:

$$_{15}^{32}\text{P} \xrightarrow[\text{14.3 days}]{T_{1/2}} \,_{16}^{32}\text{S} + \,_{-1}^{0}\beta + \tilde{\nu} + 1.7 \text{ MeV}$$

As seen in the above figure, the end point energy of the β-ray spectrum is equal to the disintegration energy and is designated by E_{max}, the maximum electron energy. Although the shape of the energy spectrum and the values for E_{max} are characteristic of the particular nuclide, the average energy of the β particles from a β emitter is approximately $E_{max}/3$.

It has been mentioned earlier that the neutrino has no charge and practically no mass. For that reason the probability of its interaction with matter is very small and its detection is extremely difficult. However, Fermi successfully presented the theoretical evidence of the existence of the neutrino and predicted the shape of the β ray spectra. Recently the existence of neutrinos has been verified by direct experiments.

---

[2] Neutrino is the generic name for the two specific particles, neutrino and antineutrino.

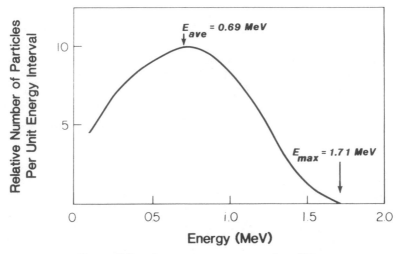

Figure 2.6. β ray energy spectrum from ^{32}P.

B.2. POSITRON EMISSION

Positron-emitting nuclides have a deficit of neutrons and their n/p ratios are lower than those of the stable nuclei of the same atomic number or neutron number (see Fig. 1.1). In order for these nuclides to achieve stability, the decay mode must result in an increase of the n/p ratio. One possible mode is the β decay involving the emission of a positive electron or positron. The overall decay reaction is as follows:

$$_Z^A X \rightarrow\ _{Z-1}^A Y +\ _{+1}^0\beta + \nu + Q$$

As in the case of the negatron emission, discussed above, the disintegration energy Q is shared by the positron, the neutrino, and any γ rays emitted by the daughter nucleus. Also, like the negatrons, the positrons are emitted with a spectrum of energies.

A specific example of positron emission is the decay of $_{11}^{22}$Na:

$$_{11}^{22}\text{Na} \xrightarrow[\text{2.60 years}]{T_{1/2}}\ _{10}^{22}\text{Ne} +\ _{+1}^0\beta + \nu + 1.82 \text{ MeV}$$

The released energy, 1.82 MeV, is the sum of the maximum kinetic energy of the positron, 0.545 MeV, and the energy of the γ ray, 1.275 MeV.

An energy level diagram for the positron decay of $_{11}^{22}$Na is shown in Fig. 2.7. It should be noted that the arrow representing β^+ decay starts from a point $2m_0c^2$ (= 1.02 MeV) below the energy state of the parent nucleus. This excess energy which is the equivalent of two electron masses must be available as part of the transition energy for the positron emission to take place. In other words, the energy levels of the parent and the daughter nucleus must be separated by more than 1.02 MeV for the β^+ decay to occur. Also, it can be shown that the energy released is given by the atomic mass difference between the parent and the daughter nuclides minus the $2m_0c^2$. It should be mentioned that the positron is unstable and eventually combines with another electron producing annihilation of the particles. This event results in two γ ray photons, each of 0.51 MeV, thus converting two electron masses into energy.

C. Electron Capture

The electron capture is a phenomenon in which one of the orbital electrons is captured by the nucleus, thus transforming a proton into a neutron:

$$_1^1p + \,_{-1}^0e \rightarrow \,_0^1n + \nu$$

The general equation of the nuclear decay is:

$$_Z^AX + \,_{-1}^0e \rightarrow \,_{Z-1}^AY + \nu + Q$$

The electron capture is an alternative process to the positron decay. The unstable nuclei with neutron deficiency may increase their n/p ratio to gain stability by electron capture. As illustrated in Fig. 2.7, $_{11}^{22}$Na decays 10% of the time by K electron capture. The resulting nucleus is still in the excited state and releases its excess energy by the emission of a γ ray photon. In general, the γ decay follows the particle emission almost instantaneously (less than 10^{-9} sec).

The electron capture process involves mostly the K shell electron because of its closeness to the nucleus. The process is then referred to as *K capture*. However, other L or M capture processes are also possible in some cases.

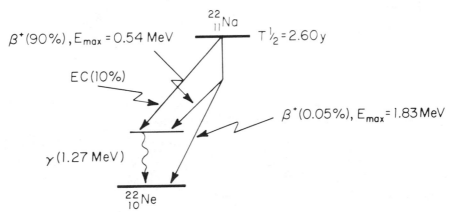

Figure 2.7.   Energy level diagram for the positron decay of $_{11}^{22}$Na to $_{11}^{22}$Ne.

The decay by electron capture creates an empty hole in the involved shell which is then filled with another outer orbit electron, thus giving rise to the characteristic x-rays. There is also the emission of *Auger electrons* which are monoenergetic electrons produced by the absorption of characteristic x-rays by the atom and re-emission of the energy in the form of orbital electrons ejected from the atom. The process can be crudely described as internal photoelectric effect (to be discussed in later chapters) produced by the inter-action of the electron capture characteristic x-rays with the same atom.

D. Internal Conversion

The emission of γ rays from the nucleus is one mode by which a nucleus left in an excited state after a nuclear transformation gets rid of excess energy. There is another competing mechanism, called internal conversion, by which the nucleus can lose energy. In this process, the excess nuclear energy is passed on to one of the orbital electrons which is then ejected from the atom. The process can be crudely likened to an internal photoelectric effect in which the γ ray escaping from the nucleus interacts with an orbital electron of the same atom. The kinetic energy of the internal conversion electron is equal to energy released by the nucleus minus the binding energy of the orbital electron involved.

As discussed in the case of the electron capture, the ejection of an orbital electron by internal conversion will create a vacancy in the involved shell, resulting in the production of characteristic photons or Auger electrons.

D.1. ISOMERIC TRANSITION

In most radioactive transformations, the daughter nucleus loses the excess energy immediately in the form of γ rays or by internal conversion. However, in the case of some nuclides, the excited state of the nucleus persists for an appreciable time. In that case, the excited nucleus is said to exist in the *metastable* state. The metastable nucleus is an *isomer* of the final product nucleus which has the same atomic and mass number but different energy state. An example of such a nuclide commonly used in nuclear medicine is ^{99m}Tc which is an isomer of ^{99}Tc. As discussed earlier (Section 2.6), ^{99m}Tc is produced by the decay of ^{99}Mo ($T_{1/2} = 67$ h) and itself decays to ^{99}Tc with a half-life of 6 h.

2.8 NUCLEAR REACTIONS

A. The α, p Reaction

The first nuclear reaction was observed by Rutherford in 1919 in an experiment in which he bombarded nitrogen gas with α particles from a radioactive source. Rutherford's original transmutation reaction can be written as:

$$^{14}_{7}\text{N} + {}^{4}_{2}\text{He} \rightarrow {}^{17}_{8}\text{O} + {}^{1}_{1}\text{H} + Q$$

where Q represents the energy released or absorbed during the nuclear reaction. If Q is positive, energy has been released and the reaction is called *exoergic*, and if Q is negative, energy has been absorbed and the reaction is called *endoergic*. Q is also called *nuclear reaction energy* or disintegration energy (as defined earlier in decay reactions) and is equal to the difference in the masses of the initial and final particles. As an example, Q may be calculated for the above reaction as follows:

Mass of Initial Particles (amu)	Mass of Final Particles (amu)
$^{14}_{7}N = 14.003074$	$^{17}_{8}O = 16.999133$
$^{4}_{2}He = \dfrac{4.002603}{18.005677}$	$^{1}_{1}H = \dfrac{1.007825}{18.006958}$

The total mass of final particles is greater than that of the initial particles.

$$\text{Difference in masses, } \Delta m = 0.001281 \text{ amu}$$

Since 1 amu = 931 MeV, we get:

$$Q = -0.001281 \times 931 = -1.19 \text{ MeV}$$

Thus, the above reaction is endoergic, that is, at least 1.19 MeV of energy must be supplied for the above reaction to take place. This minimum required energy is called the *threshold energy* for the reaction and must be available from the kinetic energy of the bombarding particle.

A reaction in which an α particle interacts with a nucleus to form a *compound nucleus* which, in turn, disintegrates immediately into a new nucleus by the ejection of a proton is called an α,p reaction. The first letter α stands for the bombarding particle and the second letter p stands for the ejected particle, in this case a proton. The general reaction of this type is written as:

$$^{A}_{Z}X + ^{4}_{2}He \rightarrow ^{A+3}_{Z+1}Y + ^{1}_{1}H + Q$$

A simpler notation to represent the above reaction is $^{A}X(\alpha, p)^{A+3}Y$. (It is not necessary to write the atomic number Z with the chemical symbol, since one can be determined by the other.)

B. The α,n Reaction

The bombardment of a nucleus by α particles with the subsequent emission of neutrons is designated as an α,n reaction. An example of this type of reaction is $^{9}Be(\alpha,n)^{12}C$. This was the first reaction employed for producing small neutron sources. A material containing a mixture of radium and beryllium has been commonly used as a neutron source in research laboratories. In this case, the α particles emitted by radium bombard the beryllium nuclei and eject neutrons.

C. Proton Bombardment

The most common reaction consists of a proton being captured by the nucleus with the emission of a γ ray. The reaction is known as p,γ. Examples are:

$$^{7}\text{Li}(p,\gamma)^{8}\text{Be and } ^{12}\text{C}(p,\gamma)^{13}\text{N}$$

Other possible reactions produced by proton bombardment are of the type p,n, p,d, and p,α. The symbol d stands for the deuteron ($_{1}^{2}\text{H}$).

D. Deuteron Bombardment

The deuteron particle is a combination of a proton and a neutron. This combination appears to break down in most deuteron bombardments with the result that the compound nucleus emits either a neutron or a proton. The two types of reactions can be written as $_{Z}^{A}X(d,n)_{Z+1}^{A+1}Y$ and $_{Z}^{A}X(d,p)_{Z}^{A+1}X$.

An important reaction which has been used as a source of high energy neutrons is produced by the bombardment of deuterons by deuterons. The equation for the reaction is

$$_{1}^{2}\text{H} + _{1}^{2}\text{H} \rightarrow _{2}^{3}\text{He} + _{0}^{1}\text{n}$$

or simply $^{2}\text{H}(d,n)^{3}\text{He}$. This process is also known as *stripping*.

E. Neutron Bombardment

Neutrons, since they possess no electric charge, are very effective in penetrating the nuclei and producing nuclear reactions. For the same reason, the neutrons do not have to possess high kinetic energies in order to penetrate the nucleus. As a matter of fact, *slow* neutrons or *thermal* neutrons (neutrons with average energy equal to the energy of thermal agitation in a material, which is about 0.025 eV at room temperature) have been found to be extremely effective in producing nuclear transformations. An example of a slow neutron capture is the n,α reaction with boron:

$$_{5}^{10}\text{B} + _{0}^{1}\text{n} \rightarrow _{3}^{7}\text{Li} + _{2}^{4}\text{He}$$

The above reaction forms the basis of neutron detection. In practice, an ionization chamber (to be discussed later in this book) is filled with boron gas such as BF_3. The α particle released by the n,α reaction with boron produces the ionization detected by the chamber.

The most common process of neutron capture is the n,γ reaction. In this case the compound nucleus is raised to one of its excited states and then immediately returns to its normal state with the emission of a γ ray photon. These γ rays, called *capture γ rays*, can be observed coming from a hydrogenous material such as paraffin used to slow down (by multiple collisions with the nuclei) the neutrons and ultimately capture some of the slow neutrons. The reaction can be written as follows:

$$_1^1H + _0^1n \rightarrow _1^2H + \gamma$$

Since the thermal neutron has negligible kinetic energy, the energy of the capture γ ray can be calculated by the mass difference between the initial particles and the product particles, assuming negligible recoil energy of $_1^2H$.

Products of the n,γ reaction, in most cases, have been found to be radioactive, emitting β particles. Typical examples are:

$$_{27}^{59}Co + _0^1n \rightarrow _{27}^{60}Co + \gamma$$

followed by

$$_{27}^{60}Co \xrightarrow[\text{5.3 years}]{T_{1/2}} _{28}^{60}Ni + _{-1}^0\beta + \gamma_1 + \gamma_2$$

$$_{79}^{197}Au + _0^1n \rightarrow _{79}^{198}Au + \gamma$$

followed by

$$_{79}^{198}Au \xrightarrow[\text{2.7 days}]{T_{1/2}} _{80}^{198}Hg + _{-1}^0\beta$$

Another type of reaction produced by neutrons, namely the n,p reaction, also yields β emitters in most cases. This process with slow neutrons has been observed in the case of nitrogen:

$$_7^{14}N + _0^1n \rightarrow _6^{14}C + _1^1H$$

followed by

$$_6^{14}C \xrightarrow[\text{5700 years}]{T_{1/2}} _7^{14}N + _{-1}^0\beta$$

The example of a fast neutron n,p reaction is the production of ^{32}P:

$$_{16}^{32}S + _0^1n \rightarrow _{15}^{32}P + _1^1H$$

followed by

$$^{32}_{15}\text{P} \xrightarrow[\text{14.3 days}]{T_{1/2}} {}^{32}_{16}\text{S} + {}^{0}_{-1}\beta$$

It should be pointed out that whether a reaction will occur with fast or slow neutrons depends on the magnitude of the mass difference between the expected product nucleus and the bombarded nucleus. For example, in the case of an n,p reaction, if this mass difference exceeds 0.000840 amu (mass difference between a neutron and a proton), then only fast neutrons will be effective in producing the reaction.

F. Photo Disintegration

An interaction of a high energy photon with an atomic nucleus can lead to a nuclear reaction and to the emission of one or more nucleons. In most cases, this process of photodisintegration results in the emission of neutrons by the nuclei. An example of such a reaction is provided by the nucleus of ^{63}Cu bombarded with a photon beam:

$$^{63}_{29}\text{Cu} + \gamma \rightarrow {}^{62}_{29}\text{Cu} + {}^{1}_{0}\text{n}$$

The above reaction has a definite threshold, 10.86 MeV. This can be calculated by the definition of *threshold energy*, namely, the difference between the rest energy of the target nucleus and that of the residual nucleus plus the emitted nucleon(s). Since the rest energies of many nuclei are known to a very high accuracy, the photodisintegration process can be used as a basis for energy calibration of machines producing high energy photons.

In addition to the γ,n reaction, other types of photodisintegration processes have been observed. Among these are γ,p, γ,d, γ,t, and γ,α, where d stands for deuteron ($^{2}_{1}\text{H}$) and t stands for triton ($^{3}_{1}\text{H}$).

G. Fission

This type of reaction is produced by bombarding certain high atomic number nuclei by neutrons. The nucleus, after absorbing the neutron, splits into nuclei of lower atomic number as well as additional neutrons. A typical example is the fission of ^{235}U with slow neutrons:

$$^{235}_{92}\text{U} + {}^{1}_{0}\text{n} \rightarrow {}^{236}_{92}\text{U} \rightarrow {}^{141}_{56}\text{Ba} + {}^{92}_{36}\text{Kr} + 3{}^{1}_{0}\text{n} + Q$$

The energy released Q can be calculated, as usual, by the mass difference between the original and the final particles and, in the above reaction, averages more than 200 MeV. This energy appears as the kinetic energy of the product particles as well as γ rays. The additional neutrons released in the process may also interact with other ^{235}U nuclei, thereby creating the possibility of *chain reaction*. However, a sufficient mass or, more technically, the *critical mass* of the fissionable material is required to produce the chain reaction.

As seen in the above instance, the energy released per fission is enormous. The process, therefore, has become a major energy source as in the case of nuclear reactors.

H. Fusion

Nuclear fusion may be considered as the reverse of nuclear fission; that is, low mass nuclei are combined to produce one nucleus. A typical reaction is:

$$^2_1H + {}^3_1H \rightarrow {}^4_2He + {}^1_0n + Q$$

Since the total mass of the product particles is less than the total mass of the reactants, energy Q is released in the process. In the above example, the loss in mass is about 0.0189 amu which gives $Q = 17.6$ MeV.

For the fusion reaction to occur, the nuclei must be brought sufficiently close together so that the repulsive Coulomb forces are overcome and the short range nuclear forces can initiate the fusion reaction. This is accomplished by heating low Z nuclei to very high temperatures (greater than 10^7 K) which are comparable to the inner core temperature of the sun. In practice, fission reactions have been used as starters for the fusion reactions.

2.9 ACTIVATION OF NUCLIDES

Elements can be made radioactive by various nuclear reactions, some of which have been described in the preceding section. The *yield* of a nuclear reaction depends on parameters such as the number of bombarding particles, the number of target nuclei, and the probability of the occurrence of the nuclear reaction. This probability is called the "*cross section*" and is usually given in units of *barns*, where a barn is 10^{-24} cm^2. The cross section of nuclear reaction depends on the nature of the target material as well as the type of the bombarding particles and their energy.

Another important aspect of activation is the *growth of activity*. It can be shown that, in the activation of isotopes, the activity of the transformed sample grows exponentially. If both the activation and decay of the material are considered, the actual growth of activity follows a net growth curve which reaches a maximum value, called *saturation activity*, after several half-lives. When that happens, the rate of activation equals the rate of decay.

As mentioned earlier, the slow (thermal) neutrons are very effective in activating nuclides. High fluxes of slow neutrons (10^{10} to 10^{14} neutrons/cm^2/ sec) are available in a nuclear reactor where neutrons are produced by fission reactions.

2.10 NUCLEAR REACTORS

In nuclear reactors, the fission process is made self-sustaining by chain reaction in which some of the fission neutrons are used to induce still more fissions. The nuclear "fuel" is usually ^{235}U, although thorium and plutonium are other possible fuels. The fuel, in the form of cylindrical rods, is arranged in a suitable lattice within the reactor core. Since the neutrons released during fission are fast neutrons, they have to be slowed down to thermal energy (about 0.025 eV) by collisions with nuclei of low Z material. Such materials are called *moderators*. Typical moderators include graphite, beryllium, water, and heavy water (water with heavy hydrogen $^{2}_{1}$H as part of the molecular structure). The fuel rods are immersed in the moderators. The reaction is "controlled" by inserting rods of material that efficiently absorbs neutrons, such as cadmium or boron. The position of these control rods in the reactor core determines the number of neutrons available to induce fission and thus control the fission rate or power output.

One of the major uses of nuclear reactors is to produce power. In this case, the heat generated by the absorption of γ rays and neutrons is used for the generation of electrical power. In addition, since reactors can provide a large and continuous supply of neutrons, they are extremely valuable for producing radioisotopes used in nuclear medicine, industry, and research.

References

1. *Radiological Health Handbook*, revised ed. United States Department of Health, Education, and Welfare, Superintendent of Documents. Washington, D. C., United States Government Printing Office, 1970.

CHAPTER 3

Production of X-Rays

X-rays were discovered by Roentgen in 1895 while studying cathode rays (stream of electrons) in a gas discharge tube. He observed that another type of radiation was produced (presumably by the interaction of electrons with the glass walls of the tube) which could be detected outside the tube. This radiation could penetrate opaque substances, produce fluorescence, blacken a photographic plate, and ionize a gas. He named the new radiation x-rays.

Following this historic discovery, the nature of x-rays was extensively studied and many other properties were unraveled. Our understanding of their nature was greatly enhanced when they were classified as one form of electromagnetic radiation (Section 1.9).

3.1 THE X-RAY TUBE

Figure 3.1 is a schematic representation of a conventional x-ray tube. The tube consists of a glass envelope which has been evacuated to high vacuum. At one end is a cathode (negative electrode) and at the other an anode (positive electrode), both hermetically sealed in the tube. The cathode is a tungsten filament which when heated emits electrons, a phenomenon known as *thermionic emission*. The anode consists of a thick copper rod at the end of which is placed a small piece of tungsten target. When a high voltage is applied between the anode and the cathode, the electrons emitted from the filament are accelerated toward the anode and achieve high velocities before striking the target. The x-rays are produced by the sudden deflection or acceleration of the electron caused by the attractive force of the tungsten nucleus. The physics of x-ray production will be discussed later in Section 3.4. The x-ray beam emerges through a thin glass window in the tube envelope. In some tubes, thin beryllium windows are used to reduce inherent filtration of the x-ray beam.

A. The Anode

The choice of tungsten as the target material in conventional x-ray tubes is based on the criteria that the target must have high atomic number and high melting point. As will be discussed in Section 3.4, the efficiency of x-ray production depends on the atomic number and for that reason tungsten with $Z = 74$ is a good target material. In addition, tungsten, which has a melting point of 3370°C, is the element of choice for withstanding intense heat produced in the target by the electronic bombardment.

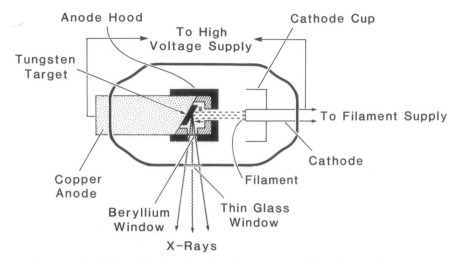

Figure 3.1.   Schematic diagram of a therapy x-ray tube with hooded anode.

Efficient removal of heat from the target is an important requirement for the anode design. This has been achieved in some tubes by conduction of heat through a thick copper anode to the outside of the tube where it is cooled by oil, water, or air. Rotating anodes have also been used in diagnostic x-rays in order to reduce the temperature of the target at any one spot. The heat generated in the rotating anode is radiated to the oil reservoir surrounding the tube. It should be mentioned that the function of the oil bath surrounding an x-ray tube is to insulate the tube housing from high voltage applied to the tube as well as absorb heat from the anode.

Some stationary anodes are *hooded* by a copper and tungsten shield to prevent stray electrons from striking the walls or other non-target components of the tube. These are secondary electrons produced from the target when it is being bombarded by the primary electron beam. Whereas, copper in the hood absorbs the secondary electrons, the tungsten shield surrounding the copper shield absorbs the unwanted x-rays produced in the copper.

An important requirement of the anode design is the optimum size of the target area from which the x-rays are emitted. This area which is called the *focal spot* should be as small as possible for producing sharp radiographic images. However, smaller focal spots generate more heat per unit area of target, and therefore limit currents and exposure. In therapy tubes, relatively larger focal spots are acceptable since the radiographic image quality is not the overriding concern.

The apparent size of the focal spot can be reduced by the principle of *line-focus*, illustrated in Fig. 3.2. The target is mounted on a steeply inclined surface of the anode. The apparent side a is equal to $A \sin \theta$, where A is the side of the actual focal spot at an angle θ with respect to the electron beam. Since the other side of the actual focal spot is perpendicular to the electron, its apparent

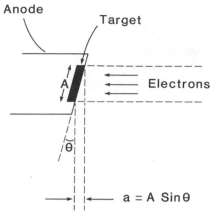

Figure 3.2. Diagram illustrating the principle of line focus. The side A of the actual focal spot is reduced to side a of the apparent focal spot. The other dimension (perpendicular to the plane of the paper) of the focal spot remains unchanged.

length remains the same as the original. The dimensions of the actual focal spot are chosen so that the apparent focal spot results in an approximate square. Therefore, by making the target angle θ small, side a can be reduced to a desired size. In diagnostic radiology, the target angles are quite small (6°–17°) to produce apparent focal spot sizes ranging from 0.1 × 0.1 to 2 × 2 mm. In most therapy tubes, however, the target angle is larger (about 30°) and the apparent focal spot ranges between 5 × 5 to 7 × 7 mm.

Since the x-rays are produced at various depths in the target, they suffer varying amounts of attenuation in the target. There is greater attenuation for x-rays coming from greater depths than those from near the surface of the target. Consequently, the intensity of the x-ray beam decreases from the cathode to the anode direction of the beam. This variation across the x-ray beam is called the *heel effect*. The effect is particularly pronounced in diagnostic tubes because of the low x-ray energy and steep target angles. The problem can be minimized by using a compensating filter to provide differential attenuation across the beam in order to compensate for the heel effect and improve the uniformity of the beam.

B. The Cathode

The cathode assembly in a modern x-ray tube (Coolidge tube) consists of a wire filament, a circuit to provide filament current and a negatively charged focusing cup. The function of the cathode cup is to direct the electrons toward the anode so that they strike the target in a well defined area, the focal spot. Since size of focal spot depends on filament size, the diagnostic tubes usually have two separate filaments to provide "dual-focus," namely one small and one large focal spot. The material of the filament is tungsten which is chosen because of its high melting point.

3.2 BASIC X-RAY CIRCUIT

The actual circuit of a modern x-ray machine is very complex. In this section, however, we will consider only the basic aspects of the x-ray circuit. For more detailed information the reader is referred to the literature.

A simplified diagram of a self-rectified therapy unit is shown in Fig. 3.3. The circuit can be divided into two parts: the high voltage circuit to provide the accelerating potential for the electrons and the low voltage circuit to supply heating current to the filament. Since the voltage applied between the cathode and the anode is high enough to accelerate all the electrons across to the target, the filament temperature or filament current controls the tube current (the current in the circuit due to the flow of electrons across the tube) and, hence, the x-ray intensity.

The filament supply for electron emission usually consists of 10 V at about 6 A. As shown in the diagram, this can be accomplished by using a step-down transformer in the AC line voltage. The filament current can be adjusted by varying the voltage applied to the filament. Since a small change in this voltage or filament current produces a large change in electron emission or the current (Fig. 3.10), a special kind of transformer is used which eliminates normal variations in line voltage.

The high voltage to the x-ray tube is supplied by the step-up transformer, as shown in Fig. 3.3. The primary of this transformer is connected to an *autotransformer* and a *rheostat*. The function of the autotransformer is to provide a stepwise adjustment in voltage. The device consists of a coil of wire wound on an iron core and operates on the principle of inductance. When an alternating line voltage is applied to the coil, potential is divided between the turns of the coil. By using a selector switch, a contact can be made to any

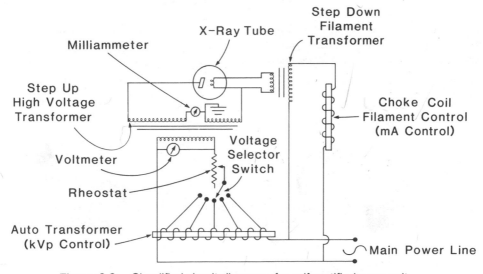

Figure 3.3.   Simplified circuit diagram of a self-rectified x-ray unit.

turn, thus varying the output voltage which is measured between the first turn of the coil and the selector contact.

The rheostat is a variable resister, *i.e.* a coil of wire wound on some cylindrical object with a sliding contact to introduce as much resistance in the circuit as desired and thus vary the voltage in a continuous manner. It may be mentioned that, whereas there is appreciable power loss in the rheostat because of the resistance of the wires, the power loss is small in the case of the inductance coil since the wires have low resistance.

The voltage input to the high tension transformer or the x-ray transformer can be read on a voltmeter in the primary part of its circuit. The voltmeter, however, is calibrated so that its reading corresponds to the kilovoltage which will be generated by the x-ray transformer secondary coil in the output part of the circuit and applied to the x-ray tube. The tube voltage can be measured by the *sphere gap* method in which the voltage is applied to two metallic spheres separated by an air gap. The spheres are slowly brought together until a spark appears. There is a mathematical relationship between the voltage, the diameter of the spheres, and the distance between them at the instant that the spark first appears.

The tube current can be read on a milliammeter in the high voltage part of the tube circuit. The meter is actually placed at the midpoint of the x-ray transformer secondary coil which is grounded. The meter, therefore, can be safely placed at the operator's console.

The alternating voltage applied to the x-ray tube is characterized by the peak voltage and the frequency. For example, if the line voltage is 220 V at 60 cycles/sec, the peak voltage will be $220\sqrt{2} = 311$ V, since the line voltage is normally expressed as the root mean square value. Thus, if this voltage is stepped up by an x-ray transformer of turn ratio 500:1, the resultant peak voltage applied to the x-ray tube, will be $220\sqrt{2} \times 500 = 155,564$ V = 155.6 kV.

Since the anode is positive with respect to the cathode only through half the voltage cycle, the tube current flows through that half of the cycle. During the next half-cycle, the voltage is reversed and the current cannot flow in the reverse direction. Thus, the tube current as well as the x-rays will be generated only during the half-cycle when the anode is positive. A machine operating in this manner is called the *self-rectified* unit. The variation with time of the voltage, tube current, and x-ray intensity[1] is illustrated in Fig. 3.4.

3.3 VOLTAGE RECTIFICATION

The disadvantage of the self-rectified circuit is that no x-rays are generated during the *inverse* voltage cycle (when the anode is negative relative to the cathode) and therefore the output of the machine is relatively low. Another problem arises when the target gets hot and emits electrons by the process of

---

[1] Intensity is defined as the time variation of energy fluence or total energy carried by particles (in this case, photons) per unit area per unit time. The term is also called energy flux density.

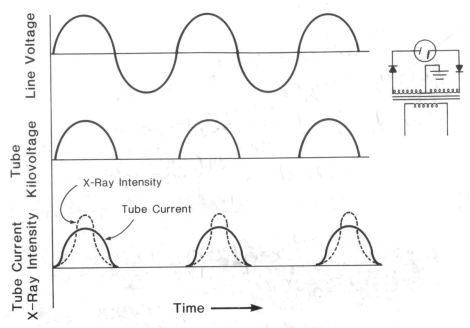

Figure 3.4. Graphs illustrating the variation with time of the line voltage, the tube kilovoltage, the tube current, and the x-ray intensity for self- or half-wave rectification. The half-value rectifier circuit is shown on the right. Rectifier indicates the direction of conventional current (opposite to the flow of electrons).

thermionic emission. During the inverse voltage cycle, these electrons will flow from the anode to the cathode and bombard the cathode filament. This can destroy the filament.

The problem of tube conduction during inverse voltage can be solved by using voltage rectifiers. Rectifiers placed in series in the high voltage part of the circuit prevent the tube from conducting during the inverse voltage cycle. The current will flow as usual during the cycle when the anode is positive relative to the cathode. This type of rectification is called *half-wave rectification* and is illustrated in Figure 3.4.

The high voltage rectifiers are either valve or solid state type. The valve rectifier is similar in principle to the x-ray tube. The cathode is a tungsten filament and the anode is a metallic plate or cylinder surrounding the filament. The current[2] flows only from anode to the cathode but the valve will not conduct during the inverse cycle even if the x-ray target gets hot and emits electrons.

A valve rectifier can be replaced by solid state rectifiers. These rectifiers consist of conductors which have been coated with certain semiconducting

---

[2] Here the current means conventional current. The electronic current will flow from the cathode to the anode.

elements such as selenium, silicon, and germanium. These semiconductors conduct electrons in one direction only and can withstand reverse voltage up to a certain magnitude. Because of their very small size, thousands of these rectifiers can be stacked in series in order to withstand the given inverse voltage.

Rectifiers can also be used to provide *full-wave* rectification. For example, four rectifiers can be arranged in the high voltage part of the circuit so that the x-ray tube cathode is negative and the anode is positive during both half-cycles of voltage. This is schematically shown in Fig. 3.5. The electronic current flows through the tube via ABCDEFGH when the transformer end A is negative and via HGCDEFBA when A is positive. Thus, the electrons flow from the filament to the target during both half-cycles of the transformer voltage. As a result of full wave rectification, the effective tube current is higher since the current flows during both half-cycles.

In addition to rectification, the voltage across the tube may be kept nearly constant by a smoothing condenser (high capacitance) placed across the x-ray tube. Such constant potential circuits are commonly used in x-ray machines for therapy.

3.4 PHYSICS OF X-RAY PRODUCTION

There are two different mechanisms by which x-rays are produced. One gives rise to *bremsstrahlung x-rays* and the other *characteristic x-rays*. These

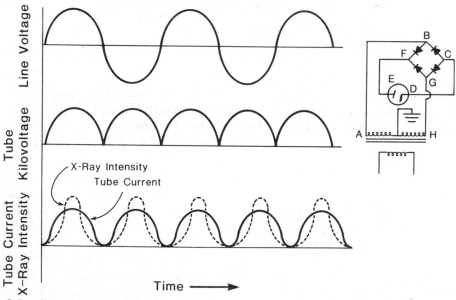

Figure 3.5. Graphs illustrating the variation with time of the line voltage, the tube kilovoltage, the tube current, and the x-ray intensity for full-wave rectification. The rectifier circuit is shown on the right. The arrow symbol of the rectifier indicates the direction of conventional current flow (opposite to the flow of electronic current).

processes were briefly mentioned earlier (Sections 1.5 and 3.1) but now will be presented in greater detail.

A. Bremsstrahlung

The process of bremsstrahlung (braking radiation) is the result of radiative "collision" (interaction) between a high speed electron and a nucleus. The electron while passing near a nucleus may be deflected from its path by the action of Coulomb forces of attraction and lose energy as bremsstrahlung, a phenomenon predicted by Maxwell's general theory of electromagnetic radiation. According to this theory, energy is propagated through space by electromagnetic fields. As the electron, with its associated electromagnetic field, passes in the vicinity of a nucleus, it suffers a sudden deflection and acceleration. As a result, a part or all of its energy is dissociated from it and propagates in space as electromagnetic radiation. The mechanism of bremsstrahlung production is illustrated in Fig. 3.6.

Since an electron may have one or more bremsstrahlung interactions in the material and an interaction may result in partial or complete loss of electron energy, the resulting bremsstrahlung photon may have any energy up to the initial energy of the electron. Also, the direction of emission of bremsstrahlung photons depends on the energy of the incident electrons (Fig. 3.7). At electron energies below about 100 keV, x-rays are emitted more or less equally in all directions. As the kinetic energy of the electrons increases, the direction of x-ray emission becomes increasingly forward. Therefore, *transmission-type targets* are used in megavoltage x-ray tubes (accelerators) in which the electrons bombard the target from one side and the x-ray beam is obtained on the other side. In the low voltage x-ray tubes, it is technically advantageous to obtain the x-ray beam on the same side of the target, *i.e.* at 90° with respect to the electron beam direction.

The energy loss per atom by electrons depends upon the square of the atomic number (Z^2). Thus, the probability of bremsstrahlung production varies with Z^2 of the target material. However the efficiency of x-ray production depends on the first power of atomic number and the voltage applied to the tube. The term efficiency is defined as the ratio of ouput energy emitted as

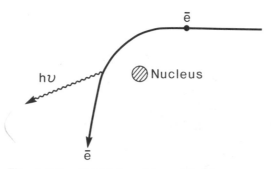

Figure 3.6. Illustration of bremsstrahlung process.

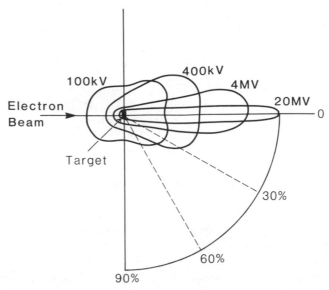

Figure 3.7. Schematic illustration of spatial distribution of x-rays around a thin target.

x-rays to the input energy deposited by electrons. It can be shown (1, 2) that:

$$\text{Efficiency} = 9 \times 10^{-10} \, ZV$$

where V is tube voltage in volts. From the above equation it can be shown that the efficiency of x-ray production with tungsten target ($Z = 74$) for electrons accelerated through 100 kV is less than 1%. The rest of the input energy (~99%) appears as heat.

B. Characteristic X-rays

Electrons incident on the target also produce characteristic x-rays. The mechanism of their production is illustrated in Fig. 3.8. An electron, with kinetic energy E_0, may interact with the atoms of the target by ejecting an orbital electron, such as a K, L, or M electron, leaving the atom *ionized*. The original electron will recede from the collision with energy $E_0 - \Delta E$, where ΔE is the energy given to the orbital electron. A part of ΔE is spent in overcoming the binding energy of the electron and the rest is carried by the ejected electron. When a vacancy is created in an orbit, an outer orbital electron will fall down to fill that vacancy. In so doing, the energy is radiated in the form of electromagnetic radiation. This is called characteristic radiation, *i.e.* characteristic of the atoms in the target and of the shells between which the transitions took place. With higher atomic number targets and the transitions involving inner shells such as K, L, M, and N, the characteristic radiations emitted are of high enough energies to be considered in the x-ray part of the elctromagnetic spectrum. Table 3.1 gives the major characteristic radiation produced in a tungsten target.

It should be noted that, unlike bremsstrahlung, characteristic radiation or x-rays are emitted at discrete energies. If the transition involved an electron descending from the L shell to the K shell, then the photon emitted will have energy $h\nu = E_K - E_L$, where E_K and E_L are the electron-binding energies of the K shell and the L shell, respectively.

The threshold energy that an incident electron must possess in order to first strip an electron from the atom is called *critical absorption energy*. These energies for some elements are given in Table 3.2.

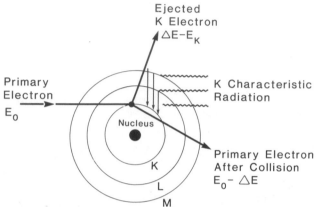

Figure 3.8. Diagram to explain the production of characteristic radiation.

Table 3.1.
Principal characteristic x-ray energies for tungsten

	Lines	Transition	Energy (keV)
K Series	$K\beta_2$	$N_{III} - K$	69.09
	$K\beta_1$	$M_{III} - K$	67.23
	$K\alpha_1$	$L_{III} - K$	59.31
	$K\alpha_2$	$L_{II} - K$	57.97
L Series	$L\gamma_1$	$N_{IV} - L_{II}$	11.28
	$L\beta_2$	$N_V - L_{III}$	9.96
	$L\beta_1$	$M_{IV} - L_{II}$	9.67
	$L\alpha_1$	$M_V - L_{III}$	8.40
	$L\alpha_2$	$M_{IV} - L_{III}$	8.33

Data from *Radiological Health Handbook* (4).

Table 3.2.
Critical absorption energies (keV)

	Element											
	H	C	O	Al	Ca	Cu	Sn	I	Ba	W	Pb	U
Level Z =	1	6	8	13	20	29	50	53	56	74	82	92
K	0.0136	0.283	0.531	1.559	4.038	8.980	29.190	33.164	37.41	69.508	88.001	115.59
L				0.087	0.399	1.100	4.464	5.190	5.995	12.090	15.870	21.753

Data from *Radiological Health Handbook* (4).

3.5 X-RAY ENERGY SPECTRA

X-ray photons produced by an x-ray machine are heterogenous in energy. The energy spectrum shows a continuous distribution of energies for the bremsstrahlung photons superimposed by characteristic radiation of discrete energies. A typical spectral distribution is shown in Fig. 3.9.

If no filtration, inherent or added, of the beam is assumed, the calculated energy spectrum will be a straight line (shown as dotted line in Fig. 3.9) and mathematically given by Kramer's equation (5):

$$I_E = KZ(E_m - E) \tag{3.1}$$

where I_E is the intensity of photons with energy E, Z is the atomic number of the target, E_m is the maximum photon energy, and K is a constant. As pointed out earlier, the maximum possible energy that a bremsstrahlung photon can have is equal to the energy of the incident electron. The maximum energy in kiloelectron volts is numerically equal to the applied kilovolts peak (kVp). However, the intensity of such photons is zero as predicted by the above equation, *i.e.* $I_E = 0$ when $E = E_m$.

The unfiltered energy spectrum discussed above is considerably modified as the photons experience inherent filtration (absorption in the target, glass walls of the tube or thin beryllium window). The inherent filtration in conventional x-ray tubes is usually equivalent to about 0.5- to 1.0-mm aluminum. Added filtration, placed externally to the tube, further modifies the spectrum. It should be noted that the filtration affects primarily the initial low energy part of the spectrum and does not affect significantly the high energy photon distribution.

The purpose of the *added filtration* is to enrich the beam with higher energy

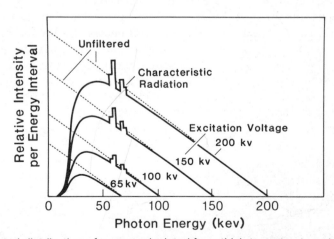

Figure 3.9. Spectral distribution of x-rays calculated for a thick tungsten target using Equation 3.1. Dotted curves are for no filtration and the solid curves are for a filtration of 1-mm aluminum. Redrawn from Johns and Cunningham (3).

photons by absorbing the lower energy components of the spectrum. As the filtration is increased, the transmitted beam *hardens, i.e.* it achieves higher average energy and therefore greater penetrating power. Thus, the addition of filtration is one way of improving the penetrating power of the beam. The other method, of course, is by increasing the voltage across the tube. Since the total intensity of the beam (area under the curves in Fig. 3.9) decreases with increasing filtration and increases with voltage, a proper combination of voltage and filtration is required to achieve desired hardening of the beam as well as acceptable intensity.

The shape of the x-ray energy spectrum is the result of the alternating voltage applied to the tube, multiple bremsstrahlung interactions within the target and filtration in the beam. However, even if the x-ray tube were to be energized with a constant potential, the x-ray beam would still be heterogeneous in energy because of the multiple bremsstrahlung processes which result in different energy photons.

Because of the x-ray beam having a spectral distribution of energies, which depends on voltage as well as filtration, it is difficult to characterize the beam quality in terms of energy, penetrating power, or degree of beam hardening. A rule of thumb is often used which states that the average x-ray energy is approximately one-third of the maximum energy or kVp. Of course, the one-third rule is a rough approximation since filtration significantly alters the average energy. Another quantity, known as *half-value layer*, has been defined to describe the quality of an x-ray beam. This topic is discussed in detail in Chapter 7.

3.6 OPERATING CHARACTERISTICS

In this section, the relationships between x-ray output, filament current, tube current, and tube voltage are briefly discussed.

The filament current affects the emission of electrons from the filament and, therefore, the tube current. Figure 3.10a shows the typical relationship between the relative exposure rate and the filament current measured in amperes (A). The figure shows that under typical operating conditions (filament current of 5 to 6 A), a small change in filament current produces a large change in relative exposure rate. This means that the constancy of filament current is critical to the constancy of the x-ray output.

The *output* of an x-ray machine can also be expressed in terms of the ionization it produces in air. This quantity, which is a measure of ionization per unit mass of air, is called *exposure*. In Fig. 3.10 (curve b), the exposure rate is plotted as a function of the tube current. There is a linear relationship between exposure rate and tube current. As the current or milliamperage is doubled, the output is also doubled.

The increase in the x-ray output with increase in voltage, however, is much greater than that given by a linear relationship. Although the actual shape of the curve (Fig. 3.10c) depends on the filtration, the output of an x-ray machine varies approximately as a square of kilovoltage.

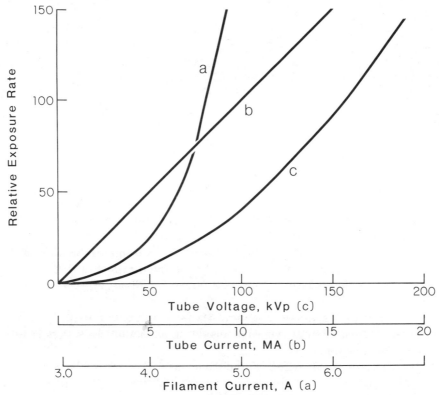

Figure 3.10.   Illustration of typical operating characteristics. Plots of relative exposure rate *vs.*: (a) filament current at a given kVp; (b) tube current at a given kVp; (c) tube voltage at a given tube current.

References

1. Botden P: Modern trends in diagnostic radiologic instrumentation. In Moseley R, Rust J (eds): *The Reduction of Patient Dose by Diagnostic Radiologic Instrumentation.* Springfield, IL, Charles C Thomas, 1964, p 15.
2. Hendee WR: *Medical Radiation Physics*, 2nd ed. Chicago, Year Book Medical Publishers, 1979.
3. Johns HE, Cunningham JR: *The Physics of Radiology*, 3rd ed. Springfield, IL, Charles C Thomas, 1969.
4. *Radiological Health Handbook*, revised ed. United States Department of Health, Education, and Welfare, Superintendent of Documents, Washington, D. C., United States Government Printing Office, 1970.
5. Kramers HA: On the theory of x-ray absorption and the continuous x-ray spectrum. *Phil Mag* 46:836, 1923.

CHAPTER **4**

Clinical Radiation Generators

4.1 KILOVOLTAGE UNITS

Up to about 1950, most of the external beam radiotherapy was carried out with x-rays generated at voltages up to 300 kVp. Subsequent development of higher energy machines and the increasing popularity of the cobalt-60 units in the 50s and the 60s resulted in a gradual demise of the conventional kilovoltage machines. However, these machines have not completely disappeared. Even in the present era of the megavoltage beams, there is still some use for the lower energy beams, especially in the treatment of superficial skin lesions.

In Chapter 3, we discussed in general the principle and operation of an x-ray generator. In this chapter, we will consider in particular the salient features of the therapy machines.

On the basis of beam quality and their use, the x-ray therapy in the kilovoltage range has been divided into subcategories (1, 2). The following ranges are more in accordance with Ref. 2.

A. Grenz-ray Therapy

The term "grenz-ray therapy" is used to describe treatment with beams of very soft (low energy) x-rays produced at potentials below 20 kV. Because of the very low depth of penetration (Fig. 4.1a), such radiations are no longer used in radiotherapy.

B. Contact Therapy

A "contact therapy" machine operates at potentials of 40–50 kV and facilitates irradiation of accessible lesions at very short source (focal spot) to surface distances (SSD). The machine operates typically at a tube current of 2 mA. Applicators available with such machines can provide an SSD of 2.0 cm or less. A filter of 0.5 to 1.0-mm thick aluminum is usually interposed in the beam to absorb the very soft component of the energy spectrum.

Because of very short SSD and low voltage, the contact therapy beam produces a very rapidly decreasing depth dose[1] in tissue. For that reason, if the beam is incident on a patient, the skin surface is maximally irradiated but

---

[1] The term dose or absorbed dose is defined as the energy absorbed per unit mass of the irradiated material.

47

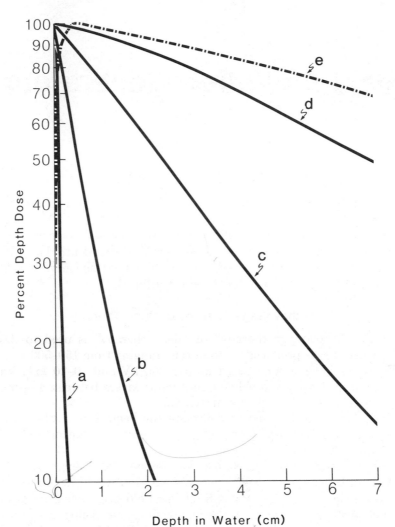

Figure 4.1.   Depth dose curves in water or soft tissues for various quality beams. [Plotted from data in Cohen M, Jones DEA, Green D (eds): *Central Axis Depth Dose Data for Use in Radiotherapy. Br J Radiol.* (Suppl 11) The British Institute of Radiology, London, 1978.] (a) Grenz rays, HVL = 0.04 mm Al, field diameter ≃ 33 cm, SSD = 10 cm. (b) Contact therapy, HVL = 1.5 mm Al, field diameter = 2.0 cm, SSD = 2 cm. (c) Superficial therapy, HVL = 3.0 mm Al, field diameter = 3.6 cm, SSD = 20 cm. (d) Orthovoltage, HVL = 2.0 mm Cu, field size = 10 × 10 cm, SSD = 50 cm. (e) Cobalt-60 γ rays, field size = 10 × 10 cm, SSD = 80 cm.

the underlying tissues are spared to an increasing degree with depth. The dose *vs.* depth curve or simply the depth dose curve of a typical contact therapy beam is shown in Fig. 4.1b. It is readily seen that this quality of radiation is useful for tumors not deeper than 1–2 mm. The beam is almost completely absorbed with 2 cm of soft tissues.

C. Superficial Therapy

The term "superficial therapy" applies to treatment with x-rays produced at potentials ranging from 50 to 150 kV. Varying thicknesses of filtration (usually 1–6-mm aluminum) are added to harden the beam to a desired degree. As mentioned in Section 3.5, the degree of hardening or beam quality can be expressed as the half-value layer (HVL). The HVL is defined as the thickness of a specified material which, when introduced into the path of the beam, reduces the exposure rate by one-half. Typical HVLs used in the superficial range are 1.0- to 8.0-mm Al.

The superficial treatments are usually given with the help of applicators or cones attachable to the diaphragm of the machine. The SSD typically ranges between 15 and 20 cm. The machine is usually operated at a tube current of 5–8 mA.

As seen in Fig. 4.1c, a superficial beam of the quality shown is useful for irradiating tumors confined to about 5-mm depth (~90% depth dose). Beyond this depth, the dose drop-off is too severe to deliver adequate depth dose without considerable overdosing of the skin surface.

D. Orthovoltage Therapy or Deep Therapy

The term "orthovoltage therapy" or "deep therapy" is used to describe treatment with x-rays produced at potentials ranging from 150–500 kV. Most orthovoltage equipment is oeprated at 200–300 kV and 10–20 mA. Various filters have been designed to achieve half-value layers between 1–4-mm Cu. An orthovoltage machine is shown in Fig. 4.2.

Although cones can be used to collimate the beam into a desired size, a movable diaphragm, consisting of lead plates, permits a continuously adjustable field size. The SSD is usually set at 50 cm.

Figure 4.1d shows a depth dose curve for a moderately filtered orthovoltage beam. Although the actual depth dose distribution would depend on many conditions such as kilovoltage, HVL, SSD, and field size, some generalizations can be made from this curve about the orthovoltage beam characteristics. The maximum dose occurs close to the skin surface, with 90% of that value occurring at about 2-cm depth. Thus, in a single field treatment, adequate dose cannot be delivered to a tumor beyond this depth. However, by increasing beam filtration or HVL and combining two or more beams directed at the tumor from different directions, one can deliver higher dose to deeper tumors. As will be discussed in further detail in Chapter 11, there are severe limitations to the use of orthovoltage beam in treating lesions deeper than 2–3 cm. The greatest limitation is the skin dose which becomes prohibitively large when adequate doses are to be delivered to deep seated tumors. In the early days of radiotherapy, when orthovoltage was the highest energy available, treatments were given until radiation tolerance of the skin was reached. Although methods were developed to use *multiple beams* and other techniques to keep the skin dose under tolerance limits, the problem of high skin dose remained an

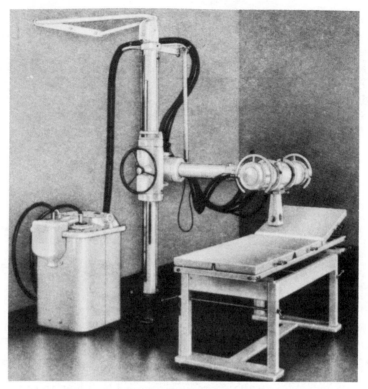

Figure 4.2.   Photograph of Sieman's Stabilapan.

overriding concern in the orthovoltage era. With the availability of cobalt
teletherapy, the *skin-sparing* properties of higher energy radiation (see Fig.
4.1e) became the major reason for the modern trend to megavoltage beams.

Although skin dose and depth dose distribution have been presented here
as two examples of the limitations posed by low energy beams, there are other
properties such as increased absorbed dose in bone and increased scattering
that make orthovoltage beams unsuitable for the treatment of tumors behind
bone.

E. Supervoltage Therapy

X-ray therapy in the range of 500–1000 kV has been designated as "high
voltage therapy" or "supervoltage therapy." In a quest for higher energy x-ray
beams, considerable progress was made during the postwar years toward
developing higher voltage machines. The major problem at that time was
insulating the high voltage transformer. It soon became apparent that conventional transformer systems were not suitable for producing potential much
above 300 kVp. However, with the rapidly advancing technology of the times,
new approaches to the design of high energy machines were found. One of

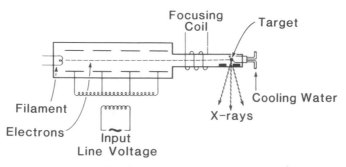

Figure 4.3. Diagram of a resonant transformer unit.

these machines is the resonant transformer, in which the voltage is stepped up in a very efficient manner.

E.1. RESONANT TRANSFORMER UNITS

Resonant transformer units have been used to generate x-rays from 300 to 2,000 kV. The schematic diagram of the apparatus is shown in Fig. 4.3. In this apparatus, the secondary of the high voltage transformer (without the iron core) is connected in parallel with capacitors distributed lengthwise inside the x-ray tube. The combination of the transformer secondary and the capacitance in parallel exhibits the phenomenon of resonance. At the resonant frequency, the oscillating potential attains very high amplitude. Thus, the peak voltage across the x-ray tube becomes very large when the transformer is tuned to resonate at the input frequency. Since the electrons attain high energies before striking the target, a transmission type target (Section 3.4) may be used to obtain the x-ray beam on the other side of the target. The electrical insulation is provided by pressurized Freon gas.

F. Megavoltage Therapy

X-ray beams of energy 1 MV or greater can be classified as megavoltage beams. Although the term strictly applies to the x-ray beams, the γ ray beams produced by radionuclides are also commonly included in this category if their energy is 1 MeV or greater. Examples of clinical megavoltage machines are accelerators such as Van de Graaff generator, linear accelerator, betatron and microton, and teletherapy γ ray units such as cobalt-60.

4.2 VAN DE GRAAF GENERATOR

The Van de Graaf machine is an electrostatic accelerator designed to accelerate charged particles. In radiotherapy, the unit accelerates electrons to produce high energy x-rays, typically at 2 MV.

Figure 4.4 shows a schematic diagram illustrating the basic principle of a Van de Graaf generator. In this machine, a charge voltage of 20–40 kV is applied across a moving belt of insulating material. A corona discharge takes

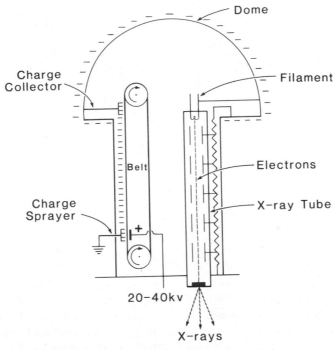

Figure 4.4. A Van de Graaff generator.

place and electrons are sprayed onto the belt. These electrons are carried to the top where they are removed by a collector connected to a spherical dome. As the negative charges collect on the sphere, a high potential is developed between the sphere and the ground. This potential is applied across the x-ray tube consisting of a filament, a series of metal rings and a target. The rings are connected to resisters in order to provide a uniform drop of potential from the bottom to the top. X-rays are produced when the electrons strike the target.

Van de Graaf machines are capable of reaching energies up to 10 MV, limited only by size and required high voltage insulation. Normally the insulation is provided by a mixture of nitrogen and CO_2. The generator is enclosed in a steel tank and is filled with the gas mixture at a pressure of about 20 atmospheres.

Van de Graaf and resonant transformer (Section 4.1E) units for clinical use are no longer produced commercially. Only about 20 units of this type still remain in operation in the United States. The reason for their demise is the emergence of technically better machines such as cobalt-60 units and linear accelerators.

4.3 LINEAR ACCELERATOR

The linear accelerator (linac) is a device which uses high frequency electro-magnetic waves to accelerate charged particles such as electrons to high energies through a linear tube. The high energy electron beam itself can be used for treating superficial tumors or it can be made to strike a target to produce x-rays for treating deep seated tumors.

There are several types of linear accelerator designs but the ones used in radiotherapy accelerate electrons either by traveling or stationary elecromagnetic waves of frequency in the microwave region (~3000 megacycles/sec). The difference between traveling wave and stationary wave accelerators is the design of the accelerator structure. Functionally, the traveling wave structures require a terminating or "dummy" load in order to absorb the residual power at the end of the structure, thus preventing a backward reflected wave. On the other hand, the standing wave structures provide maximum reflection of the waves at both ends of the structure so that the combination of forward and reverse traveling waves will give rise to stationary waves. In the standing wave design, the microwave power is coupled into the structure via side coupling cavities rather than through the beam aperture. Such a design tends to be more efficient than the traveling wave designs since axial, beam transport cavities and the side cavities can be independently optimized (3). However, it is more expensive and requires installation of a *circulator* (or isolator) between the power source and the structure to prevent reflections from reaching the power source. For further details on this subject and linear accelerator operation the reader is referred to a review article by Karzmark and Pering (3).

Figure 4.5 is a block diagram of a medical linear accelerator showing major components and auxillary systems. A *power supply* provides DC power to the *modulator* which includes the *pulse forming network* and a switch tube known as *hydrogen thyraton*. High voltage pulses from the modulator section are flat topped DC pulses of a few microseconds in duration. These pulses are delivered to the *magnetron* or *klystron*[2] and simultaneously to the electron gun. Pulsed microwaves produced in the magnetron or klystron are injected into the accelerator tube or structure via a *waveguide* system. At the proper instant electrons, produced by an *electron gun*, are also pulse-injected into the *accelerator structure.*

The accelerator structure consists of a copper tube with its interior divided by copper discs or diaphragms of varying aperture and spacing. This section is evacuated to a high vacuum. As the electrons are injected into the accelerator structure with an initial energy of about 50 keV, the electrons interact with the electromagnetic field of the microwaves. The electrons gain energy from the sinusoidal electric field by an acceleration process analogous to that of a surf rider.

As the high energy electrons emerge from the exit window of the acclerator structure, they are in the form of a pencil beam of about 3 mm in diameter. In the low energy linacs (up to 6 MV) with relatively short accelerator tube, the

---

[2] Magnetron and klystron are both devices for producing microwaves. Whereas magnetrons are generally less expensive than klystrons, the latter have a long life span. In addition, klystrons are capable of delivering higher power levels required for high energy accelerators and are preferred as the beam energy approaches 20 MeV or higher.

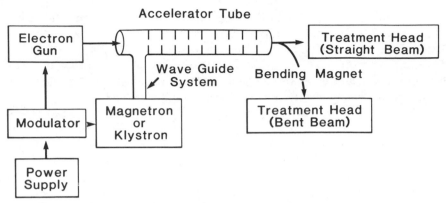

Figure 4.5. A block diagram of typical medical linear accelerator.

electrons are allowed to proceed straight on and strike a target for x-ray production. In the higher energy linacs, however, the accelerator structure is too long and, therefore, is placed horizontally or at an angle with respect to the horizontal. The electrons are then bent through a suitable angle (usually about 90° or 270°) between the accelerator structure and the target. The precision bending of the electron beam is accomplished by the *beam transport system* consisting of bending magnets, focusing coils, and other components.

A. The Linac X-ray Beam

Bremsstrahlung x-rays are produced when the electrons are incident on a target of a high Z material such as tungsten. The target is water cooled and is thick enough to absorb most of the incident electrons. As a result of bremsstrahlung type interactions (Section 3.4A), the electron energy is converted into a spectrum of x-ray energies with maximum energy equal to the incident electron energy. The average photon energy of the beam is approximately one-third of the maximum energy.

It is customary for some of the manufacturers to designate their linear accelerators that have both electron and x-ray treatment capabilities by the maximum energy of the electron beam available. For example, the Varian Clinac 18 unit produces electron beams of energy 6, 9, 12, 15, and 18 MeV and x-rays of energy 10 MV. It should be noted that the electron beam is designated by million electron volts because it is almost monoenergetic before incidence on the patient surface. The x-ray beam, on the other hand, is heterogeneous in energy and is designated by megavolts, as if the beam were produced by applying that voltage across an x-ray tube.

B. The Electron Beam

As mentioned earlier, the electron beam, as it exits the window of the accelerator tube is a narrow pencil of about 3-mm diameter. In the electron mode of linac operation, this beam, instead of striking the target, is made to strike an electron *scattering foil* in order to spread the beam as well as get a uniform electron fluence across the treatment field. The scattering foil consists of a thin metallic foil, usually of lead. The thickness of the foil is such that most of the electrons are scattered instead of suffering bremsstrahlung. However, small fraction of the total energy is still converted into bremsstrahlung and appears as x-ray contamination of the electron beam.

In some linacs, the broadening of the electron beam is accomplished by electromagnetic scanning of the electron pencil beam over a large area. Although this minimizes the x-ray contamination, some x-rays are still produced by electrons striking the collimator walls or other high atomic number materials in the electron collimation system.

C. Treatment Head

The treatment head (Fig. 4.5) consists of a thick shell of high density shielding material such as lead, tungsten, or lead-tungsten alloy. It contains an x-ray target, scattering foil, flattening filter, ion chamber, fixed and movable collimator, and light localizer system. The head provides sufficient shielding against leakage radiation in accordance with radiation protection guidelines (Section 16.7B).

D. Target and Flattening Filter

In Section 3.4A, we discussed the angular distribution of x-rays produced by electrons of various energies incident on a target. Since linear accelerators produce electrons in the megavoltage range, the x-ray intensity is peaked in the forward direction. In order to make the beam intensity uniform across the field, a *flattening filter* is inserted in the beam (Fig. 4.6A). This filter is usually

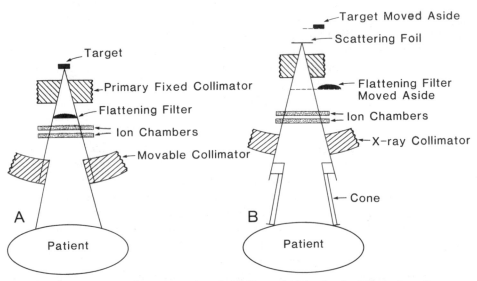

Figure 4.6. Components of treatment head. (A) X-ray therapy mode; (B) electron therapy mode.

made of lead, although tungsten, uranium, steel, and aluminum or a combination have also been used or suggested. The choice of target and flattening filter materials has been discussed by Podgorsak *et al.* (4).

E. Beam Collimation and Monitoring

The treatment beam is first collimated by a *fixed primary collimator* located immediately beyond the x-ray target or scattering foil. In the case of x-rays, the collimated beam then passes through the flattening filter. In the electron mode, the filter is moved out of the way (Fig. 4.6B).

The flattened x-ray beam or the electron beam is incident on the *dose monitoring chambers.* The monitoring system consists of several ion chambers or a single chamber with multiple plates. Although the chambers are usually transmission type, *i.e.* flat parallel plate chambers to cover the entire beam, cylindrical thimble chambers have also been used in some linacs.

The function of the ion chamber is to monitor dose rate, integrated dose, and field symmetry. Since the chambers are in a high intensity radiation field and the beam is pulsed, it is important to make sure that the ion collection efficiency of the chambers remains unchanged with changes in the dose rate. Bias voltages in the range of 300 to 1000 V are applied across the chamber electrodes, depending on the chamber design. Contrary to the beam calibration chambers, the monitor chambers in the treatment head are sealed so that their response is not influenced by temperature and pressure of the outside air. However, these chambers have to be periodically checked for leaks.

After passing through the ion chambers, the beam is further collimated by a continuously *movable x-ray collimator.* This collimator consists of two pairs of lead or tungsten blocks (jaws) which provide a rectangular opening from 0 × 0 to the maximum field size (40 × 40 cm or a little less) projected at a standard distance such as 100 cm from the x-ray source (focal spot on the target). The collimator blocks are constrained to move so that the block edge is always along a radial line passing through the target.

The field size definition is provided by a *light localizing system* in the treatment head. A combination of mirror and a light source located in the space between the chambers and the jaws projects a light beam as if emitting from the x-ray focal spot. Thus, the light field is congruent with the radiation field. Frequent checks are required to ensure this important requirement of field alignment.

Whereas the x-ray collimation systems of most medical linacs are similar, the *electron collimation systems* vary widely. Since electrons scatter readily in air, the beam collimation must be achieved close to the skin surface of the patient. There is a considerable scattering of electrons from the collimator surfaces including the movable jaws. Dose rate can change by a factor of 2 or 3 as the collimator jaws are opened to maximum field size limits. If the electrons are collimated by the same jaws as for x-rays, there will be an extremely stringent requirement on the accuracy of the jaw opening since output is so critically dependent on the surface area of the collimator. This problem has been solved by keeping the x-ray collimator wide open and attaching an auxillary collimator for electrons in the form of trimmers extended down to the skin surface. In other systems, the auxillary electron collimator consists of a set of attachable cones of various sizes.

It should be mentioned that, due to the electron scattering, the dose distribution in an electron field is significantly influenced by the collimation system provided with the machine.

F. Gantry

Most of the linear accelerators currently produced are constructed so that the source of radiation can rotate about a horizontal axis (Fig. 4.7). As the gantry rotates, the collimator axis (supposedly coincident with the central axis of the beam) moves in a vertical plane. The point of intersection of the collimator axis and the axis of rotation of the gantry is known as the *isocenter*.

The isocentric mounting of the radiation machines has advantages over the units that move only up and down. The latter units are not suitable for

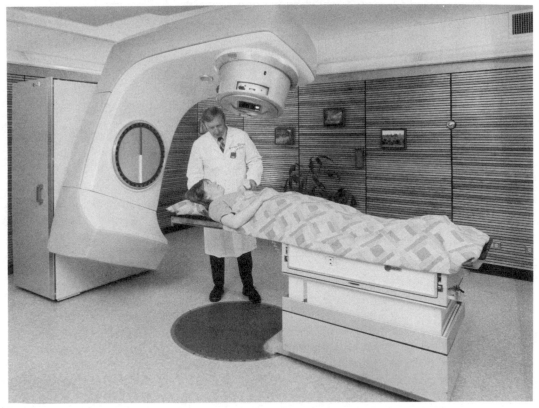

Figure 4.7. Photograph of a linear accelerator, isocentrically mounted. Courtesy of Varian Associates, Palo Alto, California.

isocentric treatment techniques in which beams are directed from different directions but intersect at the same point, the isocenter, placed inside the patient. However, the nonisocentric units are usually swivel mounted, *i.e.* the treatment head can be swiveled or rotated in any direction while the gantry can move only upward or downward. Although these units are not as flexible, they are mechanically simpler, more reliable, and less expensive than the isocentric models.

4.4 BETATRON

The operation of the betatron is based on the principle that an electron in a changing magnetic field experiences acceleration in a circular orbit. Figure 4.8 shows a schematic drawing of the machine. The accelerating tube is shaped like a hollow doughnut and is placed between the poles of an alternating current magnet. A pulse of electrons is introduced into this evacuated doughnut by an injector at the instant that the alternating current cycle begins. As the magnetic field rises, the electrons experience acceleration continuously and spin with increasing velocity around the tube. By the end of the first quarter cycle of the alternating magnetic field, the electrons have made several thousand revolutions and achieved maximum energy. At this instant or earlier, depending upon the energy desired, the electrons are made to spiral out of the orbit by an additional attractive force. The high energy electrons then strike a target to produce x-rays or a scattering foil to produce a broad beam of electrons.

Betatrons were first used for radiotherapy in the early 1950s. They preceded the introduction of linear accelerators by a few years. Although the betatrons can provide x-ray and electron therapy beams over a wide range of energies, from less than 6 to more than 40 MeV, they are inherently low electron beam current devices. The x-ray dose rates and field size capabilities of medical betatrons are low compared to medical linacs and even modern cobalt units. However, in the electron therapy mode, the beam current is adequate to provide a high dose rate. The reason for this difference between x-ray and

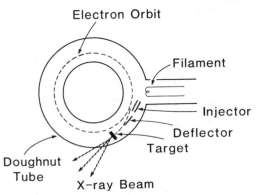

Figure 4.8. Diagram illustrating the operation of a betatron.

electron dose rates is that the x-ray production via bremsstrahlung as well as beam flattening requires a much larger primary electron beam current (about 3 orders of magnitude greater) than that required for the electron therapy beam.

The availability of medium energy linacs with high x-ray dose rates, large field sizes, and electron therapy energies up to 20 MeV, has given the linacs a considerable edge in popularity over the betatrons. Moreover, many radiotherapists regard the small field size and dose rate capabilities of the betatron as serious disadvantages to the general use of the device. Thus, a significant increase in betatron installations in this country, paralleling medical linacs, seems unlikely.

4.5 MICROTRON

The microtron is an electron accelerator which combines the principles of both the linear accelerator and the cyclotron (Section 4.6). In the microtron, the electrons are accelerated by the oscillating electric field of a single microwave cavity (Fig. 4.9). A magnetic field forces the electrons to move in a circular orbit and return to the cavity. As the electrons receive higher and higher energy by repeated passes through the cavity, they describe orbits of increasing radius in the magnetic field. The cavity voltage, frequency, and magnetic field are so adjusted that the electrons arrive each time in the correct phase at the cavity. Since the electrons travel with an approximately constant velocity (almost the speed of light), the above condition can be maintained if the path length of the orbits increases with one microwave wavelength per revolution. The microwave power source is either a klystron or a magnetron.

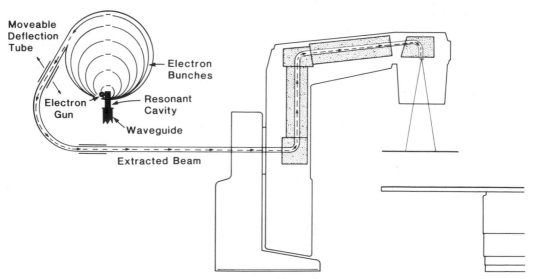

Figure 4.9. Schematic diagram of a microtron unit. (Reprinted with permission from: AB Scanditronix, Uppsala, Sweden.)

The extraction of the electrons from an orbit is accomplished by a narrow deflection tube of steel which screens the effect of the magnetic field. When the beam energy is selected, the deflection tube is automatically moved to the appropriate orbit to extract the beam.

The principal advantages of the microtron over a linear accelerator of comparable energy are its simplicity, easy energy selection, small beam energy spread, and a smaller size of the machine. Because of the low energy spread of the accelerated electrons and small beam emittance (product of beam diameter and divergence), the beam transport system is greatly simplified. These characteristics have encouraged the use of a single microtron to supply a beam to several treatment rooms.

Although the method of accelerating electrons used in the microtron was proposed as early as in 1944 by Veksler (5), the first microtron for radiotherapy (a 10-MeV unit) was described by Reistad and Brahme (6) in 1972. Later a 22-MeV microtron (7) was developed by AB Scanditronix and installed at the University of Umeå, Sweden. This particular model (MM 22) produced two x-rays beams of energy 6 or 10 and 21 MV and 10 electron beams of 2, 5, 7, 9, 11, 13, 16, 18, 20, and 22 MeV.

4.6 CYCLOTRON

The cyclotron is a charged particle accelerator, mainly used for nuclear physics research. In radiotherapy, these machines have been used as a source of high energy protons for proton beam therapy. More recently, the cyclotrons have been adopted for generating neutron beams. In the latter case the deuterons ($_{1}^{2}H^{+}$) are accelerated to high energies and then made to strike a suitable target to produce neutrons by nuclear reactions. One such reaction occurs when a beam of deuterons, accelerated to a high energy (~15–50 MeV), strikes a target of low atomic number, such as beryllium. Neutrons are produced by a process called stripping (Section 2.8D). Another important use of the cyclotron in medicine is as a particle accelerator for the production of certain radionuclides.

A schematic diagram illustrating the principle of cyclotron operation is shown in Fig. 4.10. The machine consists essentially of a short metallic cylinder

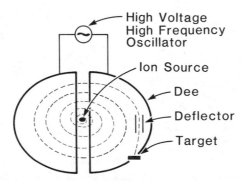

Figure 4.10.   Diagram illustrating the principle of operation of a cyclotron.

divided into two sections, usually referred to as "Ds". These Ds are highly evacuated and placed between the poles of a direct current magnet (not shown) producing a constant magnetic field. An alternating potential is applied between the two Ds. Positively charged particles such as protons or deuterons are injected into the chamber at the center of the two Ds. Under the action of the magnetic field, the particles travel in a circular orbit. The frequency of the alternating potential is adjusted so that as the particle passes from one D to the other, it is accelerated by the electric field of the right polarity. With each pass between the Ds, the particle receives an increment of energy and the radius of its orbit increases. Thus, by making many revolutions, the particle such as a deuteron achieves kinetic energy as high as 30 MeV.

There is a limit to the energy that a particle can attain by the above process. According to the theory of relativity, as the particle reaches high velocity (in the relativistic range), further acceleration causes the particle to gain in mass. This tends to slow down the particle which can then get out of step with the frequency of the alternating potential applied to the Ds. This problem has been solved in the synchrotrons where the frequency of the potential is adjusted to compensate for the decrease in particle velocity.

4.7 MACHINES USING RADIONUCLIDES

Radionuclides such as radium-226, cesium-137, and cobalt-60 have been used as sources of γ rays for teletherapy.[3] These γ rays are emitted from the radionuclides as they undergo radioactive disintegration.

Of all the radionuclides, ^{60}Co has proved to be the most suitable for external beam radiotherapy. The reasons for its choice over radium and cesium are higher possible specific activity (curies per gram), greater radiation output per curie and higher average photon energy. These characteristics for the three radionuclides are compared in Table 4.1. In addition, radium is much more expensive and has greater self-absorption of its radiation than either cesium or cobalt.

A. Cobalt-60 Unit

A.1. SOURCE

The ^{60}Co source is produced by irradiating ordinary stable ^{59}Co with neutrons in a reactor. The nuclear reaction can be represented by ^{59}Co(n,γ) ^{60}Co.

The ^{60}Co source, usually in the form of a solid cylinder, discs, or pallets, is contained inside a stainless steel capsule and sealed by welding. This capsule is placed into another steel capsule which is again sealed by welding. The double welded seal is necessary to prevent any leakage of the radioactive material.

The ^{60}Co source decays to ^{60}Ni with the emission of β particles ($E_{max} = 0.32$ MeV) and two photons per distintegration of energies 1.17 and 1.33 MeV

---

[3] Teletherapy is a general term applied to external beam treatments in which the source of radiation is at a large distance from the patient.

Table 4.1.
Teletherapy source characteristics

Radionuclide	Half-life (years)	γ Ray energy (MeV)	Γ Value* $\left(\dfrac{Rm^2}{Ci-h}\right)$	Specific activity achieved in practice (Ci/g)
Radium-226 (filtered by 0.5 mm Pt)	1622	0.83 (avg.)	0.825	~0.98
Cesium-137	30.0	0.66	0.326	~50
Cobalt-60	5.26	1.17, 1.33	1.30	~200

* Exposure rate constant (Γ) is discussed in Section 8.5. The higher the Γ value, the greater will be the exposure rate or output per curie of the teletherapy source.

(decay scheme given in Fig. 1.5). These γ rays constitute the useful treatment beam. The β particles are absorbed in the cobalt metal and the stainless steel capsules resulting in the emission of bremsstrahlung x-rays and a small amount of characteristic x-rays. However, these x-rays of average energy around 0.1 MeV do not contribute appreciably to the dose in the patient because they are strongly attenuated in the material of the source and the capsule. The other "contaminants" to the treatment beam are the lower energy γ rays produced by the interaction of the primary γ radiation with the source itself, the surrounding capsule, the source housing, and the collimator system. The scattered components of the beam contribute significantly (~10%) to the total intensity of the beam (8). All these secondary interactions thus, to some extent, result in heterogeneity of the beam. In addition, electrons are also produced by these interactions and constitute what is usually referred to as the *electron contamination* of the photon beam.

A typical teletherapy ^{60}Co source is a cylinder of diameter ranging from 1.0 to 2.0 cm and is positioned in the cobalt unit with its circular end facing the patient. The fact that the radiation source is not a point source complicates the beam geometry and gives rise to what is known as the geometric penumbra.

A.2. SOURCE HOUSING

The housing for the source is called the *sourcehead* (Fig. 4.11). It consists of a steel shell filled with lead for shielding purposes and a device for bringing the source in front of an opening in the head from which the useful beam emerges.

Also, a heavy metal alloy sleeve is provided to form an additional primary shield when the source is in the "off" position.

A number of methods have been developed for moving the source from the "off" position to the "on" position. These methods have been discussed in detail by Johns and Cunningham (9). It will suffice here to briefly mention four different mechanisms: (a) the source mounted on a rotating wheel inside the sourcehead to carry the source from the "off" position to the "on" position; (b) the source mounted on a heavy metal plus its ability to slide horizontally through a hole running through the sourcehead. In the "on" position the source

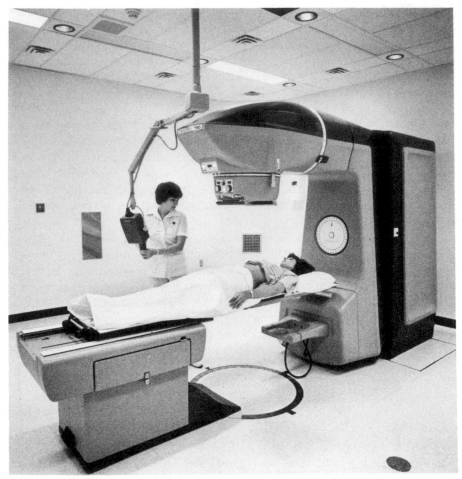

Figure 4.11. Photograph of cobalt unit, Theratron 780. (Courtesy of Atomic Energy of Canada Limited, Ottawa, Canada.)

faces the aperture for the treatment beam and in the "off" position the source moves to its shielded location and a light source mounted on the same drawer occupies the "on" position of the source; (c) mercury is allowed to flow into the space immediately below the source to shut off the beam; and (d) the source is fixed in front of the aperture and the beam can be turned on and off by a shutter consisting of heavy metal jaws. All of the above mechanisms incorporate a safety feature in which the source is returned automatically to the "off" position in case of a power failure.

A.3. BEAM COLLIMATION AND PENUMBRA

A collimator system is designed to vary the size and shape of the beam to meet the individual requirements. The simplest form of a continuously adjustable diaphragm consists of two pairs of heavy metal blocks. Each pair can be moved independently to obtain a square or a rectangle-shaped field. Some collimators are multivane type, *i.e.* multiple blocks to control the size of the beam. In either case, if the inner surface of the blocks is made parallel to the central axis of the beam, the radiation will pass through the edges of the collimating blocks resulting in what is known as the *"transmission penumbra."* The extent of this penumbra will be more pronounced for larger collimator openings because of greater obliquity of the rays at the edges of the blocks. This effect has been minimized in some designs by shaping the collimator blocks so that the inner surface of the blocks remains always parallel to the edge of the beam. In these collimators, the blocks are hinged to the top of the collimator housing so that the slope of the blocks is coincident with the included angle of the beam. Although the transmission penumbra can be minimized with such an arrangement, it cannot be completely removed for all field sizes.

The term *penumbra*, in a general sense, means the region, at the edge of a radiation beam, over which the dose rate changes rapidly as a function of distance from the beam axis (10). The transmission penumbra, mentioned above, is the region irradiated by photons which are transmitted through the edge of the collimator block.

Another type of penumbra, known as the *geometric penumbra*, is illustrated in Fig. 4.12. The geometric width of the penumbra, P_d, at any depth d from the surface of a patient can be determined by considering similar triangles

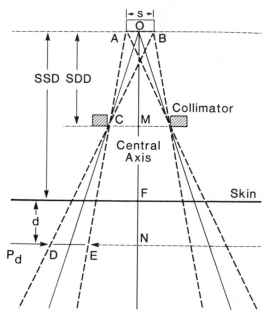

Figure 4.12.   Diagram for calculating geometric penumbra.

ABC and *DEC*. From geometry, we have:

$$\frac{DE}{AB} = \frac{CE}{CA} = \frac{CD}{CB} = \frac{MN}{OM} = \frac{OF + FN - OM}{OM} \tag{4.1}$$

If $AB = s$, the source diameter, $OM = $ SDD, the source to diaphragm distance, $OF = $ SSD, the source to surface distance, then from the above equation, the penumbra (DE) at depth d is given by

$$P_d = \frac{s \, (\mathrm{SSD} + d - \mathrm{SDD})}{\mathrm{SDD}} \tag{4.2}$$

The penumbra at the surface can be calculated by substituting $d = 0$ in Equation 4.2.

As the above equation indicates, the penumbra width increases with increase in source diameter, SSD, and depth but decreases with increase in SDD. The geometric penumbra, however, is independent of field size as long as the movement of the diaphragm is in one plane, *i.e.* SDD stays constant with increase in field size.

Since SDD is an important parameter in determining the penumbra width, this distance can be increased by extendable *penumbra trimmers*. These trimmers consist of heavy metal bars to attenuate the beam in the penumbra region, thus "sharpening" the field edges. The penumbra, however, is not eliminated completely but reduced since SDD with the trimmers extended is increased. The new SDD is equal to the source to trimmer distance. An alternative way of reducing the penumbra is to use secondary blocks, placed close to the patient, for redefining or shaping the field. As will be discussed in Chapter 13, the blocks should not be placed closer than 15 to 20 cm from the patient because of excessive electron contaminants produced by the block carrying tray.

The combined effect of the transmission and geometric penumbras is to create a region of dose variation at the field edges. A dose profile of the beam measured across the beam in air at a given distance from the source would show dosimetrically the extent of the penumbra. However, at a depth in the patient the dose variation at the field border is not only a function of geometric and transmission penumbras but also the scattered radiation produced in the patient. Thus, dosimetrically, the term *physical penumbra* width has been defined as the lateral distance between two specified isodose curves[4] at a specified depth (10).

---

[4] An isodose curve is a line passing through points of equal dose.

References

1. Paterson R: *The Treatment of Malignant Disease by Radium and X-Rays*. Baltimore, Williams and Wilkins, 1963, p 56.
2. National Council on Radiation Protection: *Medical X-Ray and Gamma Ray Protection for*

Energies up to 10 MeV. NCRP Report 34. Washington, DC, National Council on Radiation Protection and Measurements, 1970, p 31.

3. Karzmark CJ, Pering NC: Electron linear accelerators for radiation therapy: history, principles and contemporary developments. *Phys Med Biol* 18:321, 1973.
4. Podgorsak EB, Rawlinson JA, Johns HE: X-Ray depth doses from linear accelerators in the energy range from 10 to 32 MeV. *Am J Roentgenol* 123:182, 1975.
5. Veksler VJ: A new method for acceleration of relativistic particles. *Dokl Akad Nauk SSSR* 43:329, 1944.
6. Reistad D, Brahme A: The microtron, a new accelerator for radiation therapy. In *Digest of the 3rd International Conference on Medical Physics*, The Third ICMP Exec. Comm., Chalmers University of Technology, Fack, S-402 20 Götenborg, Sweden, 1972.
7. Svensson H, Johnsson L, Larsson LG, Brahme A, Lindberg B, Reistad D: A 22 MeV microtron for radiation therapy. *Acta Radiol Ther Phys Biol* 16:145, 1977.
8. Cormack DV, Johns HE: Spectral distribution of scattered radiation from a kilocurie cobalt 60 unit. *Br J Radiol* 31:497, 1958.
9. Johns HE, Cunningham JR: *The Physics of Radiology*, 3rd ed. Springfield, IL, Charles C Thomas, 1969, p 120.
10. International Commission on Radiation Units: *Determination of Absorbed Dose in a Patient Irradiated by Beams of X or Gamma Rays in Radiotherapy Procedures, ICRU Report 24.* Washington, DC, International Commission on Radiation Units and Measurements, 1976, p 54.

CHAPTER 5

Interactions of X and γ Radiations

When an x or γ ray beam passes through a medium, interaction between photons and matter can take place with the result that energy is transferred to the medium. The initial step in the energy transfer involves the ejection of electrons from the atoms of the absorbing medium. These high speed electrons transfer their energy by producing ionization and excitation of the atoms along their paths. If the absorbing medium consists of body tissues, sufficient energy may be deposited within its cells, destroying their reproductive capacity. However, most of the absorbed energy is converted into heat, producing no biological effect.

5.1 IONIZATION

The process by which a neutral atom acquires a positive or a negative charge is known as *ionization*. Removal of an orbital electron leaves the atom positively charged, resulting in an ion pair. The stripped electron, in this case, is the negative ion and the residual atom is the positive ion. In some cases, an electron may be acquired by a neutral atom and the negatively charged atom then becomes the negative ion.

Charged particles such as electrons, protons, and α particles are known as *directly ionizing radiation* provided they have sufficient kinetic energy to produce ionization by collision[1] as they penetrate matter. The energy of the incident particle is lost in a large number of small increments along the ionization track in the medium, with an occasional interaction in which the ejected electron receives sufficient energy to produce a secondary track of its own, known as a *δ ray*. If, on the other hand, the energy lost by the incident particle is not sufficient to eject an electron from the atom but is used to raise the electrons to higher energy levels, the process is termed *excitation*.

The uncharged particles such as neutrons and photons are *indirectly ionizing radiation* since they liberate directly ionizing particles from matter when they interact with matter.

Ionizing photons interact with the atoms of a material or *absorber* to produce high speed electrons by three major processes: photoelectric effect, Compton

---

[1] The process of collision is an interaction between the electromagnetic fields associated with the colliding particle and orbital electron. Actual physical contact between the particles is not required.

effect, and pair production. Before considering each process in detail, we shall discuss the mathematical aspects of radiation absorption.

5.2 BEAM DESCRIPTION

An x-ray beam emitted from a target or a γ ray beam emitted from a radioactive source consists of a large number of photons, usually with a variety of energies. A beam of photons can be described by many terms some of which are defined as follows.

(a) *Fluence:* the fluence, Φ, of photons is the quotient dN by da, where dN is the number of photons which enter an imaginary sphere of cross-sectional area da.

$$\Phi = \frac{dN}{da} \tag{5.1}$$

(b)*Fluence rate or flux density, ϕ,* is the fluence per unit time.

$$\phi = \frac{d\Phi}{dt} \tag{5.2}$$

where dt is the time interval.

(c) *Energy fluence*, Ψ, is the quotient of dE_{fl} by da, where dE_{fl} is the sum of the energies of all the photons which enter a sphere of cross-sectional area da.

$$\Psi = \frac{dE_{fl}}{da} \tag{5.3}$$

For a monoenergetic beam, dE_{fl} is just the number of photons dN times energy $h\nu$ carried by each photon:

$$dE_{fl} = dN \cdot h\nu \tag{5.4}$$

(d) *Energy fluence rate or energy flux density or intensity, ψ,* is the energy fluence per unit time:

$$\psi = \frac{d\Psi}{dt} \tag{5.5}$$

5.3 BEAM ATTENUATION

An experimental arrangement designed to measure the attenuation characteristics of a photon beam is shown in Fig. 5.1. A narrow beam of monoenergetic photons is incident upon an absorber of variable thickness. A detector is placed at a fixed distance from the source and sufficiently farther away from the absorber so that only the *primary* photons (those photons which passed through the absorber without interacting) are measured by the detector. Any photon scattered by the absorber is not supposed to be measured in this arrangement. Thus, if a photon interacts with an atom, it is either completely absorbed or scattered away from the detector.

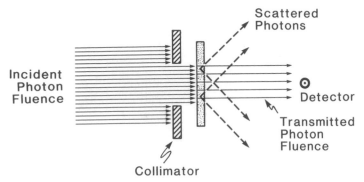

Figure 5.1.   Diagram to illustrate an experimental arrangement for studying narrow beam attenuation through absorber. Measurements under "good geometry," *i.e.* scattered photons not measured.

Under these conditions, the reduction in the number of photons, dN, is proportional to the number of incident photons, N, and to the thickness of the absorber, dx. Mathematically,

$$dN \propto Ndx$$

or

$$dN = -\mu Ndx \tag{5.6}$$

where μ is the constant of proportionality, called the *attenuation coefficient.* The minus sign indicates that the number of photons decreases as the absorber thickness increases. The above equation can also be written in terms of intensity, I:

$$dI = -\mu Idx$$

or

$$\frac{dI}{I} = -\mu dx \tag{5.7}$$

If thickness x is expressed as a length, then μ is called the *linear attenuation coefficient.* For example, if the thickness is measured in centimeters, the units of μ are 1/cm or cm^{-1}.

Equation 5.7 is identical to Equation 2.1, which describes radioactive decay, and μ is analogous to decay constant λ. As before, the differential equation for attenuation can be solved to yield the following equation:

$$I(x) = I_0 e^{-\mu x} \tag{5.8}$$

where $I(x)$ is the intensity transmitted by a thickness x and I_0 is the intensity incident on the absorber. If $I(x)$ is plotted as a function of x for a narrow monoenergetic beam, a straight line will be obtained on semilogarithmic paper

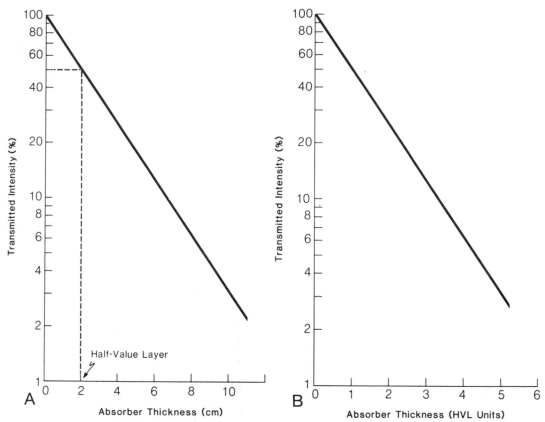

Figure 5.2. A: graph showing percent transmission of a narrow monoenergetic photon beam as a function of absorber thickness. For this quality beam and absorber material, HVL = 2 cm and μ = 0.347 cm^{-1}. B: universal attenuation curve showing percent transmission of a narrow monoenergetic beam as a function of absorber thickness in units of half-value layer (HVL).

(Fig. 5.2A), showing that the attenuation of a monoenergetic beam is described by an exponential function.

The term analogous to half-life (Section 2.4) is the *half-value layer* (HVL) defined as the thickness of an absorber required to attenuate the intensity of the beam to half its original value. That means that when x = HVL, $\dfrac{I}{I_0}$ = ½, by definition. Thus, from Equation 5.8 it can be shown that:

$$\text{HVL} = \frac{0.693}{\mu} \qquad (5.9)$$

As mentioned earlier, exponential attenuation strictly applies to a monoenergetic beam. Fig. 5.2B is a general attenuation curve for a monoenergetic beam or a beam whose half-value layer does not change with absorber thickness. Such a curve may be used to calculate the number of HVLs required to reduce the transmitted intensity to a given percentage of the incident intensity.

A practical beam produced by an x-ray generator, however, consists of a spectrum of photon energies. Attenuation of such a beam is no longer quite exponential. This effect is seen in Fig. 5.3, in which the plot of transmitted intensity on semilogarithmic paper is not a straight line. The slope of the attenuation curve decreases with increasing absorber thickness because the

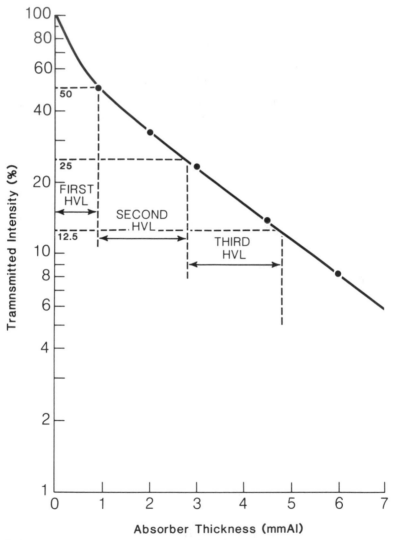

Figure 5.3. Schematic graph showing transmission of an x-ray beam with a spectrum of photon energies through an aluminum absorber. First HVL = 0.99 mm Al, second HVL = 1.9 mm Al, third HVL = 2.0 mm Al.

absorber or *filter* preferentially removes the lower energy photons. As shown in Fig. 5.3, the first HVL is defined as that thickness of material which reduces the incident beam intensity by 50%. The second HVL reduces the beam to 50% of its intensity after it has been transmitted through the first HVL. Similarly, the third HVL represents the quality of the beam after it has been transmitted through the absorber of thickness equal to two HVLs. In general, for a heterogeneous beam, the first HVL is less than the subsequent HVLs. As the filter thickness increases, the average energy of the transmitted beam increases or the beam becomes increasingly *harder*. Thus, by increasing the filtration in such an x-ray beam, one increases the penetrating power or the half-value layer of the beam.

5.4 COEFFICIENTS

A. Attenuation Coefficient

In the previous section, we discussed the linear attenuation coefficient μ which has units of cm^{-1}. In general, this coefficient depends on the energy of the photons and the nature of the material. Since the attenuation produced by a thickness x depends on the number of electrons presented in that thickness, μ is directly proportional to the density of the material. Thus, by dividing μ by density ρ, the resulting coefficient, μ/ρ, will be independent of density. μ/ρ is known as the *mass attenuation coefficient*. This is a more fundamental coefficient than the linear coefficient since the density has been factored out and its dependence on the nature of the material does not involve density but rather the atomic composition.

The mass attenuation coefficient has units of cm^2/g since $\mu/\rho = cm^{-1}/(g/cm^3)$. When using μ/ρ in the attenuation Equation 5.8, the thickness should be expressed as ρx, which has units of g/cm^2, since $\mu x = (\mu/\rho)(\rho x)$ and $\rho x = (g/cm^3)(cm)$.

In addition to the cm and g/cm^2 units, the absorber thickness can also be expressed in units of electrons/cm^2 and atoms/cm^2. The corresponding coefficients for the last two units are *electronic attenuation coefficient*, $_e\mu$, and *atomic attenuation coefficient*, $_a\mu$, respectively.

$$_e\mu = \frac{\mu}{\rho} \cdot \frac{1}{N_0} \ cm^2/electron \tag{5.10}$$

$$_a\mu = \frac{\mu}{\rho} \cdot \frac{Z}{N_0} \ cm^2/atom \tag{5.11}$$

where Z is the atomic number and N_0 is the number of electrons per gram and N_0 is given by

$$N_0 = \frac{N_A \cdot Z}{A_W} \tag{5.12}$$

where N_A is Avogadro's number and A_W is the atomic weight (see Section 1.3).

It should be emphasized that the attenuation process or the attenuation coefficient represents the fraction of photons removed per unit thickness. The transmitted intensity $I(x)$ in Equation 5.8 is due to photons that did not interact with the material. Those photons which produced interactions will transfer part of their energy to the material and result in part or all of that energy being absorbed.

B. Energy Transfer Coefficient

When a photon interacts with the electrons in the material, a part or all of its energy is converted into kinetic energy of electrons. If only a part of the photon energy is given to the electron, the photon itself is scattered with reduced energy. The scattered photon may interact again with a partial or complete transfer of energy to the electrons. Thus, a photon may experience one or multiple interactions, in which the energy lost by the photon is converted into kinetic energy of electrons.

If we consider a photon beam traversing a material, the fraction of photon energy transferred into kinetic energy of charged particles per unit thickness of absorber is given by the *energy transfer coefficient* μ_{tr}. This coefficient is related to μ as follows:

$$\mu_{tr} = \frac{\bar{E}_{tr}}{h\nu}\,\mu \tag{5.13}$$

where $\bar{E}_{tr}$ is the average energy transferred into kinetic energy of charged particles per interaction. The *mass energy transfer coefficient* is given by μ_{tr}/ρ.

C. Energy Absorption Coefficient

Most of the electrons set in motion by the photons will lose their energy by inelastic collisions (ionization and excitation) with atomic electrons of the material. A few, depending upon the atomic number of the material, will lose energy by bremsstrahlung interactions with the nuclei. The bremsstrahlung energy is radiated out of the local volume as x-rays and is not included in the calculation of locally absorbed energy.

The *energy absorption coefficient,* μ_{en}, is defined as the product of energy transfer coefficient and $(1 - g)$ where g is the fraction of the energy of secondary charged particles that is lost to bremsstrahlung in the material.

$$\mu_{en} = \mu_{tr}(1 - g) \tag{5.14}$$

As before, the mass energy absorption coefficient is given by μ_{en}/ρ.

For most interactions involving soft tissues or other low Z material in which electrons lose energy almost entirely by ionization collisions, the bremsstrahlung component is negligible. Thus, $\mu_{en} = \mu_{tr}$ under those conditions. These coefficients can differ appreciably when the kinetic energies of the secondary particles are high and material traversed has a high atomic number.

The energy absorption coefficient is an important quantity in radiotherapy since it allows the evaluation of energy absorbed in the tissues, a quantity of interest in predicting the biological effects of radiation.

5.5 INTERACTIONS OF PHOTONS WITH MATTER

Attenuation of a photon beam by an absorbing material is caused by five major types of interactions. One of these, photo disintegration, has been considered previously in Section 2.8F. This reaction between photon and nucleus is only important at very high photon energies (>10 MeV). The other four processes are coherent scattering, the photoelectric effect, the Compton effect, and the pair production. Each of these processes can be represented by its own attenuation coefficient which varies in its particular way with the energy of the photon and with the atomic number of the absorbing material. The total attenuation coefficient is the sum of individual coefficients for these processes:

$$\mu/\rho = \sigma_{coh}/\rho + \tau/\rho + \sigma_c/\rho + \pi/\rho \qquad (5.15)$$

where σ_{coh}, τ, σ_c, and π are attenuation coefficients for coherent scattering, photoelectric effect, Compton effect, and pair production, respectively.

5.6 COHERENT SCATTERING

The coherent scattering, also known as classical scattering or Rayleigh scattering, is illustrated in Fig. 5.4. The process can be visualized by considering the wave nature of electromagnetic radiation. This interaction consists of an electromagnetic wave passing near the electron and setting it into oscillation. The oscillating electron re-radiates the energy at the same frequency as the incident electromagnetic wave. These scattered x-rays have the same wavelength as the incident beam. Thus, no energy is changed into electronic motion and no energy is absorbed in the medium. The only effect is the scattering of the photon at small angles. The coherent scattering is probable in high atomic number materials and with photons of low energy. The process is only of academic interest in radiotherapy.

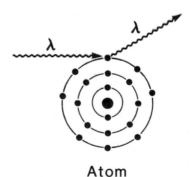

Atom

Figure 5.4. Diagram illustrating the process of coherent scattering. The scattered photon has the same wavelength as the incident photon. No energy is transferred.

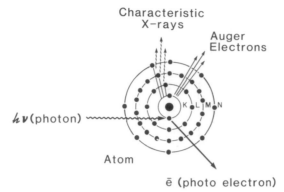

Figure 5.5. Illustration of the photoelectric effect.

5.7 PHOTOELECTRIC EFFECT

The photoelectric effect is a phenomenon in which a photon interacts with an atom and ejects one of the orbital electrons from the atom (Fig. 5.5). In this process, the entire energy, $h\nu$, of the photon is transferred to the atomic electron. The kinetic energy of the ejected electron (called the photoelectron) is equal to $h\nu - E_B$, where E_B is the binding energy of the electron. Interactions of this type can take place with electrons in the K, L, M, or N shells.

After the electron has been ejected from the atom, a vacancy is created in the shell, thus leaving the atom in an excited state. The vacancy can be filled by an outer orbital electron with the emission of characteristic x-rays (Section 3.4B). There is also the possibility of emission of Auger electrons (Section 2.7C) which are monoenergetic electrons produced by the absorption of characteristic x-rays internally by the atom. Since the K shell binding energy of soft tissues is only about 0.5 keV, the energy of the characteristic photons produced in biological absorbers is very low and can be considered to be locally absorbed. For higher energy photons and higher atomic number materials, the characteristic photons are of higher energy and may deposit energy at large distances compared to the range of the photoelectron. In such cases, the local energy absorption is reduced by the energy emitted as characteristic radiation (also called fluorescent radiation) which is considered to be remotely absorbed.

The probability of photoelectric absorption depends on the photon energy as illustrated in Fig. 5.6, where the mass photoelectric attenuation coefficient, τ/ρ, is plotted as a function of photon energy. Data are shown for water representing a low atomic number material similar to tissue, and for lead, representing a high atomic number material. Since on logarithmic paper, the graph is almost a straight line with a slope of approximately −3, we get the following relationship between τ/ρ and photon energy:

$$\tau/\rho \propto 1/E^3 \qquad (5.16)$$

The graph for lead has discontinuities at about 15 and 88 keV. These are

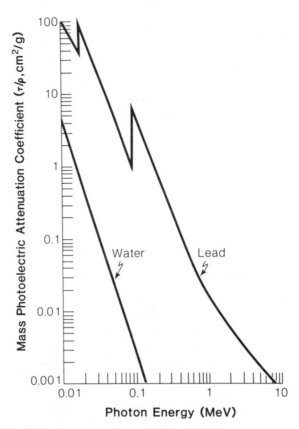

Figure 5.6. Mass photoelectric attenuation coefficient, τ/ρ, plotted against photon energy. Curves for water ($Z_{eff} = 7.42$) and lead ($Z = 82$). [Data from Grodstein (1).]

called *absorption edges* and correspond to the binding energies of L and K shells. A photon with energy less than 15 keV does not have enough energy to eject an L electron. Thus, below 15 keV, the interaction is limited to the M or higher shell electrons. When the photon has an energy that just equals the binding energy of the L shell, resonance occurs and the probability of photoelectric absorption involving the L shell becomes very high. Beyond this point, if the photon energy is increased, the probability of photoelectric attenuation decreases approximately as $1/E^3$ until the next discontinuity, the K absorption edge. At this point on the graph, the photon has 88 keV energy which is just enough to eject the K electron. As seen in Fig. 5.6, the absorption probability in lead at this critical energy increases dramatically, by a factor of about 10.

The discontinuities or absorption edges for water are not shown in the graph because the K absorption edge for water occurs at very low photon energies (~0.5 keV).

The data for varous materials indicate that photoelectric attenuation depends strongly on the atomic number of the absorbing material. The following approximate relationship holds:

$$\tau/\rho \propto Z^3 \tag{5.17}$$

This relationship forms the basis of many applications in diagnostic radiology. The difference in Z of various tissues such as bone, muscle, and fat amplifies differences in x-ray absorption, provided the primary mode of interaction is photoelectric. This Z^3 dependence is also exploited when using contrast materials such as $BaSO_4$ mix and Hypaque. In therapeutic radiology, the low energy beams produced by superficial and orthovoltage machines cause unnecessary high absorption of x-ray energy in bone due to this Z^3 dependence. This problem will be discussed later in Section 5.10. By combining Equations 5.16 and 5.17, we have:

$$\tau/\rho \propto Z^3/E^3 \tag{5.18}$$

The angular distribution of electrons emitted in a photoelectric process depends on the photon energy. For a low energy photon, the photoelectron is emitted most likely at 90° relative to the direction of the incident photon. As the photon energy increases, the photoelectrons are emitted in a more forward direction.

5.8 COMPTON EFFECT

In the Compton process, the photon interacts with an atomic electron as though it were a "free" electron. The term "free" here means that the binding energy of the electron is much less than the energy of the bombarding photon. In this interaction, the electron receives some energy from the photon and is emitted at an angle θ (Fig. 5.7). The photon, with reduced energy, is scattered at an angle ϕ.

The Compton process can be analyzed in terms of a collision between two

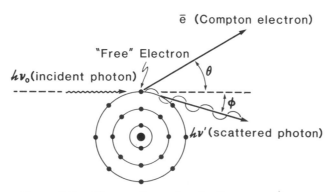

Figure 5.7. Diagram illustrating the Compton effect.

particles, a photon and an electron. By applying the laws of conservation of energy and momentum, one can derive the following relationships.

$$E = h\nu_0 \frac{\alpha(1 - \cos \phi)}{1 + \alpha(1 - \cos \phi)} \tag{5.19}$$

$$h\nu' = h\nu_0 \frac{1}{1 + \alpha(1 - \cos \phi)} \tag{5.20}$$

$$\cot \theta = (1 + \alpha)\tan \phi/2 \tag{5.21}$$

where $h\nu_0$, $h\nu'$, and E are the energies of the incident photon, scattered photon, and electron, respectively and, $\alpha = h\nu_0/m_0c^2$, where m_0c^2 is the rest energy of the electron (0.511 MeV). If $h\nu_0$ is expressed in MeV, then $\alpha = h\nu_0/0.511$.

A. Special Cases of Compton Effect

A.1. DIRECT HIT

If a photon makes a direct hit with the electron, the electron will travel forward ($\theta = 0°$) and the scattered photon will travel backward ($\phi = 180°$) after the collision. In such a collision, the electron will receive maximum energy E_{max} and the scattered photon will be left with minimum energy $h\nu'_{min}$. One can calculate E_{max} and $h\nu'_{min}$ by substituting $\cos \phi = \cos 180° = -1$ in Equations 5.19 and 5.20.

$$E_{max} = h\nu_0 \frac{2\alpha}{1 + 2\alpha} \tag{5.22}$$

$$h\nu'_{min} = h\nu_0 \frac{1}{1 + 2\alpha} \tag{5.23}$$

A.2. GRAZING HIT

If a photon makes a grazing hit with the electron, the electron will be emitted at right angles ($\theta = 90°$) and the scattered photon will go in the forward direction ($\phi = 0°$). By substituting $\cos \phi = \cos 0° = 1$ in Equations 5.19 and 5.20, one can show that for this collision $E = 0$ and $h\nu' = h\nu_0$.

A.3. 90° PHOTON SCATTER

If a photon is scattered at right angles to its original direction ($\phi = 90°$), one can calculate E and $h\nu'$ from Equations 5.19 and 5.20 by substituting $\cos \phi = \cos 90° = 0$. The angle of the electron emission in this case will depend on α according to Equation 5.21.

Examples. Some useful examples will now be given to illustrate application of the Compton effect to practical problems.

(a) Interaction of a low energy photon. If the incident photon energy is much less than the rest energy of the electron, only a small part of its energy is

imparted to the electron resulting in a scattered photon of almost the same energy as the incident photon. For example, suppose $h\nu_0 = 51.1$ keV; then $\alpha = h\nu_0/m_0 c^2 = 0.0511$ MeV/0.511 MeV $= 0.1$. From Equations 5.19 and 5.20,

$$E_{max} = 51.1 \text{ (keV) } \frac{2(0.1)}{1 + 2(0.1)} = 8.52 \text{ keV} \tag{5.24}$$

$$h\nu'_{min} = 51.1 \text{ (keV) } \frac{1}{1 + 2(0.1)} = 42.58 \text{ keV} \tag{5.25}$$

Thus, for a low energy photon beam, the Compton scattered photons have approximately the same energy as the original photons. Indeed, as the incident photon energy approaches zero, the Compton effect becomes the classical scattering process described in Section 5.6.

(b) *Interaction of a high energy photon.* If the incident photon has a very high energy (much greater than the rest energy of the electron), the photon loses most of its energy to the Compton electron and the scattered photon has much less energy. Suppose $h\nu_0 = 5.11$ MeV; then $\alpha = 10.0$. From Equations 5.19 and 5.20,

$$E_{max} = 5.11 \text{ (MeV) } \frac{2(10)}{1 + 2(10)} = 4.87 \text{ MeV} \tag{5.26}$$

$$h\nu'_{min} = 5.11 \text{ (MeV) } \frac{1}{1 + 2(10)} = 0.24 \text{ MeV} \tag{5.27}$$

In contrast to Example a above, the scattered photons produced by high energy photons carry away only a small fraction of the initial energy. Thus, at high photon energy, the Compton effect causes a large amount of energy absorption compared to the Compton interactions involving low energy photons.

(c) *Compton scatter at $\phi = 90°$ and $180°$.* In designing radiation protection barriers (walls) to attenuate scattered radiation, one needs to know the energy of the photons scattered at different angles. The energy of the photons scattered by a patient under treatment at 90° with respect to the incident beam is of particular interest in calculating barrier or wall thicknesses against scattered radiation.

By substituting $\phi = 90°$ in Equation 5.20, we obtain:

$$h\nu' = \frac{h\nu_0}{1 + \alpha} \tag{5.28}$$

For high energy photons with $\alpha \gg 1$, the above equation reduces to

$$h\nu' \approx \frac{h\nu_0}{\alpha} \tag{5.29}$$

or

$$h\nu' = m_0 c^2 = 0.511 \text{ MeV}$$

Similar calculations for scatter at $\phi = 180°$ will indicate $h\nu' = 0.255$ MeV. Thus, if the energy of the incident photon is high ($\alpha \gg 1$), we have the following important generalizations: (i) the radiation scattered at right angles is independent of incident energy and has a maximum value of 0.511 MeV; (ii) the radiation scattered backwards is independent of incident energy and has a maximum value of 0.255 MeV.

The maximum energy of radiation scattered at angles between 90° and 180° will lie between the above energy limits. However, the energy of the photons scattered at angles less than 90° will be greater than 0.511 MeV and will approach the incident photon energy for the condition of forward scatter. Since the energy of the scattered photon plus that of the electron must equal the incident energy, the electron may acquire any energy between 0 and E_{max} (given by Equation 5.22).

B. Dependence of Compton Effect on Energy and Atomic Number

It was mentioned earlier that the Compton effect is an interaction between a photon and a "free" electron. Practically, this means that the energy of the incident photon must be large compared to the electron binding energy. This is in contrast to the photoelectric effect which becomes most probable when the energy of the incident photon is equal to or slightly greater than the binding energy of the electron. Thus, as the photon energy increases beyond the binding energy of the K electron, the photoelectric effect decreases rapidly with energy (Equation 5.16 and Fig. 5.6) and the Compton effect becomes more and more important. However, as shown in Fig. 5.8, the Compton effect also *decreases with increasing photon energy.*

Since the Compton interaction involves essentially free electrons in the absorbing material, *it is independent of atomic number Z.* It follows that the Compton mass attenuation coefficient, σ/ρ, is independent of Z and depends only on the number of electrons per gram. Although the number of electrons per gram of elements decreases slowly but systematically with atomic number, most materials except hydrogen can be considered as having approximately the same number of electrons per gram (see Table 5.1). Thus, σ/ρ *is nearly the same for all materials.*

From the above discussion, it follows that if the energy of the beam is in the region where the Compton effect is the only possible mode of interaction, approximately the same attenuation of the beam will occur in any material of equal density thickness,[2] expressed as g/cm^2. For example, in the case of a ^{60}Co γ ray beam which interacts by Compton effect, the attenuation per g/cm^2 for bone is nearly the same as that for soft tissue. However, 1 cm of bone will attenuate more than 1 cm of soft tissue because bone has a higher electron

---

[2] Density thickness is equal to the linear thickness multiplied by density, *i.e* cm × g/cm^3 = g/cm^2.

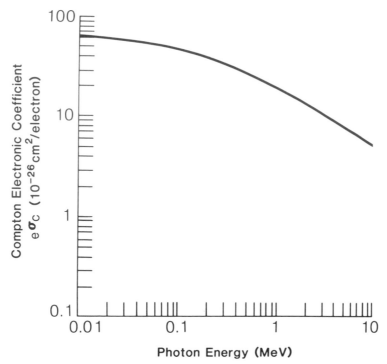

Figure 5.8. A plot of Compton electronic coefficient e^{σ} against photon energy. The mass coefficient, σ/ρ, is obtained by multiplying the electronic coefficient with the number of electrons per gram for a given material. [Data from Hubbell (2).]

Table 5.1.
Number of electrons per gram of various materials

Material	Density (g/cm³)	Atomic number	Number of electrons per gram
Hydrogen	0.0000899	1	6.00×10^{23}
Carbon	2.25	6	3.01×10^{23}
Oxygen	0.001429	8	3.01×10^{23}
Aluminum	2.7	13	2.90×10^{23}
Copper	8.9	29	2.75×10^{23}
Lead	11.3	82	2.38×10^{23}
		Effective atomic number	
Fat	0.91	5.92	3.48×10^{23}
Muscle	1.00	7.42	3.36×10^{23}
Water	1.00	7.42	3.34×10^{23}
Air	0.001293	7.64	3.01×10^{23}
Bone	1.85	13.8	3.00×10^{23}

Data from Johns and Cunningham (3).

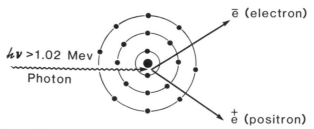

Figure 5.9.   Diagram illustrating the pair production process.

density,[3] ρ_e (number of electrons per cm^3), which is given by density times the number of electrons per gram. If the density of bone is assumed to be 1.85 g/cm^3 and that of soft tissue 1 g/cm^3, then the attenuation produced by 1 cm of bone will be equivalent to that produced by 1.65 cm of soft tissue:

$$(1 \text{ cm}) \frac{(\rho_e)_{\text{bone}}}{(\rho_e)_{\text{muscle}}} = (1 \text{ cm}) \times \frac{1.85 \text{ (g/cm}^3) \times 3.00 \times 10^{23} \text{ (electrons/g)}}{1.00 \text{ (g/cm}^3) \times 3.36 \times 10^{23} \text{ (electrons/g)}}$$

$$= 1.65 \text{ cm}$$

5.9 PAIR PRODUCTION

If the energy of the photon is greater than 1.02 MeV, the photon may interact with matter through the mechanism of pair production. In this process (Fig. 5.9), the photon interacts strongly with the electromagnetic field of an atomic nucleus and gives up all its energy in the process of creating a pair consisting of a negative electron (e^-) and a positive electron (e^+). Since the rest mass energy of the electron is equivalent to 0.51 MeV, a minimum energy of 1.02 MeV is required in order to create the pair of electrons. Thus, the *threshold energy* for the pair production process is 1.02 MeV. The photon energy in excess of this threshold is shared between the particles as kinetic energy. The total kinetic energy available for the electron-positron pair is given by ($h\nu$ − 1.02) MeV. The particles tend to be emitted in the forward direction relative to the incident photon.

The most probable distribution of energy is for each particle to acquire half the available kinetic energy, although any energy distribution is possible. For example, in an extreme case, it is possible that one particle may receive all the energy while the other receives no energy.

✳ The pair production process is an example of an event in which energy is converted into mass, as predicted by Einstein's equation, $E = mc^2$. The reverse process, namely, the conversion of mass into energy, takes place when a positron combines with an electron to produce two photons, called the annihilation radiation.

---

[3] In the literature, the term electron density has been defined both as the number of electrons per gram and the number of electrons per cm^3. The reader should be aware of this possible source of confusion.

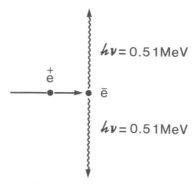

Figure 5.10. Diagram illustrating the production of annihilation radiation.

A. Annihilation Radiation

The positron created as a result of pair production process loses its energy as it traverses the matter by the same type of interactions as an electron does, namely, by ionization and excitation and bremsstrahlung. Near the end of its range, the slowly moving positron combines with one of the free electrons in its vicinity to give rise to two annihilation photons each having 0.51 MeV energy. Since momentum is conserved in the process, the two photons are ejected in opposite directions (Fig. 5.10).

B. Variation of Pair Production with Energy and Atomic Number

Since the pair production results from an interaction with the electromagnetic field of the nucleus, the probability of this process increases rapidly with atomic number. The attenuation coefficient for pair production (Π) varies with Z^2 per atom, Z per electron, and approximately Z per gram. In addition, for a given material, the likelihood of this interaction increases as the logarithm of the incident photon energy above the threshold energy. These relationships are shown in Fig. 5.11. To remove the major dependence of the pair production process on atomic number, the coefficients per atom have been divided by Z^2 before plotting. For energies up to about 20 MeV, the curves are almost coincident for all materials, indicating that $_a\Pi \propto Z^2$. At higher energies, the curves for higher Z materials fall below the low Z materials because of the screening of the nuclear charge by the orbital electrons.

5.10 RELATIVE IMPORTANCE OF VARIOUS TYPES OF INTERACTIONS

The total mass attenuation coefficient (μ/ρ) is the sum of the four individual coefficients:

$$\underset{\text{Total}}{(\mu/\rho)} = \underset{\text{Photoelectric}}{(\tau/\rho)} + \underset{\text{Coherent}}{(\sigma_{\text{coh}}/\rho)} + \underset{\text{Compton}}{(\sigma/\rho)} + \underset{\text{Pair}}{(\Pi/\rho)} \quad (5.30)$$

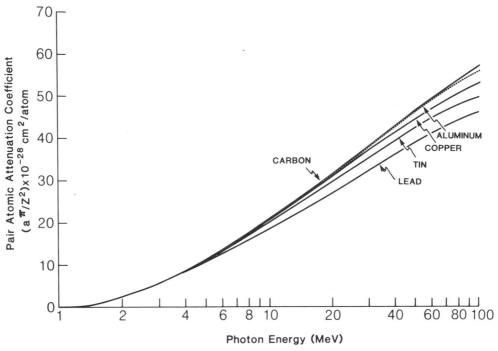

Figure 5.11. Plot of pair atomic attenuation coefficient divided by the square of the atomic number as a function of photon energy for carbon ($Z = 6$), and lead ($Z = 82$). The mass attenuation coefficient can be obtained by multiplying $a\tau/Z^2$ obtained from the graph, first by Z^2 and then by the number of atoms per gram of the absorber. [Data from Hubbell (2).]

As noted earlier, coherent scattering is only important for very low photon energies (<10 keV) and high Z materials. At therapeutic energies, it is often omitted from the sum.

Figure 5.12 is the plot of total coefficient $(\mu/\rho)_{total}$ $vs.$ energy for two different materials, water and lead, representative of low and high atomic number materials. The mass attenuation coefficient is large for low energies and high atomic number media because of the predominance of photoelectric interactions under these conditions.

The attenuation coefficient decreases rapidly with energy until the photon energy far exceeds the electron binding energies and the Compton effect becomes the predominant mode of interaction. In the Compton range of energies, the μ/ρ of lead and water do not different greatly since this type of interaction is independent of atomic number. The coefficient, however, decreases with energy until pair production begins to become important. The dominance of pair production occurs at energies much greater than the threshold energy of 1.02 MeV.

The relative importance of various types of interaction is presented in a tabular form in Table 5.2. These data for water will also be true for soft tissue.

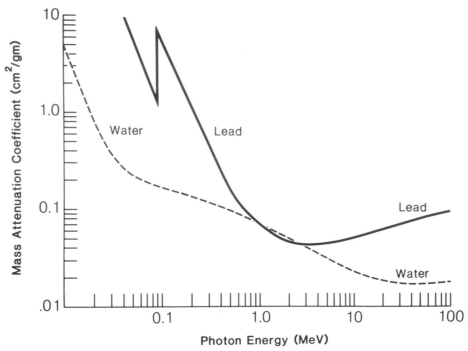

Figure 5.12. Plot of total mass attenuation coefficient, μ/ρ, as a function of photon energy for lead and water. [Reprinted with permission from: Johns and Cunningham (3).]

Table 5.2.
Relative importance of photoelectric (τ), Compton (σ), and pair production (Π) processes in water

Photon energy (MeV)	Relative number of interactions (%)		
	τ	σ	Π
0.01	95	5	0
0.026	60	50	0
0.060	7	93	0
0.150	0	100	0
4.00	0	94	6
10.00	0	77	23
24.00	0	50	50
100.00	0	16	84

Data from Johns and Cunningham (3).

It should be noted that the photon energies listed in column 1 represent monoenergetic beams. As was discussed in Chapter 3, an x-ray tube operating at a given peak voltage produces radiation of all energies less than the peak energy. As a rough approximation and for the purposes of the above table, one may consider the average energy of an x-ray beam to be equivalent to ⅓ of the peak energy. Thus, a 30-keV monoenergetic beam in column 1 should be considered as equivalent to an x-ray beam produced by an x-ray tube operated at about 90 kVp. Of course, the accuracy of this approximation is limited by the effects of filtration on the energy spectrum of the beam.

References

1. Grodstein, GW: *X-ray Attenuation Coefficients from 10 keV to 100 MeV.* Washington, DC, United States National Bureau of Standards, 1957, Publication No. 583.
2. Hubbel JH: *Photon Cross Sections Attenuation Coefficients and Energy Absorption Coefficients from 10 keV to 100 GeV.* Washington, DC, United States National Bureau of Standards, 1969, Publication No. 29.
3. Johns HE, Cunningham JR: *The Physics of Radiology*, 3rd ed. Springfield, Il, Charles C Thomas, 1969.

CHAPTER 6

Measurement of Ionizing Radiation

6.1 INTRODUCTION

In the early days of x-ray usage for diagnosis and therapy, attempts were made to measure ionizing radiation on the basis of their chemical and biological effects. For instance, radiation effects on photographic emulsions, changes in the color of some chemical compounds, and reddening of the human skin could be related to the amount of radiation absorbed. However, these effects were poorly understood at the time and could only provide crude estimation of radiation dose. For example, in radiotherapy, a unit called skin erythema dose (SED) was defined as that amount of x- or γ radiation that just produced reddening of the human skin. However, the unit has many drawbacks. Skin erythema depends on many conditions such as the type of skin, the quality of radiation, the extent of skin exposed, dose fractionation (dose per fraction and time interval between fractions), and differences between early and delayed skin reactions.

Although the SED was later discarded in favor of a more precisely measurable unit such as the roentgen, the skin erythema was used by physicians as an approximate index of response to the radiation treatments. This happened in the orthovoltage era when the skin was the limiting organ to the delivery of tumorcidal doses. The reliance on skin reaction for the assessment of radiation response had to be abandoned when megavoltage beams with the skin sparing properties became the main tools of radiotherapy.

In 1928, the International Commission on Radiological Units and Measurements (ICRU) adopted the roentgen as the unit of measuring x- and γ radiation exposure. The unit is denoted by R.

6.2 THE ROENTGEN

The roentgen is a unit of exposure. The quantity *exposure* is a measure of ionization produced in air by photons. The ICRU (12) defines exposure, X, as the quotient of dQ by dm where dQ is the absolute value of the total charge of the ions of one sign produced in air when all the electrons (negatrons and positrons) liberated by photons in air of mass dm are completely stopped in air.

$$X = \frac{dQ}{dm} \qquad (6.1)$$

87

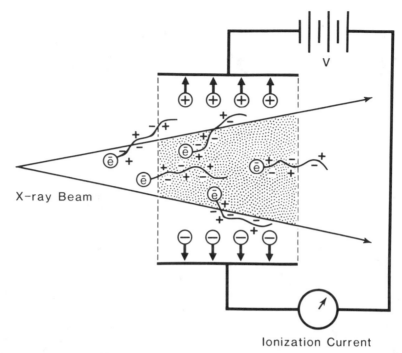

Figure 6.1.   Diagram illustrating electronic equilibrium in a free-air chamber.

The SI (Systems Internationale d'Unites) unit for exposure is coulomb per kilogram (C/kg) but the special unit is roentgen (R).[1]

$$1R = 2.58 \times 10^{-4} \text{ C/kg air}$$

The definition of roentgen is illustrated in Fig. 6.1. An x-ray beam in passing through air sets in motion electrons by photoelectric, Compton, or pair production. These high speed electrons produce ionization along their tracks. Because of the electric field produced by the voltage applied across the ion collection plates, the positive charges move toward the negative plate and the negative charges move toward the positive plate. This constitutes a current. The collected charge of either sign can be measured by an electrometer.

According to the definition of roentgen, the electrons produced by photons in a specified volume (shaded in the figure) must spend all their energies by ionization in air enclosed by the plates (region of ion collection) and the total ionic charge of either sign should be measured. However, some electrons

---

[1] Roentgen was originally defined as $1R = 1$ electrostatic unit (esu)/cm³ air at standard temperature and pressure (STP) (0°C, 760 mm Hg). The current definition of $1R = 2.58 \times 10^{-4}$ C/kg air is equivalent to the original if the charge is expressed in coulombs (1 esu = 3.333×10^{-10}C) and the volume of air is changed to mass (1 cm³ of air at STP weighs 1.293×10^{-6} kg).

produced in the specified volume deposit their energy outside the region of ion collection and thus are not measured. On the other hand, electrons produced outside the specified volume may enter the ion-collecting region and produce ionization there. If the ionization loss is compensated by the ionization gained, a condition of *electronic equilibrium* exists. Under this condition, the definition of roentgen is effectively satisfied. This is the principle of free-air ionization chamber, described below.

6.3 FREE-AIR IONIZATION CHAMBER

The free-air or standard ionization chamber is an instrument employed in the measurement of the roentgen according to its definition. Generally, such a primary standard is used only for the calibration of secondary instruments designed for field use. The free-air chamber installations are thus confined principally to some of the national standards laboratories.

A free-air chamber is represented schematically in Fig. 6.2. An x-ray beam, originating from a focal spot S, is defined by the diaphragm D and passes centrally between a pair of parallel plates. A high voltage (field strength of the order of 100 V/cm) is applied between the plates to collect ions produced in the air between the plates. The ionization is measured for a length L defined by the limiting lines of force to the edges of the collection plate C. The lines of force are made straight and perpendicular to the collector by a guard ring G.

As discussed earlier, electrons produced by the photon beam in the specified

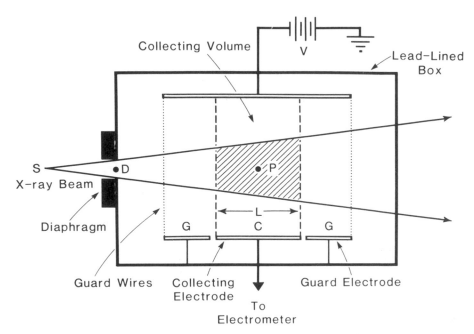

Figure 6.2. A schematic diagram of a free-air chamber.

volume (shaded in the figure) must spend all their energy by ionization of air between the plates. Such a condition can exist only if the range of the electrons liberated by the incident photons is less than the distance between each plate and the specified volume. In addition, for electronic equilibrium to exist, the beam intensity (photon fluence per unit time) must remain constant across the length of the specified volume, and the separation between the diaphragm and the ion collecting region must exceed the electron range in air.

If ΔQ is the charge collected in coulombs and ρ is the density (kg/m^3) of air, then the exposure X_p at the center of the specified volume (point P) is

$$X_p = \frac{\Delta Q}{\rho \cdot A_p \cdot L} \cdot \frac{1}{2.58 \times 10^{-4}} \text{ roentgens} \tag{6.2}$$

where A_p is the cross-sectional area (m^2) of the beam at point P and L (m) is the length of the collecting volume. In practice, it is more convenient to state the exposure, X, at the position of the diaphgragm. Suppose f_1 and f_2 are the distances of the x-ray source to the diaphragm and point P, respectively. Since the intensity at point P and at the diaphragm are related by an inverse square law factor $(f_1/f_2)^2$ which also relates the area of the beams at the diaphragm and at point P, exposure X_D at the diaphragm is given by:

$$X_D = \frac{\Delta Q}{\rho \cdot A_D \cdot L} \cdot \frac{1}{2.58 \times 10^{-4}} \text{ roentgens} \tag{6.3}$$

where A_D is the diaphragm aperture area.

Accurate measurements with a free-air ionization chamber require considerable care. A few corrections that are usually applied include: 1) correction for air attenuation; 2) correction for recombination of ions; 3) correction for the effects of temperature, pressure, and humidity on the density of air; and 4) correction for ionization produced by scattered photons. For details of various corrections the reader is referred to National Bureau of Standards handbook (1).

There are limitations on the design of a free-air chamber for the measurement of roentgens for high energy x-ray beams. As the photon energy increases, the range of the electrons liberated in air increases rapidly. This necessitates an increase in the separation of the plates to maintain electronic equilibrium. Too large a separation, however, creates problems of nonuniform electric field and greater ion recombination. Although the plate separation can be reduced by using air at high pressures, the problems still remain with regard to air attenuation, photon scatter, and reduction in the efficiency of ion collection. Because of these problems, there is an upper limit on the photon energy above which the roentgen cannot be accurately measured. This limit occurs at about 3 MeV.

6.4 THIMBLE CHAMBERS

Free-air ionization chambers are too delicate and bulky for routine use. Their main function is in the standarizing laboratories where they can be used to calibrate field instruments such as a thimble chamber.

The principle of the thimble chamber is illustrated in Fig. 6.3. In Fig. 6.3A, a spherical volume of air is shown with an air cavity at the center. Suppose this sphere of air is irradiated uniformly with a photon beam. Also, suppose that the distance between the outer sphere and the inner cavity is equal to the maximum range of electrons generated in air. If the number of electrons entering the cavity is the same as that leaving the cavity, electronic equilibrium exists. Suppose also that we are able to measure the ionization charge produced in the cavity by the electrons liberated in the air surrounding the cavity. Then by knowing the volume or mass of air inside the cavity, we can calculate the charge per unit mass or the beam exposure at the center of the cavity. Now if the air wall in Fig. 6.3A is compressed into a solid shell as in B, we get a thimble chamber. Although the thimble wall is solid, it is air-equivalent, *i.e.* its effective atomic number is the same as that of air. In addition, the thickness of the thimble wall is such that the electronic equilibrium occurs inside the cavity, just as it did in Fig. 6.3A. As before, it follows that the wall thickness must be equal to or greater than the maximum range of the electrons liberated in the thimble wall.

Since the density of the solid air-equivalent wall is much greater than that of free air, the thicknesses required for electronic equilibrium in the thimble chamber are considerably reduced. For example, in the 100 to 250 kVp x-ray

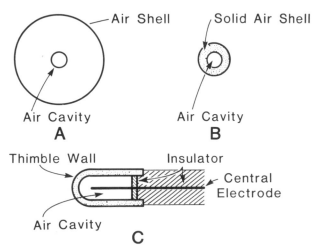

Figure 6.3. Schematic diagram illustrating the nature of the "thimble" ionization chamber. A, air shell with air cavity; B, solid air shell with air cavity; C, the "thimble" chamber.

range, the wall thickness of the thimble (assuming unit density) is about 1 mm and in the case of ^{60}Co γ rays (average $h\nu \approx 1.25$ MeV) it is approximately 5 mm. In practice, however, a thimble chamber is constructed with wall thicknesses of 1 mm or less and this is supplemented with close-fitting caps of Plexiglas or other plastic to bring the total wall thickness up to that needed for electronic equilibrium for the radiation in question.

A. Chamber Wall

Figure 6.3C shows a typical thimble ionization chamber. The wall is shaped like a sewing thimble—hence the name. The inner surface of the thimble wall is coated by a special material to make it electrically conducting. This forms one electrode. The other electrode is a rod of low atomic number material such as graphite or aluminum held in the center of the thimble but electrically insulated from it. A suitable voltage is applied between the two electrodes to collect the ions produced in the air cavity.

As mentioned earlier, most of the ionization produced in the cavity air arises from electrons liberated in the surrounding wall (for at least up to 2 MeV photons). In order for the thimble chamber to be equivalent to a free-air chamber, the thimble wall should be air equivalent. This condition would ensure that the energy spectrum of electrons liberated in the thimble wall is similar to that in air.

In order for the thimble chamber to be air equivalent, the effective atomic number of the wall material and the central electrode must be such that the system as a whole behaves like a free-air chamber. Most commonly used wall materials are made either of graphite (carbon), Bakelite, or a plastic coated on the inside by a conducting layer of graphite or of a conducting mixture of Bakelite and graphite. The effective atomic number of the wall is generally a little less than that of air. It is closer to that of carbon ($Z = 6$). As a consequence, such a wall should give rise to less ionization in the air cavity than a free-air wall. However, the usually greater atomic number of the central electrode, its dimensions, and placement geometry within the thimble can provide compensation for the lower atomic number of the wall.

B. Effective Atomic Number

It is instructive to discuss the term effective atomic number, $\bar{Z}$, in a greater detail. $\bar{Z}$ is the atomic number of an element with which photons interact the same way as with the given composite material. Since photoelectric effect is highly Z dependent (Section 5.7), $\bar{Z}$ is considered for photoelectric interactions. Mayneord (2) has defined the effective atomic number of a compound as follows:

$$\bar{Z} = (a_1 Z_1^{2.94} + a_2 Z_2^{2.94} + a_3 Z_3^{2.94} + \ldots + a_n Z_n^{2.94})^{1/2.94} \qquad (6.4)$$

where $a_1, a_2, a_3, \ldots a_n$ are the fractional contributions of each element to the total number of electrons in the mixture.

EXAMPLE 1: CALCULATION OF $\bar{Z}$ FOR AIR

Composition by weight: nitrogen 75.5%, oxygen 23.2%, and argon 1.3%

Number of electrons/g of air: $\dfrac{N_A Z}{A_w} \times$ (fraction by weight)

$$\text{Nitrogen} = \frac{6.02 \times 10^{23} \times 7}{14.007} \times 0.755 = 2.27 \times 10^{23}$$

$$\text{Oxygen} = \frac{6.02 \times 10^{23} \times 8}{15.999} \times 0.232 = 0.7 \times 10^{23}$$

$$\text{Argon} = \frac{6.02 \times 10^{23} \times 18}{39.94} \times 0.013 = 0.04 \times 10^{23}$$

Total number of electrons/g of air = 3.01×10^{23} (check Table 5.1)

$$a_1 \text{ for nitrogen} = \frac{2.27}{3.01} = 0.753$$

$$a_2 \text{ for oxygen} = \frac{0.70}{3.01} = 0.233$$

$$a_3 \text{ for argon} = \frac{0.04}{3.01} = 0.013$$

$$\bar{Z}_{air} = ((0.753) \times 7^{2.94} + (0.233) \times 8^{2.94} + (0.013) \times 18^{2.94})^{1/2.94}$$

$$= 7.64$$

C. Chamber Calibration

A thimble chamber could be used directly to measure exposure if (a) it were air equivalent, (b) its cavity volume were accurately known, and (c) its wall thickness was sufficient to provide electronic equilibrium. Under the above conditions, the exposure X is given by:

$$X = \frac{Q}{\rho \cdot v} \cdot \frac{1}{A} \tag{6.5}$$

where Q is the ionization charge liberated in the cavity air of density ρ and volume v; A is the fraction of the energy fluence transmitted through the air equivalent wall of equilibrium thickness. The factor A is slightly less than 1.00 and is used here to calculate the exposure for the energy fluence that would exist at the point of measurement in the absence of the chamber.

There are practical difficulties in designing a chamber that would rigorously satisfy the conditions of Equation 6.5. It is almost impossible to construct a thimble chamber that is exactly air equivalent, although with a proper combination of wall material and the central electrode one can achieve acceptable air equivalence in a limited photon energy range. In addition, it is difficult to

accurately determine the chamber volume directly. Therefore, in actual practice, the thimble chambers are always calibrated against a free-air chamber
for x-rays up to a few hundred kilovolts (1). At higher energies (up to ^{60}Co γ
rays), the thimble chambers are calibrated against a standard cavity chamber
with nearly air-equivalent walls (*e.g.*, graphite) and accurately known volume
(9). In any case, the exposure calibration of a thimble chamber removes the
need for knowing its cavity volume (see Section 8.3).

Although adequate wall thickness is necessary to achieve electronic equilibrium, the wall produces some attenuation of the photon flux. Figure 6.4 shows
the effect of wall thickness on the chamber response. When the wall thickness
is much less than that required for equilibrium or maximum ionization, too
few electrons are generated in the wall and thus the chamber response is low.
Beyond the equilibrium thickness, the chamber response is again reduced
because of increased attenuation of the beam in the wall. The true exposure
(without attenuation) can be obtained by extrapolating linearly the attenuation
curve beyond the maximum back to zero thickness, as shown in Figure 6.4. If
the chamber response is normalized to the maximum reading, then the extrapolated value for zero wall thickness gives the correction factor $1/A$ used in
Equation 6.5. The correction for zero wall thickness, however, is usually
allowed for in the exposure calibration of the chamber and is inherent in the
calibration factor. Thus, when the calibration factor is applied to the chamber
reading (corrected for changes in temperature and pressure of cavity air), it
converts the value into true exposure in free air (without chamber). The
exposure value thus obtained is free from the wall attenuation or the perturbing
influence of the chamber.

D. Desirable Chamber Characteristics

A practical ion chamber for exposure measurement should have the following characteristics.

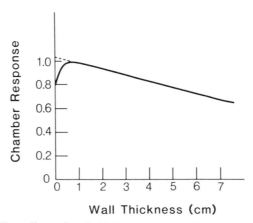

Figure 6.4.   The effect of wall thickness on chamber response (schematic).

1) There should be minimal variation in sensitivity or exposure calibration factor over a wide range of photon energies.

2) There should be suitable volume to allow measurements for the expected range of exposures. The sensitivity (charge measured per roentgen) is directly proportional to the chamber sensitive volume. For example, the reading obtained for a given exposure with a 30-cc chamber will be approximately 50 times higher than that obtained with a 0.6-cc chamber. However, the ratio may not be exactly 50, since a chamber response also depends on the chamber design, as discussed earlier.

3) There should be minimal variation in sensitivity with the direction of incident radiation. Although this kind of variation can be minimized in the design of the chamber, care is taken to use the chamber in the same configuration with respect to the beam as specified under chamber calibration conditions.

4) There should be minimal stem "leakage." A chamber is known to have stem leakage if it records ionization produced anywhere other than its sensitive volume. The problem of stem leakage is discussed later in this chapter.

5) The chamber should have been calibrated for exposure against a standard instrument for all radiation qualities of interest.

6) There should be minimal ion recombination losses. If the chamber voltage is not high enough or regions of low electric field strength occur inside the chamber such as in the vicinity of sharply concave surfaces or corners, ions may recombine before contributing to the measured charge. The problem becomes severe with high intensity or pulsed beams.

6.5 PRACTICAL THIMBLE CHAMBERS

A. Condenser Chambers

A condenser chamber is a thimble ionization chamber connected to a condenser. Fig. 6.5 shows a Victoreen condenser chamber, manufactured by Victoreen Instrument Company. The thimble at the right-hand end consists of an approximately air equivalent wall (Bakelite, nylon, or other composition) with a layer of carbon coated on the inside to make it electrically conducting. The conducting layer makes contact with the metal stem. The central electrode

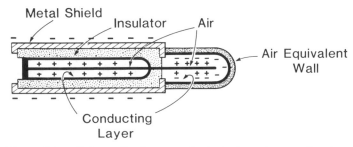

Figure 6.5.   Schematic diagram of a typical condenser chamber.

(aluminum rod) is connected to a conducting layer of carbon coated on the inside of a hollow polystyrene insulator. This arrangement of an outer metal shield and an inner conducting layer with an insulator in between constitutes an electrical condenser, capable of storing charge. The central wire and the thimble's inner conducting surface together also act as a condenser. Thus, the chamber has a total capacitance C between the central electrode and the outer metal sheath which is given by

$$C = C_c + C_t \qquad (6.6)$$

where C_c and C_t are the capacitance of the condenser and thimble, respectively. Usually C_c is much greater than C_t.

The device for charging the condenser chamber and measuring its charge is an electrometer (described later in this section). When fully charged, the potential difference between the carbon layer of the thimble wall and the central electrode is of the order of 400 V. When the chamber is exposed to radiation, electrons are generated in the thimble wall and produce ionization of the air in the thimble cavity. The negative ions are attracted to the positive central electrode and the positive ions are attracted to the negative inner wall. As ions are collected, the charge on the electrodes is reduced. The reduction in charge is proportional to the exposure.

In general, all the ionization measured is produced in the air volume within the thimble. Although the ionization is also produced in the air within the hollow portion of the stem, these ions recombine since they are in a field free region.

Figure 6.6 shows several Victoreen condenser chambers designed with different sensitivities. The chambers are designated by the maximum exposure that can be measured. For example, a 100-R chamber is capable of measuring exposures up to 100 R. This chamber has a sensitive volume of about 0.45 cm³. A 25-R chamber has a volume of about 1.8 cm³, which is four times that of 100-R chamber and therefore about four times as sensitive since chamber sensitivity is directly proportional to sensitive volume (Equation 6.11).

A.1. CHAMBER SENSITIVITY

Suppose a chamber with volume v is given an exposure X. The charge Q collected is given by

$$Q = X \cdot \rho_{\text{air}} \cdot v \qquad (6.7)$$

where ρ_{air} is the density of air and $\rho_{\text{air}} \cdot v$ is the mass of the air volume. The above equation is in accordance with the definition of exposure, given by Equation 6.1, as well as Equation 6.5 if A is assumed equal to 1. Using appropriate units,

$$Q \text{ (coulombs)} = X(R) \cdot (2.58 \times 10^{-4} \text{ C/kg}_{\text{air}}) \cdot \rho_{\text{air}}(\text{kg/m}^3) \cdot v(\text{m}^3)$$

If air is assumed to be at standard temperature and pressure (0°C and 760 mm

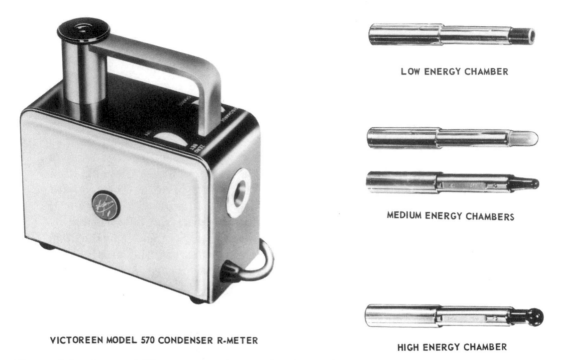

LOW ENERGY CHAMBER

MEDIUM ENERGY CHAMBERS

HIGH ENERGY CHAMBER

VICTOREEN MODEL 570 CONDENSER R-METER

Figure 6.6. A set of Victoreen condenser chambers with a string electrometer. (Courtesy of Victoreen, Inc., Melbourne, Florida.)

Hg), $\rho_{\text{air}} = 1.29$ kg/m^3. Then,

$$Q = 3.33 \times 10^{-4} X \cdot v \tag{6.8}$$

If C is the total capacitance of the chamber (Equations 6.6) in farads, then the voltage drop V across the chamber is:

$$V = \frac{Q}{C} = \frac{3.33 \times 10^{-4} X \cdot v}{C} \tag{6.9}$$

The voltage drop per roentgen is

$$\frac{V}{X} = 3.33 \times 10^{-4} \frac{v}{C} \tag{6.10}$$

The voltage drop per roentgen is known as the *sensitivity* of the chamber. Thus, the chamber sensitivity is directly proportional to the chamber volume and inversely to the chamber capacitance.

If the chamber is connected to an electrometer of capacitance C_e used to measure the charge, then the sensitivity of the chamber is modified:

$$\frac{V}{X} = \frac{3.33 \times 10^{-4} v}{C + C_e} \tag{6.11}$$

A.2. STEM EFFECT

Figure 6.7 shows an arrangement used for measuring exposure with a condenser chamber. A chamber is oriented with the axis of the chamber at a right angle to the direction of the beam. Different lengths of the chamber stem are included in the field, depending upon the field size. However, the calibration of the thimble chamber against a standard chamber is performed with a fixed field which may cover the entire stem or only a small portion of the stem. If the irradiation of the stem gives rise to ionization that can be measured by the chamber, the chamber reading will depend upon the amount of the stem in the beam. Thus, a correction will be necessary whenever the length of the stem irradiated differs from that irradiated at the time of the chamber calibration.

Stem effect can be caused by two problems: (i) measureable ionization in the body of the stem; and (ii) ionization of the air between the end of the chamber and the metal cap. As discussd earlier, the ionization produced in air in the central hollow portion of the stem is normally not measured since this is a field free region and the ions produced there recombine. However, electrons ejected from the metal stem and the insulator could reach the central electrode and reduce its charge. This kind of stem leakage is usually small and occurs only with high energy radiation (~2 MeV or higher). The stem leakage due to ionization of the air surrounding the stem end is eliminated or minimized by a metal cap which fits over the end of the chamber and covers up the central electrode. In addition, the end cap attenuates the radiation and reduces the stem ionization. This cap must be in place during irradiation (Fig. 6.6). If the cap does not fit properly over the chamber end, some charge can be collected

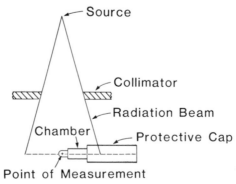

Figure 6.7. Geometry of exposure measurements with a condenser chamber.

in the air adjacent to the end of the electrode, thus causing stem leakage. Correction for the stem effect may be as large as 10%. For further details concerning condenser chamber stem leakage, see Reference 3.

The stem correction may be determined as illustrated in Fig. 6.8. Measurements are made with the chamber oriented in each of the two positions shown. A number of points in the field are selected for such measurements and correction factors are obtained as a function of the stem length exposed relative to the amount of the stem exposed during calibration. Figure 6.9 presents data for a particular chamber which had been calibrated for ^{60}Co exposure with the center of the chamber sensitive volume at the center of a 10×10 cm field. It appears that in this case the major stem effect is occurring at the stem end where the protective cap seals the chamber.

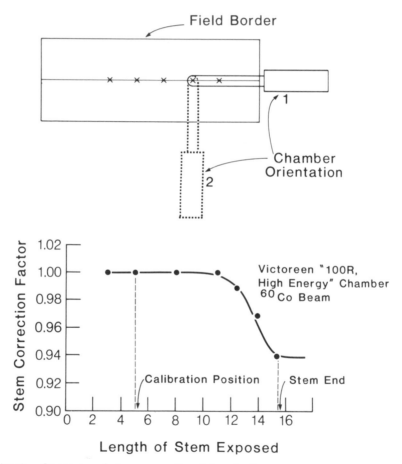

Figure 6.8 (top). Geometry of stem correction determination.
Figure 6.9 (bottom). Plot of stem correction factor (multiplicative) as a function of stem length, measured from center of sensitive volume.

B. Farmer Chamber

Condenser chambers are suitable for measuring exposure rate in air for relatively lower energy beams (≤2 MeV). Although there are no basic limitations to their use for higher energy radiation, the design of the stem and excessive stem leakage create dosimetric problems, especially when making measurements in phantoms. In 1955, Farmer (4) designed a chamber which provided a stable and reliable secondary standard for x-rays and γ rays for all energies in the therapeutic range. This chamber connected to a specific electrometer (to measure ionization charge) is known as the Baldwin-Farmer substandard dosimeter.

The original design of the Farmer chamber was later modified by Aird and Farmer (5) to provide better (flatter) energy response characteristics and more constancy of design from one chamber to another. This chamber is shown schematically in Fig. 6.10. Actual dimensions of the thimble and the central electrode are indicated on the diagram. The thimble wall is made of pure graphite and the central electrode is of pure aluminum. The insulator consists of polytrichlorofluorethylene. The collecting volume of the chamber is nominally 0.6 cc.

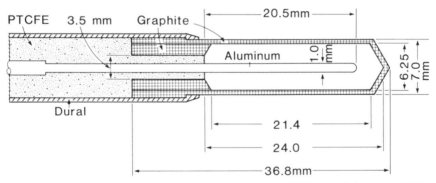

Figure 6.10.   Farmer graphite/aluminum chamber. Nominal air volume, 0.6 cc. PTCFE, polytrichlorofluorethylene. (Redrawn from Reference 5.)

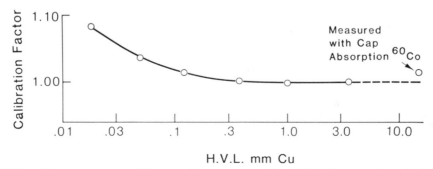

Figure 6.11.   Energy response of the chamber shown in Fig. 6.10. (Redrawn from Reference 5.)

The energy response of the chamber designed by Aird and Farmer is shown in the form of a plot of calibration factor as a function of beam half-value layer (Fig. 6.11). The response is almost constant from 0.3 mm Cu HVL upwards and within 4% from 0.05 mm Cu upwards. The above authors found the total stem leakage of this chamber to be about 0.4% when irradiated with 4-MV x-rays with the whole stem in the beam.

Farmer chambers, like the one described above and other Farmer-type chambers are commercially available. The latter chambers are constructed similar to the original Farmer chamber but vary with respect to the composition of the wall material or the central electrode. The user of any such chamber is cautioned against using a chamber whose characteristics have not been evaluated and found acceptable. For further details of chamber design and characteristics the reader is referred to Boag (6).

6.6 ELECTROMETERS

A. String Electrometer

The electrometer is basically a charge measuring device. The string electrometer is a type of electrometer that operates on the principle of a gold leaf electroscope. Such electrometers are commonly used for the measurement of charge on a condenser chamber. Figure 6.12 shows the mechanism of a string

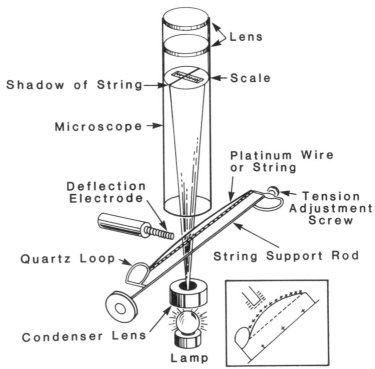

Figure 6.12.   Schematic diagram of Victoreen electrometer. (Adopted from diagram by Victoreen, Inc.)

electrometer used in a Victoreen R meter. The device consists of a string (platinum wire) stretching along a support rod and maintained under tension by a quartz loop attached at one end of the rod. A deflection electrode is mounted near the middle of the string. When the support rod and the platinum wire are positively charged, a negative charge is induced on the deflection electrode. The deflection electrode attracts the wire which moves a distance that depends on the amount of charge on the wire. The deflection of the wire is viewed through a small microscope which shows a shadow of the wire projected on an illuminated scale.

To operate the instrument, the condenser chamber is inserted into the electrometer. This connects the central electrode of the chamber with the support rod and the wire. The chamber and the electrometer are then charged until the shadow of the wire coincides with the zero end of the scale (fully charged position). The voltage across the chamber electrodes at this instant is about 400 V. The chamber is then removed from the electrometer and exposed to radiation. The ionization produced in the thimble air of the chamber reduces the charge on the central electrode. As the chamber is reconnected to the electrometer, the reduction in charge is shared by the chamber and the electrometer. The attraction between the wire and the deflection electrode is decreased and the string shadow moves upscale. The reading on the scale reflects the amount of radiation received by the chamber. The exposure in roentgens can be calculated by multiplying the reading with several correction factors such as temperature and pressure correction, chamber calibration factor for the given quality of radiation, and stem correction.

B. Other Electrometers

The condenser chambers described earlier are detached from the electrometer during exposure and then reattached to measure the charge. Other exposure measuring devices are available in which the chamber remains connected to the electrometer during exposure. The cable is long enough so that the electrometer is placed outside the room at the control console of the radiation generator. This arrangement is more convenient than that of the detachable condenser chamber in which the operator must carry the chamber to the room, return to the control console, operate the machine, and then go back in the room to retrieve the chamber for charge measurement. In calibrating a radiation unit, this amounts to a large number of trips, going in and out of the room.

There are many dosimetry systems (chambers and electrometers) with thimble chambers connected to electrometers via long shielded cables. The general principles of such a system are shown in Fig. 6.13. The instrument can operate either in the integrate mode or the rate mode. In the integrate mode, the central electrode of the chamber is connected to one plate of condenser C and the chamber wall is connected through a battery to the other plate of the condenser. The voltage supplied by the battery should be high enough to provide better than 99% ion collection efficiency (see Section 6.8).

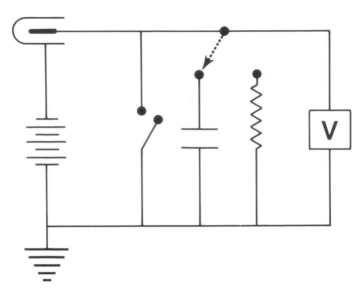

Figure 6.13. Schematic circuit diagram of a dosimetry system capable of measuring exposure in the integrate mode or the rate mode.

As the chamber is irradiated, the charge due to ionization begins to accumulate in the condenser. At the end of the radiation, a charge Q is accumulated and the voltage V generated across the condenser is given by Q/C, where C is the condenser capacity. Measurement of this voltage is essentially the measurement of ionization charge and hence the exposure. Since the magnitude of the charge liberated is very small, complex electronics circuitry is used to measure it accurately.

In the rate mode, the condenser is replaced by a resistance R. Irradiation of the chamber causes an ionization current I to flow through the circuit, generating a voltage $V = IR$ across the resistance. The measurement of this voltage reflects the magnitude of the current or the charge liberated per unit time or the radiation exposure rate. Again, due to the smallness of the ionization current, its measurement is difficult. Special electrometer circuits have been designed to accurately measure ionization currents, even as low as 10^{-15} A. Some of these instruments are described in Reference 7.

Several combinations of chambers and electrometers are commercially available. Figure 6.14 shows one of such systems. A Farmer 0.6-cc ion chamber is connected through a long shielded cable to a Keithley 616 electrometer. The system can be used to measure integrated charge or ionization current. Both the chamber and the electrometer are calibrated so that the reading can be converted into exposure.

6.7 SPECIAL CHAMBERS

A cylindrical thimble chamber is most often used for exposure calibration of radiation beams where the dose gradient across the chamber volume is

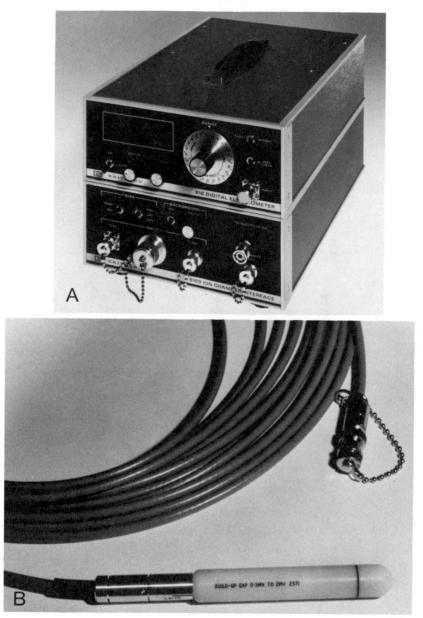

Figure 6.14. A photograph of a Farmer 0.6-cc ion chamber with a Keithley 616 electrometer. (Courtesy of Keithley Instruments, Inc., Cleveland, Ohio.)

minimal. It is not suitable for surface dose measurements. As will be discussed in Chapter 13, high energy photon beams exhibit a *dose build-up* effect, *i.e.* a rapid increase of dose with depth in the first few millimeters. In order to measure the dose at a point in this build-up region or at the surface, the detector must be very thin so that there is no dose gradient across its sensitive volume. In addition, the chamber must not significantly perturb the radiation field. Special chambers have been designed to achieve the above requirements.

A. Extrapolation Chamber

Failla (11) designed an ionization chamber for measuring surface dose in an irradiated phantom in 1937. He called this chamber an extrapolation chamber (Fig. 6.15). The beam enters through a thin foil which is carbon coated to form the upper electrode. The lower or the collecting electrode is a small coin-shaped region surrounded by a guard ring and is connected to an electrometer. The electrode spacing can be varied accurately by micrometer screws. By measuring the ionization per unit volume as a function of electrode spacing, one can estimate the superficial dose by extrapolating the ionization curves to zero electrode spacing.

The extrapolation chambers of the type described above have been used for special dosimetry, *e.g.* the measurement of dose in the superficial layers of a medium and the dosimetry of electrons and β particles.

B. Parallel-Plate Chambers

These chambers are similar to the extrapolation chambers except for the variable electrode spacing. The electrode spacing of the parallel plate chambers is small (~2 mm) but fixed. A thin wall or window (*e.g.* foils of 0.01 to 0.03 mm thick Mylar, polystyrene, or mica) allows measurements practically at the surface of a phantom without significant wall attenuation. By adding layers of phantom material on top of the chamber window, one can study the variation in dose as a function of depth, at shallow depths where cylindrical chambers are unsuitable because of their larger volume.

The small electrode spacing in a parallel plate chamber minimizes cavity perturbations in the radiation field. This feature is especially important in the dosimetry of electron beams where cylindrical chambers may produce significant perturbations in the electron field.

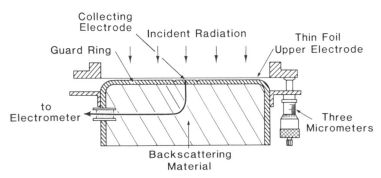

Figure 6.15. Extrapolation ion chamber by Failla. (Redrawn from Reference 6.)

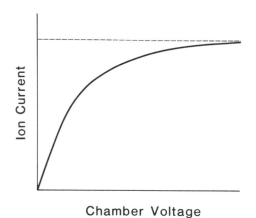

Figure 6.16.   Saturation curve for an ion chamber.

6.8 ION COLLECTION

A. Saturation

As the voltage difference between the electrodes of an ion chamber, exposed to radiation, is increased, the ionization current increases at first almost linearly and later more slowly. The curve finally approaches a saturation value for the given exposure rate (Fig. 6.16). The initial increase of ionization current with voltage is due to incomplete ion collection at low voltages. The negative and the positive ions tend to recombine unless they are quickly separated by the electric field. This recombination can be minimized by increasing the field strength (V/cm).

If the voltage is increased much beyond saturation, the ions, accelerated by the electric field, can gain enough energy to produce ionization by collision with gas molecules. This results in a rapid multiplication of ions and the current, once again, becomes strongly dependent on the applied voltage. The chamber should be used in the saturation region so that small changes in the voltage do not result in changes in the ionic current.

B. Collection Efficiency

As discussed above, the maximum field that can be applied to the chamber is limited by the onset of ionization by collision. Depending upon the chamber design and the ionization intensity, a certain amount of ionization loss by recombination can be expected. Especially at very high ionization intensity such as possible in the case of pulsed beams, significant loss of charge by recombination may occur even at maximum possible chamber voltages. Under these conditions, the *recombination losses* may have to be accepted and the correction applied for these losses.

The *collection efficiency*, defined as the ratio of the number of ions collected to the number produced, may be determined either by calculation (6, 8) or by measurements (8). Experimentally, the measured current is plotted against the inverse of the polarizing voltage in the region of losses below 5%. The "ideal" saturation current is then determined by linear interpolation of the curve to infinite polarizing voltage. Another simpler method, called the two-voltage testing technique, has been described by Boag and Currant (10) for determining the efficiency of ion collection. In this method, measurements are made at two different voltages, one given working voltage and the other much lower voltage. By combining the two readings in accordance with the theoretical formula by Boag and Currant (10), one can obtain the collection efficiency at the given voltage.

Whenever possible, the voltage on the chamber should be arranged to give less than 1% loss of charge by recombination, *i.e.* collection efficiency of better than 99%. In a 0.6-cc Farmer-type chamber, this is generally achieved if the collection voltage is about 300 V or higher and a dose per pulse in the chamber cavity is 0.1 rad or less.

6.9 CHAMBER POLARITY EFFECTS

It is sometimes found that for a given exposure the ionic charge collected by an ion chamber changes in magnitude as the polarity of the collecting voltage is reversed. There are many possible causes of such polarity effects, some of which have been reviewed by Boag (6). With the chamber operating under saturation conditions, major causes of the polarity effects include the following.

1) High energy electrons such as Compton electrons ejected by high energy photons constitute a current (also called the "Compton current") independent of gas ionization. This may add or reduce the collector current depending upon the polarity of the collecting electrode. In addition, some of these electrons may stop in the collector but may not be entirely balanced by ejection of recoil electrons from the collector. The above effects are minimized by making the central electrode very thin. Errors due to these causes are likely to be appreciable for parallel plate chambers with small electrode spacing. However, the true ionization current in this case can be determined by taking the mean of two currents obtained by reversing the chamber polarity.

2) "Extracameral" current, *e.g.* current collected outside the sensitive volume of the chamber, may cause the polarity effect. Such current may be collected at inadequately screened collector circuit points. Also, irradiation of the cable connecting the chamber with the electrometer can cause extracameral current as well as the "Compton" current discussed above. The errors caused by these effects can be minimized but not eliminated by reversing the chamber polarity and taking the mean value of the collector current.

In general, the chamber polarity effects are relatively more severe for measurements in electron beams than photon beams and, in addition, the effect increases with decreasing electron energy. Therefore, it is important to determine polarity effects of a chamber at various depths in a phantom.

Many of the polarity effects and stem leakage can be minimized in the design of the chamber and the associated circuitry. Also, the adequacy of chamber voltage is an important factor in minimizing some of the other polarity effects [not mentioned here but discussed by Boag (6)]. Finally, it is recommended that the difference between the ionization currents measured at positive and negative polarizing potential should be less than 0.5% for any radiation beam quality.

6.10 ENVIRONMENTAL CONDITIONS

If the ion chamber is not sealed, its response is affected by air temperature, pressure, and relative humidity. In fact, most chambers are unsealed and communicate to the outside atmosphere. Since the density of air depends on the temperature and pressure, in accordance with the gas laws, the density of air in the chamber volume will likewise depend on these atmospheric conditions. The density or the mass of air in the chamber volume will increase as the temperature decreases or pressure increases. Since exposure is given by the ionization charge collected per unit mass of air (Section 6.2), the chamber reading for a given exposure will increase as the temperature decreases or as the pressure increases.

Standard laboratories calibrate chambers under the conditions present at the time of calibration. This factor is then converted to specific atmospheric conditions, namely, 760 mm Hg pressure and 22°C temperature. The correction, $C_{T,P}$, for conditions other than the above reference conditions can be calculated.

$$C_{T,P} = \left(\frac{760}{P}\right) \times \left(\frac{273 + t}{295}\right) \tag{6.12}$$

where P is the pressure in mm Hg and t is temperature in °C. The second bracketed term gives the ratio of temperature t to the reference temperature (22°C), both converted to the absolute scale of temperature (in degrees Kelvin) by adding 273 to the Celsius temperatures.

For extreme accuracy, a correction may also be made for relative humidity. This correction is due to differences in electron densities and the energy W needed to produce an ion pair for air $vs.$ water vapor. Suppose the vapor pressure is P_1 mm Hg; then the combined correction factor, $C_{T,P,H}$ for temperature, pressure, and relative humidity is given by (1)

$$C_{T,P,H} = \frac{760}{P - 0.238\,P_1} \times \frac{273 + t}{295} \tag{6.13}$$

The correction for relative humidity is usually less than 1% and can be neglected in most situations.

6.11 MEASUREMENT OF EXPOSURE

Exposure in units of roentgen can be measured with a thimble chamber having an exposure calibration factor, N_C, traceable to the National Bureau of Standards, for a given quality of radiation. The chamber is held at the desired point of measurement in the same configuration as used in the chamber calibration (*e.g.* Fig. 6.7). Precautions are taken to avoid media, other than air, in the vicinity of the chamber which might scatter radiation. Suppose a reading M is obtained for a given exposure. This can be converted to roentgens as follows:

$$X = M \cdot N_C \cdot C_{T,P} \cdot C_s \cdot C_{st} \qquad (6.14)$$

where $C_{T,P}$ is the correction for temperature and pressure (Equation 6.12), C_s is the correction for loss of ionization due to recombination (Section 6.8), and C_{st} is the stem leakage correction (Section 6.5). The quantity X given by Equation 6.14 above is the exposure that would be expected in free air at the point of measurement in the absence of the chamber. In other words, the correction for any perturbation produced in the beam by the chamber is inherent in the chamber calibration factor N_C.

For lower energy radiation such as in the superficial and orthovoltage range, the thimble chambers are usually calibrated and used without a build-up cap. For higher energies such as cobalt-60, a Lucite build-up cap is used unless the chamber wall is already thick enough to provide electronic equilibrium (*e.g.* Victoreen high energy chambers). In either case, the correction to zero wall thickness (Section 6.4) is inherent in the chamber calibration factor N_C.

References

1. Wyckoff, HO, Attix FH: *Design of Free-Air Ionization Chambers.* Washington, DC, National Bureau of Standards Handbook 64, US Government Printing Office, 1957.
2. Mayneord WV: The significance of the Röntgen. In *Acta of the International Union against Cancer*, vol. 2. 1937, p. 271.
3. Adams GD: On the use of thimble chambers in phantoms. *Radiology* 78:77, 1962.
4. Farmer FT: A substandard x-ray dose-meter. *Br J Radiol* 28:304, 1955.
5. Aird EGA, Farmer FT: The design of a thimble chamber for the farmer dosemeter. *Phys Med Biol* 17:169, 1972.
6. Boag JW: Ionization chambers. In Attix FH, Roesch WC (eds): *Radiation Dosimetry*, vol II. New York, Academic Press, 1969, p. 1.
7. Johns HE, Cunningham JR: *The Physics of Radiology*, 3rd ed. Springfield, IL, Charles C Thomas, 1969.
8. International Commission on Radiological Units and Measurements (ICRU) Report No. 10b: *Physical Aspects of Irradiation.* Washington, DC, NBS Handbook 85, 1964.
9. Loftus TP, Weaver JT: Standardization of ^{60}Co and ^{137}Cs gamma-ray beams in terms of exposure. *J Res Natl Bur Stand (US)* 78A (Phys. and Chem.): 465, 1974.
10. Boag JW, Currant J: Current collection and ionic recombination in small cylindrical ionization chambers exposed to pulsed radiation. *Br J Radiol* 53:471, 1980.
11. Failla G: The measurement of tissue dose in terms of the same unit for all ionizing radiations. *Radiology* 29:202, 1937.
12. ICRU Report No. 33: *Radiation Quantities and Units.* Washington, DC, International Commission on Radiation Units and Measurements, 1980.

CHAPTER 7

Quality of X-ray Beams

In Chapter 5, we described x-ray beam in terms of photon fluence and energy fluence. Such a description requires the knowledge of the number and energy of the photons in the beam. In this chapter, we will characterize an x-ray beam in terms of its ability to penetrate materials of known composition. The penetrating ability of the radiation is often described as the *quality* of the radiation.

An ideal way to describe the quality of an x-ray beam is to specify its spectral distribution, *i.e.* energy fluence in each energy interval as shown in Fig. 3.9. However, spectral distributions are difficult to measure and, furthermore, such a complete specification of the beam quality is not necessary in most clinical situations. Since the biological effects of x-rays are not very sensitive to the quality of the beam, in radiotherapy one is interested primarily in the penetration of the beam into the patient rather than its detailed energy spectrum. Thus, a crude but simpler specification of the beam quality is often used, namely, the *half-value layer*.

7.1 HALF-VALUE LAYER

As defined earlier (Section 5.3), the term half-value layer (HVL) is the thickness of an absorber of specified composition required to attenuate the intensity of the beam to half its original value. Although all beams can be described in terms of their HVL, the quality of a γ ray beam is usually stated in terms of the energy of the γ rays or its nuclide of origin which has a known emission spectrum. For example, the quality of a γ ray beam emitted from a ^{60}Co source can be stated in terms of 1.17 and 1.33 MeV (average 1.25 MeV) or simply cobalt-60 beam. Since all x-ray beams produced by radiation generators are heterogeneous in energy, *i.e.* possess continuous energy spectra which depend on the peak voltage, target material, and beam filtration, they are usually described by the HVL, a single parameter specifying the overall penetrating ability of the beam.

In the case of low energy x-ray beams (below megavoltage range), it is customary to describe quality in terms of HVL together with kVp, although HVL alone is adequate for most clinical applications. On the other hand, in the megavoltage x-ray range, the quality is specified by the peak energy and rarely by the HVL. The reason for this convention is that in the megavoltage range the beam is so heavily filtered through the transmission type target and the flattening filter that any additional filtration does not significantly alter the beam quality or its HVL. Thus, for a "hard" beam with a fixed filtration, the x-ray energy spectrum is a function primarily of the peak energy and so is the beam quality. The average energy of such a beam is approximately one-third of the peak energy.

7.2 FILTERS

In Section 3.5, we briefly discussed the energy spectrum of an x-ray beam. The x-rays produced by an x-ray generator show a continuous distribution of energies of bremsstrahlung photons upon which is superimposed discrete lines of characteristic radiation (Fig. 7.1). Curve A in Fig. 7.1 schematically represents the energy spectrum of a 200 kVp x-ray beam filtered by a 1-mm thick aluminum filter. This distribution includes the effects of attenuation in the glass envelope of the x-ray tube, the surrounding oil, and the exit window of the tube housing as well. This so-called *inherent filtration* is equivalent to about 1 mm Al in most x-ray tubes.

The K characteristic x-rays produced in the tungsten target possess discrete energies between 58 and 69 keV (see Table 3.1). Other emission lines of tungsten, however, have much lower energies and are not shown in the figure since they are effectively removed by the inherent filtration as well as the added filtration.

The energy fluence of the K lines of tungsten can be preferentially reduced using a tin filter. Since the K absorption edge of tin is at about 29.2 keV (Table 3.2), it strongly absorbs photons above 29.2 keV by the photoelectric process. However, lower energy photons cannot eject the K electrons. As seen in curve B, the energy fluence in the region from 30 to 70 keV is considerably reduced relative to either the higher energy part of the spectrum or the spectrum below 29 keV. Since the L absorption edge of tin is only 4.5 keV,

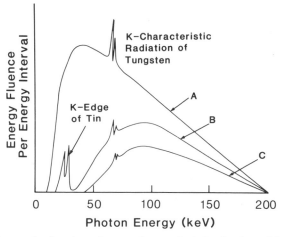

Figure 7.1. Schematic graph showing changes in spectral distribution of 200 kVp x-ray beam with various filters. Curve A is for Al, Curve B is for Sn + Al, and Curve C is for Sn + Cu + Al.

there is little reduction in the spectrum below 29 keV. In addition to the above effects, tin produces its own characteristic radiation by the photoelectric process involving the K shell and these lines are superimposed on the spectrum below the tin absorption edge.

In order to preferentially absorb the energy fluence below the K edge of tin including the characteristic x-rays of tin, a copper filter is quite efficient. The K edge of copper is at 9 keV and therefore the photons below 29 keV are strongly absorbed by the copper filter as seen in curve C. The very low energy characteristic x-rays produced by copper can be effectively absorbed by adding an aluminum filter next to the copper filter.

Combination filters containing plates of tin, copper, and aluminum have been designed to increase the resulting half-value layer of the orthovoltage beams without reducing the beam intensity to unacceptably low values. Such filters are called *Thoraeus filters* (1) and are described in Table 7.1. It is important that the combination filters be arranged in the proper order, with the highest atomic number material nearest the x-ray target. Thus, a Thoraeus filter is inserted with tin facing the x-ray tube and the aluminum facing the patient, with the copper sandwiched between the tin and the aluminum plates.

In the diagnostic and superficial x-ray energy range (Section 4.1), primarily aluminum filters are used to harden the beam. The half-value layers of these beams are also expressed in terms of millimeters of aluminum. In the orthovoltage range, however, combination filters are often used to obtain half-value layers in the range of about 1–4 mm Cu. For cesium and cobalt teletherapy machines, on the other hand, filters are not needed since the beams are almost monoenergetic.

Although a megavoltage x-ray beam has a spectrum of energies, the beam is hardened by the inherent filtration of the transmission target as well as by transmission through the flattening filter. Thus, no additional filtration is required to improve the beam quality. It may be mentioned that the primary purpose of the flattening filter is to make the beam intensity uniform in cross section rather than to improve the beam quality.

7.3 MEASUREMENT OF BEAM QUALITY PARAMETERS
A. Half-Value Layer

As discussed earlier in Section 5.3, the half-value layer of a beam is related to the linear attenuation coefficient (μ) by the following equation:

$$\text{HVL} = \frac{0.693}{\mu} \tag{7.1}$$

Table 7.1.
Thoraeus filters used with orthovoltage x-rays

Filter	Composition
Thoraeus I	0.2 mm Sn + 0.25 mm Cu + 1 mm Al
Thoraeus II	0.4 mm Sn + 0.25 mm Cu + 1 mm Al
Thoraeus III	0.6 mm Sn + 0.25 mm Cu + 1 mm Al

Like the attenuation coefficient, the half-value layer must be measured under narrow-beam or "good" geometry conditions. Such a geometry can be achieved by using a narrow beam and a large distance between the absorber and the detector such as an ion chamber (Fig. 5.1). Under these conditions, the exposure reading is mainly due to the photons that are transmitted through the absorber without interaction and practically no scattered photons are detected by the chamber. The attenuation data are obtained by measuring transmitted exposure through absorbers of varying thickness but constant composition. These data are then plotted on a semilogarithmic graph paper to determine HVL. If the beam has a low filtration or contains an appreciable amount of low energy component in the spectrum, the slope of the attenuation curve decreases with increasing absorber thickness (Fig. 5.3). Thus, different half-value layer beams can be obtained from such a beam by using different filters. In general, the HVL increases with increasing filter thickness as the beam becomes increasingly "harder," *i.e.* contains a greater proportion of higher energy photons. Beyond a certain thickness, however, additional filtration may result in "softening" of the beam by Compton scattering.

Since an increase in filtration is accompanied by a reduction in the available exposure rate, the filtration is carefully chosen to obtain a suitable HVL as well as acceptable beam output. In addition, as discussed in the previous section, certain filters are more efficient than others in selectively removing low energy photons from the beam including characteristic x-rays which are undesirable for therapy because of their low energy.

B. Peak Voltage

Neither the HVL nor the tube potential nor both provide sufficient information regarding the spectral distribution of the radiation. However, for most clinical purposes, these two parameters give an appropriate specification of radiation quality. It has been recommended (2) that the quality of the clinical beams in the superficial and orthovoltage range be specified by the HVL and the kVp in preference to the HVL alone.

The determination of x-ray tube potential is difficult since the high tension circuits of most x-ray equipment are sealed and hence are not easily accessible for direct voltage measurement. Indirect methods therefore are often used to measure the kVp without approach to the high tension circuits. However, if access to the high voltage terminals can be achieved, direct measurements can be made by precision voltage dividers or a sphere-gap apparatus.

B.1. DIRECT MEASUREMENT

Voltage Divider. If the high tension leads of the x-ray tube are accessible, then the effective voltage across the tube can be measured directly by a voltage divider. The voltage divider is a circuit in which several high resistances are connected in series to form a resistance tower which is placed across the high tension leads. The total potential is thus divided among the separate resisters. The effective voltage between any two points is given by the effective current through the tower times the resistance between the two points. The ratio of total resistance to the output resistance between two selected points gives the calibration factor which when multiplied by the observed output voltage across those points gives the total voltage across the voltage divider. For further details of the method, the reader is referred to References 3 and 4.

Sphere-Gap Method. This is one of the oldest methods of determining the kVp. Each high voltage lead of the x-ray tube is connected to a polished metallic sphere by a cable adapter. The distance between the two spheres is reduced until an electric spark passes between them. By knowing the critical distance, corrected for air density and humidity, one can calculate the peak voltage across the x-ray tube.

B.2. INDIRECT MEASUREMENT

Fluorescence Method. This method (5) is based on two principles. First, the peak photon energy is given by the peak potential, *i.e.* $h\nu_{max}$ in keV is numerically equal to the kVp. Second, K edge absorption is a threshold phenomenon in which K orbit fluorescence (characteristic x-ray production) occurs when the photon energy is just equal to or greater than the binding energy of the K

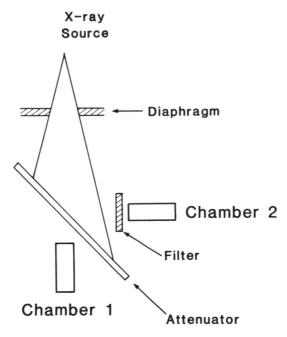

Figure 7.2. Experimental arrangement for measuring tube voltage by K fluorescence method. Chamber 1 measures radiation transmitted through the attenuator and Chamber 2 measures characteristic as well as scattered x-rays. The filter in front of Chamber 2 absorbs most of the scattered radiation from the attenuator.

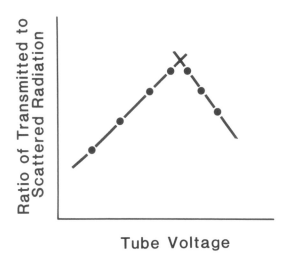

Figure 7.3. Plot of the transmitted (Chamber 1 reading) to scattered radiation (Chamber 2 reading) as a function of tube kilovoltage. The discontinuity occurs in the curve at the tube voltage numerically equal to the K edge threshold of the attenuator.

shell electron. Hence, by using materials of several different K absorption edges, one can calibrate the kVp dial on the machine.

Figure 7.2 illustrates an experimental arrangement for the procedure. A secondary radiator (attenuator) whose K absorption edge is accurately known, is placed at an angle of 45° to the central axis of the beam. While one ionization chamber, placed behind the radiator, measures the transmitted x-rays, a second chamber, placed at an angle of 90° to the beam axis, measures scattered and fluorescent radiation. This chamber is well shielded to prevent the reception of radiation other than that from the radiator. Also a differential filter (low Z absorber) is used in front of this chamber to minimize the effect of low energy scattered x-rays.

When the tube voltage is below the K edge, both the transmitted and the scattered radiation increase at a faster rate. Due to a sudden increase in absorption at and beyond the K edge, the transmitted radiation decreases and the secondary radiation increases due to the production of characteristic fluorescent radiation. Thus, if the ratio of the transmitted to the secondary radiation is plotted against the tube potential, a break in the curve is observed at the K edge threshold (Fig. 7.3). The applied kVp at that point is numerically equal to the K edge absorption energy expressed in keV.

Attenuation Method. This method, described by Morgan (6) and by Newell and Henny (7), is based on the observation that the slope of the transmission curve of an x-ray beam at high filtration depends on the peak kilovoltage. The apparatus consists of a detector such as an ion chamber with two caps of copper or aluminum of different thicknesses. The instrument is first calibrated by determining the ratio of the detector response with the two caps in place as a function of kVp of x-ray beams produced by a generator of accurately known peak potentials. Accordingly, an unknown kVp of an x-ray beam can be estimated from the calibration curve by determining the ratio of the detector response for the same two caps. This method, however, has a limited accuracy and depends strongly on the wave form of the x-ray tube potential.

Penetrameter. The operation of this device consists of comparing transmission through two materials whose x-ray absorptions change differently with photon energy. The original penetrameter was designed by Benoist (8) in 1901. The design was optimized in 1966 by Stanton *et al.* (9). Their device consists of a rectangular central reference block of polyethylene, on both sides of which are identical metal step wedges. Aluminum wedges are recommended for the low kV range and brass wedges for the higher kV. The central polyethylene block is surrounded on its sides by lead scatter shields.

For kilovoltage measurement, the penetrameter is radiographed in the beam with heavy filtration and scatter shielding. The optical density ratios of adjacent wedge and reference areas are used to obtain the "matching step position." If the instrument has been calibrated against known potentials, the desired peak voltage can be read from the calibration curve.

Another penetrameter, known as the Ardran-Crooks cassette, has been described by Ardran and Crooks (10). This device consists of a film which is covered partly with a slow intensifying screen and partly with a fast screen. A copper step system is superimposed on the fast screen, while the slow screen is kept uncovered to serve as a reference. A sheet of lead allows only small (0.5-cm diameter) beam to pass through each copper step and the uncovered slow screen. When a radiograph is taken, the match of a step density with the reference depends on the kV. By using an appropriate calibration curve, one can determine the desired kV. A commercial version of the Ardran-Crooks penetrameter is known as the Wiscon Test Cassette.[1]

C. Effective Energy

Since x-ray beams used in radiology are always heterogeneous in energy, it is convenient sometimes to express the quality of an x-ray beam in terms of the effective energy. The *effective (or equivalent) energy* of an x-ray beam is the energy of photons in a monoenergetic beam which is attenuated at the same rate as the radiation in question. Since the attenuation curve for a given material is characterized by the slope or the linear attenuation coefficient, μ, the effective energy is determined by finding the energy of monoenergetic photons which have the same μ as the given beam. In general, however, the μ or the effective energy of a heterogeneous beam varies with the absorber thickness (see Fig. 5.3).

Since μ and HVL are interrelated (Equation 7.1), the effective energy may

---

[1] Available at Radiation Measurements, Inc., Middleton, Wisconsin.

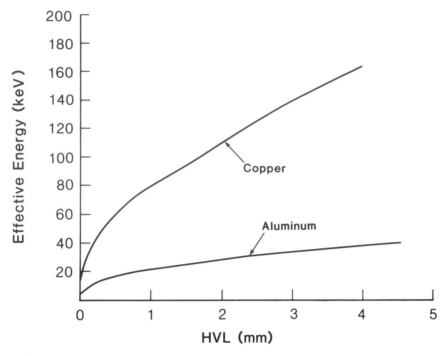

Figure 7.4. Plot of effective energy as a function of half-value layer. Data calculated from attenuation coefficients of monoenergetic photon beams.

also be defined as the energy of a monoenergetic photon beam having the same HVL as the given beam. Figure 7.4 shows the relationship between effective energy and half-value layer for x-ray beams in the superficial and orthovoltage range. These data were calculated by using Equation 7.1 to obtain μ and finding the energy of a monoenergetic photon beam with the same μ given in the Appendix.

Although lead is commonly used to express half-value layers for the megavoltage beams, it is not necessarily the best choice for characterizing the beam quality in this energy range. It has been shown that the low atomic number materials such as water are more sensitive to changes in spectral quality of megavoltage x-rays than the high atomic number materials such as lead (17). This can be seen in Fig. 7.5 in which HVL is plotted as a function of peak photon energy. It may also be noted that the HVL in terms of lead begins to decrease with increase in energy beyond about 20 MV. This is because the mass attenuation coefficient of lead first decreases and then increases with increase in energy whereas for water it monotonically decreases (see Section 5.10).

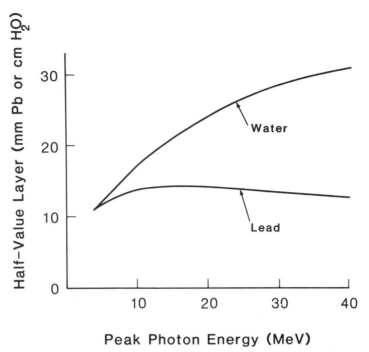

Figure 7.5. Half-value layer as a function of peak photon energy for water and lead. Data are from Nath and Schulz (17). *Note:* since these data were calculated from thin-target Schiff (11) spectra, HVL values plotted here are slightly lower than those measured in practical radiotherapy machines.

D. Mean Energy

A more accurate but complex way of characterizing the x-ray beam energy is by the *mean energy,* $\bar{E}$. This can be calculated from the distribution of photon fluence Φ_E with respect to photon energy E.

$$\bar{E} = \frac{\int_0^{E_{max}} \Phi_E E \cdot dE}{\int_0^{E_{max}} \Phi_E \cdot dE} \qquad (7.2)$$

The mean energy can also be calculated from the energy fluence Ψ_E distribution.

$$\bar{E} = \frac{\int_0^{E_{max}} \Psi_E E \cdot dE}{\int_0^{E_{max}} \Psi_E dE} \qquad (7.3)$$

The above two expressions, however, lead to different values of $\bar{E}$ since $\Phi_E \neq \Psi_E$. Thus, it is important to specify the type of distribution used in calculating the mean energy.

7.4 MEASUREMENT OF MEGAVOLTAGE BEAM ENERGY

The complete energy spectrum of a megavoltage x-ray beam can be obtained by calculation (11) (thin target bremsstrahlung spectra), scintillation spectrometry (12, 13), and photoactivation (14). However, for the characterization of a megavoltage x-ray beam by a single energy parameter, namely, by its maximum energy, one needs to determine the energy of the electron beam before incidence on the target. Several methods for determining this energy are discussed later in Chapter 14.

The most practical method of determining the megavoltage beam energy is by measuring percent depth dose distribution, tissue-air ratios, or tissue-maximum ratios (Chapter 10) and comparing them with the published data such as those in Reference 15. Although clinically relevant, the method is only approximate since depth dose distributions are relatively insensitive to small changes in the peak energy.

A sensitive method of monitoring x-ray beam spectral quality has been proposed by Nath and Schulz (16) and is referred to as the *photoactivation ratio (PAR)* method. The basic procedure involves irradiating a pair of foils which can be activated by the photodisintegration process (Section 2.8F). The choice of foils must be such that one of them is sensitive to higher energies than the other in the energy spectrum of the x-ray beam. After irradiation, the induced radioactivity in the foils is measured using a scintillation counter. The ratio of induced activities gives the PAR which can be related to the peak photon energy. The PAR method provides a more sensitive method of meas-

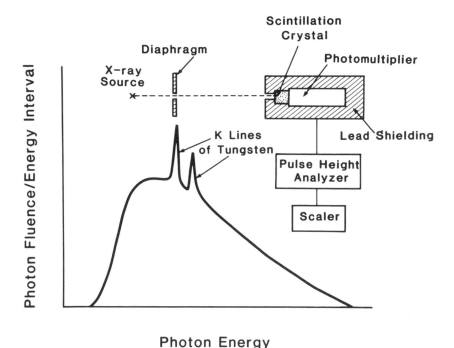

Figure 7.6.   Energy spectrum of an x-ray beam determined by scintillation spectrometer (shown in the inset).

uring x-ray spectral quality than the conventional method of measuring HVL in water.

7.5 MEASUREMENT OF ENERGY SPECTRUM

Although the HVL is a practical parameter characterizing therapeutic beams, it is only approximate and cannot be used in systems which are sensitive to spectral distribution of photons. For example, some radiation detectors show a large variation in response with different photon energies (*e.g.* film, diodes) and even ion chambers are more or less energy dependent, depending upon their design. In such instances, spectral distribution is the relevant parameter of beam quality. In this and other investigative work, it is important to experimentally determine spectral distributions of photon beams. There are many references dealing with spectrometry (11–14) and the interested reader is referred to those papers. Only one method, namely scintillation spectrometry, will be briefly described here.

The scintillation spectrometer consists of a crystal or phosphor, usually sodium iodide, attached to a photomultiplier tube (Fig. 7.6). When a photon beam is incident on the crystal, electrons are ejected which travel in the crystal and produce ionization and excitation of the crystal atoms. As a result, photons of energy in the optical or ultraviolet region are produced along the electron tracks. These light photons, on striking the photosensitive surface (photocathode) of a photomultiplier tube, eject low energy photoelectrons which are collected and multiplied about a million times by the photomultiplier dynodes. This results in an output pulse which is proportional to the energy of the original x-ray photon entering the crystal. A multichannel pulse height analyzer is used to electronically sort out different size pulses. Each channel corresponds to a particular input photon energy and accumulates counts or number of photons with a particular energy. The spectrum is then displayed in terms of photons per unit energy interval as a function of photon energy (Fig. 7.6).

References

1. Thoraeus R: A study of the ionization method for measuring the intensity and absorption of x-rays and of different filters used in therapy. *Acta Radiol* (Suppl 15), 1932.
2. International Commission on Radiological Units and Measurements (ICRU): *Report 10b.* Washington, DC, United States National Bureau of Standards, 1962.
3. Gilbertson JD, Fingerhut AG: Standardization of diagnostic x-ray generators. *Radiology* 93:1033, 1969.
4. Giarratano JC, Waggener RG, Hevezi JM, Shalek RJ: Comparison of voltage-divider, modified Ardran-Crooks cassette and Ge (Li) spectrometer methods to determine the peak kilovoltage (kVp) of diagnostic x-ray units. *Med Phys* 3:142, 1976.
5. Greening J: The measurement of ionization methods of the peak kilovoltage across x-ray tubes. *Br J Appl Phys* 6:73, 1955.
6. Morgan R: A simple method of measuring peak voltage in diagnostic Roentgen equipment. *Am J Roentgenol* 52:308, 1944.
7. Newell RR, Henny GC: Inferential kilovoltmeter: measuring x-ray kilovoltage by absorption in two filters. *Radiology* 64:88, 1955.
8. Glasser O, Quimby EH, Taylor LS, Weatherwax JL, Morgan RH: *Physical Foundations of Radiology*, 3rd ed. New York, Paul B. Hoeber, 1961, p 241.

9. Stanton L, Lightfoot DA, Mann S: A penetrameter method for field kV calibration of diagnostic x-ray machines. *Radiology* 87:87, 1966.
10. Ardran GM, Crooks HE: Checking diagnostic x-ray beam quality. *Br J Radiol* 41:193, 1968.
11. Schiff LI: Energy-angle distribution of thin target bremsstrahlung. *Phys Rev* 83:252, 1951.
12. Skarsgard LD, Johns HE: Spectral flux density of scattered and primary radiation generated at 250 kV. *Radiat Res* 14:231, 1961.
13. Epp ER, Weiss H: Experimental study of the photon energy spectrum of primary diagnostic x-rays. *Phys Med Biol* 11:225, 1966.
14. Nath R, Schulz RJ: Determination of high energy x-ray spectra by photoactivation. *Med Phys* 3:133, 1976.
15. Hospital Physicist's Association: Central axis depth dose data for use in radiotherapy. *Br J Radiol* (Suppl 11), 1978.
16. Nath R, Schulz RJ: Photoactivation ratios for specification of high-energy x-ray quality: part I and II. *Med Phys* 4:36, 1977.
17. Nath R, Schulz RJ: On the choice of material for half-value-layer measurements for megavoltage x-rays. *Med Phys* 4:132, 1977.

CHAPTER 8

Measurement and Calculation of Absorbed Dose

8.1 RADIATION ABSORBED DOSE

In Chapter 6, the quantity exposure and its unit, the roentgen, were discussed. It was then pointed out that the roentgen applies only to x and γ radiations, is a measure of ionization in air only, and cannot be used for photon energies above about 3 MeV. The quantity absorbed dose has been defined to describe the quantity of radiation for all types of ionizing radiation, including charged and uncharged particles, all materials, and all energies. Absorbed dose is a measure of the biologically significant effects produced by ionizing radiation.

The current (1) definition of *absorbed dose*, or simply *dose*, is the quotient $d\bar{\epsilon}/dm$, where $d\bar{\epsilon}$ is the mean energy imparted by ionizing radiation of material of mass dm. The most common unit of dose is *rad* (an acronym for radiation absorbed dose) and represents the absorption of 100 ergs of energy per gram of absorbing material.

$$1 \text{ rad} = 100 \text{ ergs/g} = 10^{-2} \text{ J/kg} \tag{8.1}$$

The *SI unit* for absorbed dose is called *gray* (Gy) and is defined as

$$1 \text{ Gy} = 1 \text{ J/kg} \tag{8.2}$$

Thus, the relationship between gray and rad is

$$1 \text{ Gy} = 100 \text{ rad} \tag{8.3}$$

or

$$1 \text{ rad} = 10^{-2} \text{ Gy} \tag{8.4}$$

Since gray is a larger unit than rad, there is a practical difficulty in switching from rad to grays. For instance, if a patient receives treatments of 175 rad/day, the dose will have to be recorded as 1.75 grays. Since most people prefer numbers without decimals as well as a common resistance to change to the metric system in this country, the adoption of the SI system has been delayed. However, for some, the change is inevitable and the rad is routinely converted into grays. A subunit, centigray (cGy), has often been used as being equivalent to rad.

8.2 CALCULATION OF DOSE FROM EXPOSURE

A. Absorbed Dose in Air

In Chapter 6, the quantity exposure was defined as dQ/dm where dQ is the total charge of the ions of one sign produced in air when all the electrons (negatrons and positrons) liberated by photons in air of mass dm are completely stopped in air. Since the energy, in general, is not deposited in the same mass of air that the secondary electrons come from, the exposure can be measured only if a state of electronic equilibrium exists in the volume element of mass dm. Under equilibrium conditions, the energy deposited in each mass dm is the same and, thus, the above definition of exposure is effectively satisfied.

It is possible to relate exposure and the energy absorbed in air under equilibrium conditions as follows:

The mean energy required to produce an ion pair in air is almost constant for all electron energies and has a value of $\bar{W}_{air} = 33.85$ eV/ion pair (2). If e is the electronic charge (= 1.602×10^{-19} C), then $\dfrac{\bar{W}_{air}}{e}$ is the average energy absorbed per unit charge of ionization produced. Since 1 eV = 1.6×10^{-19} J, $\dfrac{\bar{W}_{air}}{e} = 33.85$ J/C.[1] Thus, the mean energy absorbed, $d\bar{\epsilon}$, in producing a charge dQ in air of mass dm is given by

$$d\bar{\epsilon} = dQ \cdot \frac{\bar{W}_{air}}{e}$$

or

$$\frac{d\bar{\epsilon}}{dm} = \frac{dQ}{dm} \cdot \frac{\bar{W}_{air}}{e}$$

Since absorbed dose is the energy absorbed per unit mass or $\dfrac{d\bar{\epsilon}}{dm}$ and exposure, X, is given by $\dfrac{dQ}{dm}$, the above equation gives the absorbed dose in air, D_{air}.

$$D_{air} = X \cdot \frac{\bar{W}_{air}}{e} \qquad (8.5)$$

---

[1] The currently recommended value of W/e for dry air is 33.85 J/C (2). This value has been used in this text instead of the old value of 33.7 J/C (42).

Since $1R = 2.58 \times 10^{-4}$ C/kg,

$$D_{air} \text{ (J/kg)} = X(R) \cdot 2.58 \times 10^{-4} \left(\frac{C/kg}{R}\right) \cdot 33.85 \text{ (J/C)}$$

$$= 0.873 \times 10^{-2} \cdot \left(\frac{J/kg}{R}\right) \cdot X(R)$$

Since $1 \text{ rad} = 10^{-2}$ J/kg,

$$D_{air} \text{ (rad)} = 0.873 \left(\frac{rad}{R}\right) \cdot X(R) \tag{8.6}$$

From Equation 8.6 it is seen that the *roentgen-to-rad conversion factor* for air is 0.873.

B. Absorbed Dose in any Medium

In the presence of charged particle equilibrium, the absorbed dose, D, in a medium can be calculated from the energy fluence ψ and the weighted mean mass energy absorption coefficient, $\bar{\mu}_{en}/\rho$.

$$D = \psi \cdot \bar{\mu}_{en}/\rho \tag{8.7}$$

Suppose ψ_{air} is the energy fluence at a point in air and ψ_{med} is the energy fluence at the same point when a material other than air (medium) is interposed in the beam. Then, under conditions of electronic equilibrium in either case, the dose in air is related to the dose in the medium by the following relationship:

$$\frac{D_{med}}{D_{air}} = \frac{(\bar{\mu}_{en}/\rho)_{med}}{(\bar{\mu}_{en}/\rho)_{air}} \cdot A \tag{8.8}$$

where A is a transmission factor which equals the ratio ψ_{med}/ψ_{air} at the point of interest.

From Equations 8.5 and 8.8, we obtain the relationship between exposure in air to absorbed dose in a medium.

$$D_{med} = X \cdot \frac{\bar{W}_{air}}{e} \cdot \frac{(\bar{\mu}_{en}/\rho)_{med}}{(\bar{\mu}_{en}/\rho)_{air}} \cdot A \tag{8.9}$$

Again, if we express X in roentgens and D_{med} in rad, we have:

$$D_{med} = \left[0.873 \frac{(\bar{\mu}_{en}/\rho)_{med}}{(\bar{\mu}_{en}/\rho)_{air}}\right] \cdot X \cdot A \tag{8.10}$$

The quantity in brackets has frequently been represented by the symbol f_{med} so that

$$D_{med} = f_{med} \cdot X \cdot A \tag{8.11}$$

where

$$f_{\text{med}} = 0.873 \frac{(\bar{\mu}_{\text{en}}/\rho)_{\text{med}}}{(\bar{\mu}_{\text{en}}/\rho)_{\text{air}}} \tag{8.12}$$

The quantity f_{med} or simply the *f factor* is sometimes called the *roentgen-to-rad conversion factor*. As the above equation suggests, this factor depends on the mass energy absorption coefficient of the medium relative to the air. Thus, the *f* factor is a function of the medium composition as well as the photon energy.

A list of *f* factors for water, bone, and muscle as a function of photon energy is given in Table 8.1. Since for materials with an atomic number close to that of air, *e.g.* water and soft tissue, the ratio $(\bar{\mu}_{\text{en}}/\rho)_{\text{med}}/(\bar{\mu}_{\text{en}}/\rho)_{\text{air}}$ varies slowly with photon energy (~10% variation from 10 keV and 10 MeV), the *f* factor for these materials does not vary much over practically the whole therapeutic range of energies. However, bone with a high effective atomic number not only has a much larger *f* factor between 10 and 100 keV, but the *f* factor drops sharply from its maxium value of 4.24 at 30 keV to about 1.0 at 175 keV. This high peak value and rapid drop of the *f* factor are due to the photoelectric process for which the mass energy absorption coefficient varies approximately as Z^3 and $1/E^3$ (see Equation 5.18). At higher photon energies where the Compton process is the only mode of interaction possible, the *f* factors are approximately the same for all materials.

Table 8.1.
f Factors for water, bone, and muscle under conditions of charged particle equilibrium

Photon energy (keV)	f Factor					
	Water		Bone		Muscle	
	(Gy kg/C)	(rad/R)	(Gy kg/C)	(rad/R)	(Gy kg/C)	(rad/R)
10	35.3	0.911	134	3.46	35.7	0.921
15	34.9	0.900	149	3.85	35.7	0.921
20	34.6	0.892	158	4.07	35.6	0.919
30	34.3	0.884	164	4.24	35.6	0.918
40	34.4	0.887	156	4.03	35.7	0.922
50	34.9	0.900	136	3.52	36.0	0.929
60	35.5	0.916	112	2.90	36.3	0.937
80	36.5	0.942	75.1	1.94	36.8	0.949
100	37.1	0.956	56.2	1.45	37.1	0.956
150	37.5	0.967	41.2	1.06	37.2	0.960
200	37.6	0.969	37.9	0.978	37.2	0.961
300	37.6	0.970	36.5	0.941	37.3	0.962
400	37.6	0.971	36.2	0.933	37.3	0.962
600	37.6	0.971	36.0	0.928	37.3	0.962
1000	37.6	0.971	35.9	0.927	37.3	0.962
2000	37.6	0.971	35.9	0.927	37.3	0.962

Data from Ref. 3. Calculations are based on energy absorption coefficient data from Hubbell (25).

Strictly speaking, in the Compton range of energies, the f factor varies as a function of the number of electrons per gram. Since the number of electrons per gram for bone is slightly less than for air, water, or fat, the f factor for bone is also slightly lower than for the latter materials in the Compton region of the megavoltage energies. Of course, the f factor is not defined beyond 3 MeV since the roentgen is not defined beyond this energy.

C. Dose Calibration with Ion Chamber in Air

As discussed earlier in Chapter 6, a cavity ion chamber is exposure calibrated against a free-air ion chamber or a standard cavity chamber, under conditions of electronic equilibrium. For lower energy radiations such as x-ray beams in the superficial or orthovoltage range, the chamber walls are usually thick enough to provide the desired equilibrium and, therefore, the chamber calibration is provided without a buildup cap. However, in the case of higher energy radiations such as from cobalt-60, a buildup cap is used over the sensitive volume of the chamber so that the combined thickness of the chamber wall and the buildup cap is sufficient to provide the required equilibrium. This buildup cap is usually made up of acrylic (same as Plexiglas, Lucite, or Perspex) and must be in place when measuring exposure.

Suppose the chamber is exposed to the beam (Fig. 8.1a) and the reading M is obtained (corrected for air temperature and pressure, stem leakage, collection efficiency, etc.). The exposure X is then given by:

$$X = M \cdot N_c \tag{8.13}$$

where N_c is the exposure calibration factor for the given chamber and the given beam quality. The exposure thus obtained is the exposure at point P (center of the chamber sensitive volume) in free air in the absence of the

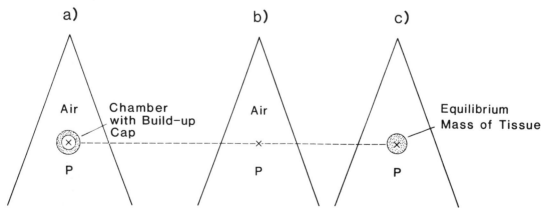

Figure 8.1. a, Chamber with buildup cap is placed in a radiation beam at point P in air and reading M is obtained. b, Exposure in free air at P is calculated, using Equation 8.13. c, Dose in free space at P is calculated, using Equation 8.14.

chamber (Fig. 8.1b). In other words, the perturbing influence of the chamber is removed once the chamber calibration factor is applied.

Consider a small amount of soft tissue at point P that is just large enough to provide electronic equilibrium at its center (Fig. 8.1c). The dose at the center of this equilibrium mass of tissue is referred to as the *"dose in free space."* The term dose in free space was introduced by Johns and Cunningham (4) who related this quantity to the dose in an extended tissue medium by means of tissue air ratios (to be discussed in Chapter 9).

Equation 8.11 can be used to convert exposure into dose in free space, $D_{f.s.}$.

$$D_{f.s.} = f_{tissue} \cdot X \cdot A_{eq} \tag{8.14}$$

where A_{eq} is the transmission factor representing the ratio of the energy fluence at the center of the equilibrium mass of tissue to that in free air at the same point. Thus, A_{eq} represents the ratio of the energy fluence at point P in Fig. 8.1c to that at the same point in Fig. 8.1b. For cobalt-60 beam, A_{eq} is close to 0.99 (4) and its value approaches 1.000 as the beam energy decreases to the orthovoltage range.

D. Dose Calibration with Ion Chamber in a Medium

Equations 8.13 and 8.14 provide the basis for absorbed dose calculation in any medium from exposure measurement in air. Similar procedure is valid when the measurement is made with the chamber imbedded in a medium. Figure 8.2a shows an arrangement in which the chamber with its buildup cap is surrounded by the medium and exposed to a photon energy fluence ψ_b at

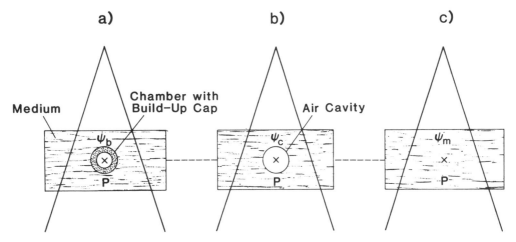

Figure 8.2. a, Chamber with buildup cap with its center at point P in a medium, exposed to a photon beam whose energy fluence is ψ_b at P. Reading M is obtained. b, Exposure at P in air cavity of size equal to the external dimensions of the buildup cap is calculated. Energy fluence at P is ψ_c. c, Absorbed dose at point P in the medium is calculated by Equation 8.15. ψ_m is the energy fluence at P.

the center of the chamber (point P). If the energy of the beam incident on the chamber is such that a state of electronic equilibrium exists within the air cavity, then the exposure at point P, with the chamber and the buildup cap removed, is given by

$$X = M \cdot N_c$$

The exposure thus measured is defined in free air at point P due to energy fluence ψ_c that would exist at P in the air-filled cavity of the size equal to the external dimensions of the buildup cap (Fig. 8.2b). In order to convert this exposure to absorbed dose at P in the medium, the air in the cavity must be replaced by the medium (Fig. 8.2c) and the following equation is applied:

$$D_{\text{med}} = X \cdot f_{\text{med}} \cdot A_m$$

or

$$D_{\text{med}} = M \cdot N_c \cdot \frac{\bar{W}}{e} \cdot \left(\frac{\bar{\mu}_{\text{en}}}{\rho} \right)_{\text{air}}^{\text{med}} \cdot A_m \qquad (8.15)$$

where A_m is the transmission factor for the photon energy fluence at point P when the cavity in Fig. 8.2b is replaced by the medium. If ψ_m is the energy fluence at P in the medium, the factor A_m is given by ψ_m/ψ_c and has been called a displacement factor.

The above equation is similar to Equation 8.14 except that A_m is used instead of A_{eq}. However, the difference between A_m and A_{eq} is small for a tissue equivalent medium since the equilibrium mass of tissue to which A_{eq} applies is only slightly smaller than the mass of the medium displaced by a typical small ion chamber with its buildup cap.

An interesting question arises with regard to the necessity of the buildup cap being left on the chamber when making measurements in a medium. If the chamber has been calibrated for exposure in air with its buildup cap on (to achieve electronic equilibrium) and if a significant part of the cavity ionization is due to electrons produced in the buildup cap, then replacing the buildup cap with the medium could, in general, alter the chamber reading. This substitution of a layer of medium for the buildup cap could change the electronic and photon fluence incident on the chamber wall by virtue of differences in the composition of the medium and the material of the buildup cap. However, in practical calibration measurements, no significant differences have been observed when exposing the chamber in water with and without the Lucite buildup cap. Day et al. (41) added Perspex sheaths up to 5 mm in thickness to a Baldwin-Farmer ionization chamber irradiated at a depth of 5 cm in a water phantom using radiations from ^{137}Cs to 6 MV. The readings differed by less than 0.5%.

8.3 THE BRAGG-GRAY CAVITY THEORY

Calculation of absorbed dose from exposure is subject to some major limitations. For instance, it may not be used for photons above 3 MeV and may not be used in cases where electronic equilibrium does not exist. The reason for these limitations is that the quantity exposure is not truly defined under these conditions, and, therefore, absorbed dose cannot be calculated from a measurement of exposure. In addition, the term exposure applies only to x and γ radiations and for that reason methods of Section 8.2 are not valid for particle dosimetry. The Bragg-Gray cavity theory, on the other hand, may be used without such restrictions to calculate dose directly from ion chamber measurements in a medium.

According to the Bragg-Gray theory (5, 6), the ionization produced in a gas-filled cavity placed in a medium is related to the energy absorbed in the surrounding medium. When the cavity is sufficiently small so that its introduction into the medium does not alter the number or distribution of the electrons that would exist in the medium without the cavity, then the following Bragg-Gray relationship is satisfied:

$$D_{\text{med}} = J_g \cdot \frac{\overline{W}}{e} \cdot (\overline{S}/\rho)_g^{\text{med}} \tag{8.16}$$

where D_{med} is the absorbed dose in the medium, J_g is the ionization charge of one sign produced per unit mass of the cavity gas, and $(\overline{S}/\rho)_g^{\text{med}}$ is a weighted mean ratio of the mass stopping power of the medium to that of the gas for the electrons crossing the cavity. The product $J_g\left(\dfrac{\overline{W}}{e}\right)$ is the energy absorbed per unit mass of the cavity gas.

The basic Bragg-Gray relationship has been carefully examined by many investigators and several modifications of the theory have been proposed (7–10). These refinements resulted in more detailed considerations of what is appropriate to use for the mass stopping power ratio in Equation 8.16.

A. Stopping Power

The term *stopping power* refers to the energy loss by electrons per unit path length of a material (for greater details, see Section 14.1). An extensive set of calculated values of mass stopping powers has been published by Berger and Seltzer (11, 12). As mentioned earlier, in order to use stopping power ratios in the Bragg-Gray formula, it is necessary to determine a weighted mean of the stopping power ratios for the electron spectrum set in motion by the photon spectrum in the materials concerned. Methods for calculating average stopping powers, $\overline{S}$, for photon beams are described in Reference 13.

Several authors have worked out the theory of the stopping power ratio for an air-filled cavity in a medium such as water under electron irradiation. A good approximation is provided by the Spencer-Attix formulation (7, 14):

$$\overline{L}/\rho = \frac{\Delta\int^{E_0} \phi(E)\cdot L/\rho(E)dE}{\Delta\int^{E_0} \phi(E)dE} \tag{8.17}$$

where $\phi(E)$ is the distribution of electron fluence in energy and L/ρ is the *restricted mass collision stopping power* with Δ as the cutoff energy.

The "primary electrons" (original electrons or electrons generated by photons) give rise to ionization as well as "secondary electrons" or δ-rays. The effects of the latter are accounted for in the Spencer-Attix formulation by using an arbitrary energy limit, Δ, below which energy transfers are considered dissipative, that is, the secondary electron of energy less than Δ is assumed to dissipate its energy near the site of its release. Thus, when the integration is performed (Equation 8.17) to obtain the energy deposited in the cavity by the electron fluence, the lower energy limit should be Δ, greater than zero. For ion chambers it must have a value of the order of the energy of an electron that will just cross the cavity. The value of Δ for most cavity applications in ion chambers will lie between 10 and 20 keV.

The Spencer-Attix formulation of the Bragg-Gray cavity theory uses the following relationship:

$$D_{\text{med}} = J_g \cdot \frac{\overline{W}}{\rho} \cdot \left(\frac{\overline{L}}{\rho}\right)_g^{\text{med}} \tag{8.18}$$

where $\dfrac{\overline{L}}{\rho}$ is the average restricted mass collisional stopping power of electrons.

Tables A.1–A.5 in the Appendix give the $\dfrac{\overline{L}}{\rho}$ for various media and various photon and electron energies.

B. Chamber Volume

The quantity J_g in Equation 8.18 can be determined for a chamber of known volume or known mass of air in the cavity if the chamber is connected to a charge-measuring device. However, the chamber volume is usually not known to an acceptable accuracy. An indirect method of measuring J_{air} is to make use of the exposure calibration of the chamber for ^{60}Co γ-ray beam. This in effect determines the chamber volume.

Consider an ion chamber that has been calibrated with a buildup cap for ^{60}Co exposure. Suppose the chamber with this buildup cap is exposed in air to a ^{60}Co beam and that electronic equilibrium exists at the center of the chamber. Also assume initially that the chamber wall and the buildup cap are composed of the same material (m). Now, if the chamber (plus the buildup cap) is replaced by a homogeneous mass of material m with outer dimensions equal to that of the cap, the dose D_m at the center of this mass can be calculated by two methods: (a) the exposure method (Equation 8.15) and (b) the Bragg-Gray cavity method (Equation 8.18).

$$D_m = M \cdot N_c \cdot \left(\frac{\overline{W}}{e}\right) \cdot \left(\frac{\bar{\mu}_{\text{en}}}{\rho}\right)_{\text{air}}^m \cdot A_m \tag{8.19}$$

where M is the charge measured in coulombs, N_c is the ^{60}Co exposure calibration factor in R/C, $\dfrac{\overline{W}}{e}$ is the average energy absorbed per unit charge of ionization produced in air $\left(\dfrac{\overline{W}}{e} = 33.85 \text{ J/C} = 0.873 \text{ rad/R in air}\right)$, $\left(\dfrac{\bar{\mu}_{en}}{\rho}\right)^m_{air}$ is the ratio of weighted mean mass energy absorption coefficient of material m to that of air, and A_m is the displacement factor. This factor A_m is the ratio of photon energy fluence at the center of the mass to that at the same point in free air.

Also,

$$D_m = J_{air} \cdot \left(\frac{\overline{W}}{e}\right) \cdot \left(\frac{\overline{L}}{\rho}\right)^m_{air} \cdot A_2 \tag{8.20}$$

where J_{air} is the ionization charge produced per unit mass of the cavity air, $\left(\dfrac{\overline{L}}{\rho}\right)^m_{air}$ is the $m/$air ratio of the mean restricted mass collision stopping powers for the electrons crossing the cavity, A_2 is a correction for the change in electron fluence when the chamber cavity is filled by material m. (In Equation 8.18, the cavity is assumed to be so small that $A_2 \simeq 1.00$.)

Comparing Equations 8.19 and 8.20,

$$J_{air} = M \cdot N_c \cdot A_c \cdot \left(\frac{\bar{\mu}_{en}}{\rho}\right)^m_{air} \cdot \left(\frac{\overline{L}}{\rho}\right)^{air}_m \tag{8.21}$$

where $A_c = \dfrac{A_m}{A_2}$. For a common practical small chamber with a Lucite buildup cap, $A_c \simeq 0.99$ for ^{60}Co γ-rays.

Now consider a more realistic situation in which the chamber has a wall of material wl and buildup cap of material b. Then according to the two-component model of Almond and Svensson (15), let α be the fraction of cavity ionization due to electrons generated in the wall and the remaining $(1 - \alpha)$ from the buildup cap. Equation 8.21 can now be written as

$$J_{air} = M \cdot N_c \cdot A_c \cdot \left[\alpha \left(\frac{\bar{\mu}_{en}}{\rho}\right)^{wl}_{air} \cdot \left(\frac{\overline{L}}{\rho}\right)^{air}_{wl} + (1 - \alpha) \left(\frac{\bar{\mu}_{en}}{\rho}\right)^{b}_{air} \cdot \left(\frac{\overline{L}}{\rho}\right)^{air}_{b}\right] \tag{8.22}$$

or

$$J_{air} = M \cdot N_c \cdot A_c \cdot A_\alpha \tag{8.23}$$

where A_α is the quantity in the brackets of Equation 8.22 and represents a function whcih takes into account the modification of J_{air} due to the chamber wall and buildup cap composition. The fraction α has been determined experimentally by dose buildup measurements for various wall thicknesses (Fig.

8.3). In addition, it has been shown (16) that α is independent of wall composition or buildup cap, as long as they are of low atomic number materials.

Since J_{air} is the charge produced per unit mass of the cavity air,

$$J_{air} = \frac{M}{\rho_{air} \cdot V_c} \tag{8.24}$$

where M is the chamber reading or the charge produced and V_c is the cavity volume. Comparing Equations 8.23 and 8.24

$$V_c = \frac{1}{N_c \cdot \rho_{air} \cdot A_c \cdot A_\alpha} \tag{8.25}$$

Here ρ_{air} should correspond to the conditions which apply to the calibration factor N_c, e.g. 760 mm Hg and 22°C.

For example, using appropriate units and $\rho_{air} = 1.1966$ kg/m^3 at 760 mm Hg and 22°C,

$$V_c(\text{m}^3) = \frac{1}{N_c(\text{R/C})} \cdot \frac{(\text{R})}{2.58 \times 10^{-4}(\text{C/kg})} \cdot \frac{1}{1.1966(\text{kg/m}^3)} \cdot \frac{1}{A_c \cdot A_\alpha}$$

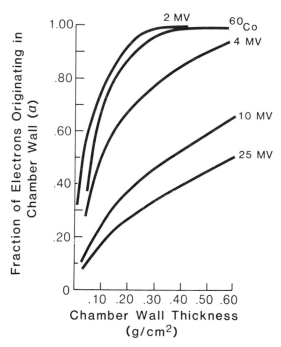

Figure 8.3. The fraction, α, of cavity ionization due to electrons generated in the chamber wall, plotted as a function of wall thickness. [Reprinted with permission from: Lempert *et al.* (16).]

or

$$V_c(\text{m}^3) = \frac{3.239 \times 10^3}{N_c(\text{R/C}) \cdot A_c \cdot A_\alpha} \qquad (8.26)$$

Assuming $A_c \simeq 0.99$ and $A_\alpha = 0.98$ (for a Farmer chamber with carbon wall and Lucite buildup cap, assuming $\alpha = 0.40$ for ^{60}Co γ-rays), the above equation reduces to:

$$V_c(\text{m}^3) = \frac{3.338 \times 10^3}{N_c(\text{R/C})} \qquad (8.27)$$

8.4 DETERMINATION OF ABSORBED DOSE IN A MEDIUM USING CHAMBER AS A BRAGG-GRAY CAVITY

In this section, we will discuss the application of the Bragg-Gray cavity theory to the problem of absorbed dose determination in a medium using a heterogeneous chamber, *i.e.* a chamber with wall material different than the surrounding medium. It will be assumed that the chamber with its buildup cap is calibrated for cobalt-60 exposure and this provides the basis for the determination of cavity volume, V_c, as discussed in Section 8.3C. Although the chamber volume will cancel out from the final expressions, it is instructive to use it conceptually in developing this formalism.

A. The C_λ and C_E Methods

PHOTON BEAMS

Suppose the chamber, with its buildup cap removed (it is recommended not to use buildup cap for in-phantom dosimetry), is placed in a medium and irradiated by a photon beam of quality λ. The charge measured per unit mass of the cavity air or J_{air} is given by

$$J_{\text{air}} = \frac{M_\lambda}{\rho_{\text{air}} \cdot V_c} \qquad (8.28)$$

where M_λ is the charge measured in the photon beam. The absorbed dose, D_{air}, at point P at the center of the cavity air is given by

$$D_{\text{air}} = J_{\text{air}} \cdot \frac{\overline{W}}{e} = \frac{M_\lambda}{\rho_{\text{air}} \cdot V_c} \cdot \frac{\overline{W}}{e} \qquad (8.29)$$

From Equations 8.25 and 8.29

$$D_{\text{air}} = M_\lambda \cdot [N_c \cdot A_c \cdot A_\alpha]_{\text{Co}} \cdot \frac{\overline{W}}{e} \qquad (8.30)$$

The subscript Co stands for ^{60}Co as the chamber calibration beam.

If the electrons crossing the cavity arise entirely from photons interacting with the wall material, we have from the Bragg-Gray theory:

$$D_{wl} = D_{air}\left[\left(\frac{\bar{L}}{\rho}\right)^{wl}_{air}\right]_{\lambda} \cdot p_1 \tag{8.31}$$

where D_{wl} is the dose to point P if cavity air is replaced by the wall material and p_1 is a factor that accounts for the difference in the electron fluence. Dose to point P if medium replaces the wall material is given by

$$D_{med} = D_{wl} \cdot \left[\left(\frac{\bar{\mu}_{en}}{\rho}\right)^{med}_{wl}\right]_{\lambda} \cdot p_2 \tag{8.32}$$

where p_2 accounts for the change in the photon energy fluence.

Thus, combining Equations 8.31 and 8.32,

$$D_{med} = D_{air} \cdot \left[\left(\frac{\bar{L}}{\rho}\right)^{wl}_{air} \cdot \left(\frac{\bar{\mu}_{en}}{\rho}\right)^{med}_{wl}\right]_{\lambda} \cdot p_\lambda \tag{8.33}$$

where $p_\lambda = p_1 \cdot p_2$, a factor which accounts for change in the photon energy fluence and the electron fluence at point P when the medium replaces the chamber.

On the other hand, if all the electrons crossing the cavity arise from the medium, we effectively have a case of a chamber with medium equivalent walls. Then

$$D_{med} = D_{air} \cdot \left[\left(\frac{\bar{L}}{\rho}\right)^{med}_{air}\right]_{\lambda} \cdot p_\lambda \tag{8.34}$$

But in practice, a fraction α of the ionization arises from electrons released in the wall and a fraction $(1 - \alpha)$ from electrons released in the medium. Thus, for the two-component model:

$$D_{med} = D_{air} \cdot \left[\alpha\left(\frac{\bar{L}}{\rho}\right)^{wl}_{air}\left(\frac{\bar{\mu}_{en}}{\rho}\right)^{med}_{wl} + (1 - \alpha)\left(\frac{\bar{L}}{\rho}\right)^{med}_{air}\right]_{\lambda} \cdot p_\lambda \tag{8.35}$$

By combining Equations 8.30 and 8.35, we obtain the final equation:

$$D_{med} = M_\lambda \cdot \frac{\bar{W}}{e} \cdot [N_c \cdot A_c \cdot A_\alpha]_{Co} \cdot \left[\alpha\left(\frac{\bar{L}}{\rho}\right)^{wl}_{air}\left(\frac{\bar{\mu}_{en}}{\rho}\right)^{med}_{wl} + (1 - \alpha)\left(\frac{\bar{L}}{\rho}\right)^{med}_{air}\right]_{\lambda} \cdot p_\lambda \tag{8.36}$$

If Equation 8.36 is rewritten as

$$D_{med} = M_\lambda \cdot N_c \cdot C_\lambda \tag{8.37}$$

Then the *general* expression for C_λ becomes

$$C_\lambda(\text{general}) = A_c \cdot \frac{\overline{W}}{e} \cdot \left[\alpha \left(\frac{\bar{\mu}_{en}}{\rho} \right)_{air}^{wl} \cdot \left(\frac{\overline{L}}{\rho} \right)_{wl}^{air} \right.$$

$$+ (1 - \alpha) \left(\frac{\bar{\mu}_{en}}{\rho} \right)_{air}^{b} \cdot \left(\frac{\overline{L}}{\rho} \right)_{b}^{air} \Bigg]_{Co} \left[\alpha \left(\frac{\overline{L}}{\rho} \right)_{air}^{wl} \left(\frac{\bar{\mu}_{en}}{\rho} \right)_{wl}^{med} \right. \qquad (8.38)$$

$$+ (1 - \alpha) \left(\frac{\overline{L}}{\rho} \right)_{air}^{med} \Bigg]_{\lambda} \cdot p_\lambda$$

Approximate C_λ values (18) assume buildup cap, wall, and medium to be water equivalent. Also p_λ is considered equal to unity and unrestricted stopping power $\frac{\overline{S}}{\rho}$ is used instead of $\frac{\overline{L}}{\rho}$. Thus, for a water medium,

$$C_\lambda(\text{approx.}) = A_c \cdot \frac{\overline{W}}{e} \cdot \left[\left(\frac{\bar{\mu}_{en}}{\rho} \right)_{air}^{water} \cdot \left(\frac{\overline{S}}{\rho} \right)_{water}^{air} \right]_{Co} \cdot \left[\left(\frac{\overline{S}}{\rho} \right)_{air}^{water} \right]_{\lambda}$$

Table 8.2 gives the approximate C_λ values for various photon beam energies. The difference between the general C_λ and $C_\lambda(\text{approx.})$ will depend on the chamber (*e.g.* composition of wall, buildup cap) and photon energy.

ELECTRON BEAMS

Suppose the chamber without its buildup cap is placed in a medium and irradiated by an electron beam of average energy $\overline{E}_Z$ at the point of measure-

Table 8.2.
Approximate values of C_λ in rad/R for photon beams in water

Radiation	$C_\lambda(\text{approx.})$
[137]Cs	0.95
[60]Co	0.95
x-rays (MV)	
2	0.95
4	0.94
6	0.94
8	0.93
10	0.93
12	0.92
14	0.92
16	0.91
18	0.91
20	0.90
25	0.90
30	0.89
35	0.88

Data from Greene and Massey (17) and recommended by Reference 18.

ment. The charge measured per unit mass of the cavity air will be

$$J_{\text{air},E} = \frac{M_E}{\rho_{\text{air}} \cdot V_c} \qquad (8.39)$$

where M_E is the charge measured in the electron beam.

$$D_{\text{air}} = J_{\text{air},E} \cdot \frac{\bar{W}}{e}$$

$$= \frac{M_E}{\rho_{\text{air}} \cdot V_c} \cdot \frac{\bar{W}}{e} \qquad (8.40)$$

From Equations 8.25 and 8.40

$$D_{\text{air}} = M_E [N_c \cdot A_c \cdot A_\alpha]_{\text{Co}} \cdot \frac{\bar{W}}{e} \qquad (8.41)$$

The dose, D_{med}, can be calculated from D_{air} using the Bragg-Gray relationship:

$$D_{\text{med}} = D_{\text{air}} \left[\left(\frac{\bar{L}}{\rho} \right)^{\text{med}}_{\text{air}} \right]_{\bar{E}_z} \cdot p_E \qquad (8.42)$$

where p_E is the perturbation correction for the change in the electron fluence when the chamber is replaced by the medium.

By combining Equations 8.41 and 8.42, we have

$$D_{\text{med}} = M_E \cdot \frac{\bar{W}}{e} \cdot [N_c \cdot A_c \cdot A_\alpha]_{\text{Co}} \cdot \left[\left(\frac{\bar{L}}{\rho} \right)^{\text{med}}_{\text{air}} \right]_{\bar{E}_z} \cdot p_E \qquad (8.43)$$

If Equation 8.43 is rewritten as

$$D_{\text{med}} = M_E \cdot N_C \cdot C_E \qquad (8.44)$$

then the *general* expression for C_E becomes

$$C_E(\text{general}) = A_c \cdot \frac{\bar{W}}{e} \cdot \left[\alpha \left(\frac{\bar{\mu}_{\text{en}}}{\rho} \right)^{wl}_{\text{air}} \cdot \left(\frac{\bar{L}}{\rho} \right)^{\text{air}}_{wl} \right.$$

$$\left. + (1 - \alpha) \left(\frac{\bar{\mu}_{\text{en}}}{\rho} \right)^{b}_{\text{air}} \cdot \left(\frac{\bar{L}}{\rho} \right)^{\text{air}}_{b} \right]_{\text{Co}} \cdot \left[\left(\frac{\bar{L}}{\rho} \right)^{\text{med}}_{\text{air}} \right]_{\bar{E}_z} \cdot p_E \qquad (8.45)$$

Approximate C_E values (19) assume that the chamber is air equivalent and that $\alpha = 1$ when the chamber is exposed to ^{60}Co. In addition, it is assumed that the chamber wall is so thin that it does not introduce any perturbation to the electron fluence. The perturbation correction p_E accounts for the change in fluence only due to the presence of the air cavity within the medium. Also, unrestricted stopping powers are used instead of restricted $\frac{\bar{L}}{\rho}$. Thus, the C_E

values listed in Reference 19 are based on the relationship:

$$C_E(\text{approx.}) = \frac{\overline{W}}{e} \cdot A_c \cdot \left[\left(\frac{\overline{S}}{\rho}\right)^{\text{water}}_{\text{air}}\right]_{\overline{E}_Z} = 0.87 \cdot 0.985 \cdot \left[\left(\frac{\overline{S}}{\rho}\right)^{\text{water}}_{\text{air}}\right]_{\overline{E}_Z} (\text{rad/R})$$

Table 8.3 gives the approximate C_E values for electrons of different energies. The perturbation correction, p_E, is applied separately (Table 8.4).

B. The N_{gas} Method

A new protocol for the dosimetry of photons and electrons has been prepared by Task Group 21 of the AAPM Radiation Therapy Committee (21). This protocol recommends that the response of an ionization chamber be characterized by a parameter, N_{gas}, which is a function of a variety of chamber-dependent parameters in addition to the ^{60}Co exposure calibration. This method is equivalent to the C_λ and C_E method provided general expressions for these quantities (Equations 8.38 and 8.45) are used.

Table 8.3.
Values of C_E(approx.) in rad/R for electron beams in water

Depth in water (cm)	Initial electron energy									
	5	10	15	20	25	30	35	40	45	50
1	0.922	0.877	0.843	0.823	0.808	0.795	0.784	0.775	0.768	0.762
2		0.893	0.858	0.835	0.819	0.806	0.795	0.786	0.778	0.771
3		0.915	0.871	0.848	0.830	0.816	0.804	0.794	0.786	0.778
4		0.947	0.886	0.859	0.840	0.824	0.812	0.801	0.792	0.785
5		0.963	0.901	0.871	0.847	0.831	0.819	0.809	0.799	0.791
6			0.933	0.885	0.856	0.839	0.825	0.815	0.806	0.798
7			0.965	0.902	0.867	0.846	0.832	0.821	0.812	0.803
8				0.941	0.882	0.854	0.839	0.827	0.816	0.808
9				0.959	0.898	0.865	0.847	0.832	0.820	0.814
10				0.926	0.917	0.878	0.856	0.840	0.827	0.819
11					0.946	0.890	0.866	0.848	0.834	0.823
12					0.939	0.906	0.879	0.857	0.841	0.829
13						0.926	0.890	0.867	0.848	0.835
14						0.959	0.907	0.877	0.857	0.842
15						0.933	0.924	0.890	0.866	0.849
16							0.954	0.903	0.876	0.857
17							0.929	0.919	0.887	0.864
18								0.940	0.900	0.874
19								0.936	0.915	0.883
20									0.935	0.895
21									0.943	0.908
22									0.921	0.924
23										0.945
										0.918

Data from Reference 19. The chamber perturbation correction, p_E, is assumed to be unity.

Table 8.4.
Perturbation correction factor, p_E, for ionization chambers of internal radius, r, in water for various mean electron energies $\bar{E}_z$

$\bar{E}_z$ (MeV)	$r = 0.25$ cm	$r = 0.5$ cm	$r = 0.8$ cm
1	0.947		
2	0.970	0.958	
3	0.978	0.970	0.962
4	0.984	0.977	0.972
5	0.986	0.981	0.977
10	0.992	0.989	0.987
11	0.997	0.995	0.993

Calculated values by Reference 20.

N_{gas} is defined as the dose absorbed in the cavity gas per unit charge or reading

$$N_{gas} = \frac{D_{gas}}{M}$$

N_{gas} is unique to each ionization chamber, is applicable to all ionizing radiation, and does not depend on the composition of the dosimetry phantom. Conceptually, N_{gas} represents calibration of the cavity gas in terms of absorbed dose in the gas per unit charge. Once N_{gas} is known, the chamber can be used as a calibrated Bragg-Gray cavity. The theoretical details of this formalism have been discussed by Loevinger (22).

For an air ionization chamber which has been calibrated with a buildup cap, b, for exposure in a ^{60}Co beam, N_{gas} can be obtained from Equation 8.22.

$$N_{gas} = \frac{D_{air}}{M} = \frac{J_{air} \cdot \dfrac{\overline{W}}{e}}{M}$$

or

$$N_{gas} = N_c \cdot A_c \cdot \frac{\overline{W}}{e} \left[\alpha \left(\frac{\bar{\mu}_{en}}{\rho} \right)^{wl}_{air} \cdot \left(\frac{\overline{L}}{\rho} \right)^{air}_{wl} + (1 - \alpha) \left(\frac{\bar{\mu}_{en}}{\rho} \right)^{b}_{air} \cdot \left(\frac{\overline{L}}{\rho} \right)^{air}_{b} \right]_{Co} \qquad (8.46)^2$$

If this chamber, without its buildup cap, is placed in a medium to measure absorbed dose, D_{med}, in a photon beam of any quality, λ,

$$D_{med} = M_\lambda \cdot N_{gas} \cdot \left[\alpha \left(\frac{\overline{L}}{\rho} \right)^{wl}_{air} \left(\frac{\bar{\mu}_{en}}{\rho} \right)^{med}_{wl} + (1 - \alpha) \left(\frac{\overline{L}}{\rho} \right)^{med}_{air} \right]_\lambda \cdot p_\lambda \qquad (8.47)$$

---

[2] N_{gas} may be further corrected for ion collection efficiency and β, the quotient of absorbed dose by collision fraction kerma (22) in the chamber wall. The latter correction arises from the fact that if complete electronic equilibrium is not established, β is different from unity, e.g. $\beta < 1$ in the electronic buildup region near the surface and $\beta > 1$ in the region of transient electron equilibrium.

(see Equation 8.35). Similarly, D_{med} in an electron beam is given by

$$D_{med} = M_E \cdot N_{gas} \cdot \left[\left(\frac{\bar{L}}{\rho} \right)^{med}_{air} \right]_{\bar{E}_z} \cdot p_E \tag{8.48}$$

(see Equation 8.42).

EXAMPLE 1

A Farmer chamber with graphite walls is used to measure absorbed dose to water in a water phantom irradiated by 4-MV x-rays. After a given irradiation, a reading of 2.734×10^{-8} C is obtained. Calculate the dose at the point of measurement, using the C_λ and N_{gas} methods, given the following data: temperature (of cavity air) = 26°C; pressure = 752 mm Hg; chamber calibration factor for ^{60}Co exposure with Lucite buildup cap = 46.86×10^8 R/C. Assume ion collection efficiency = 1.

(a) Approximate C_λ: from Table 8.2, approximate $C_\lambda = 0.94$ cGy/R.

Temperature and pressure correction, $C_{T,P} = \dfrac{760}{752} \times \dfrac{26 + 273}{295} = 1.024$.

$$D_{water} = \text{reading} \times C_{T,P} \times N_c \times C_\lambda$$

or

$$D_{water} = (2.734 \times 10^{-8} \ C) \times 1.024 \times (46.86 \times 10^8 \ \text{R/C}) \times 0.94 \ \text{cGy/R}$$

$$= 123.3 \ \text{cGy}$$

(b) Generalized C_λ: by consulting relevant tables in the Appendix and Fig. 8.3, the following values are substituted in Equation 8.38

$$A_c \simeq 0.99, \ \frac{\bar{W}}{e} = 0.873 \ \text{cGy/R}$$

$$\left[\alpha \simeq 0.4, \ \left(\frac{\bar{\mu}_{en}}{\rho} \right)^{wl}_{air} = 1.001, \ \left(\frac{\bar{L}}{\rho} \right)^{air}_{wl} = 0.990, \right.$$

$$\left. \left(\frac{\bar{\mu}_{en}}{\rho} \right)^{b}_{air} = 1.081, \ \left(\frac{\bar{L}}{\rho} \right)^{air}_{b} = 0.907 \right]_{Co}$$

$$\left[\alpha \simeq 0.2, \ \left(\frac{\bar{L}}{\rho} \right)^{wl}_{air} = 1.007, \ \left(\frac{\bar{\mu}_{en}}{\rho} \right)^{med}_{wl} = 1.114, \ \left(\frac{\bar{L}}{\rho} \right)^{med}_{air} = 1.131 \right]_{\lambda}$$

$$p_\lambda \simeq 0.995$$

$$C_\lambda = 0.99 \times 0.873 \ \text{cGy/R} \times [0.4 \times 1.001$$

$$\times 0.990 + 0.6 \times 1.081 \times 0.907]$$

$$\times [0.2 \times 1.007 \times 1.114 + 0.8 \times 1.131] \times 0.995$$

$$= 0.99 \times 0.873 \text{ cGy/R} \times [0.985] \times [1.129] \times 0.995$$

$$= 0.956 \text{ cGy/R}$$

$$D_{\text{water}} = (2.734 \times 10^{-8} \text{ C} \times 1.024) \times (46.86 \times 10^8 \text{ R/C}) \times 0.956 \text{ cGy/R}$$

$$= 125.4 \text{ cGy}$$

(c) N_{gas} method: substituting values from the above example in Equation 8.46,

$$N_{\text{gas}} = 46.86 \times 10^8 \text{ R/C} \times 0.99 \times 0.873 \text{ cGy/R} \, [0.4 \times 1.001$$

$$\times 0.990 + 0.6 \times 1.081 \times 0.907]$$

$$= 39.88 \text{ cGy/C}$$

From Equation 8.47,

$$D_{\text{water}} = (2.734 \times 10^{-8} \text{ C} \times 1.024) \times 39.88 \text{ cGy/C}$$

$$\times [0.2 \times 1.007 \times 1.114 + 0.8 \times 1.131] \times 0.995$$

$$= 125.4 \text{ cGy}$$

As seen in Equation 8.46, N_{gas}/N_c is a function only of the chamber wall composition and its buildup cap. Table 8.5 lists ratios of N_{gas}/N_c for a group of commonly employed chambers.

Table 8.5.
Ratios of N_{gas}/N_c for commonly employed chambers

Chamber	A_c	α	N_{gas}/N_c (Gy/R)
Capintec-Farmer 0.6 cm³, graphite wall, acrylic cap	0.990	0.42	8.52×10^{-3}
Capintec 0.1 cm³, graphite wall, acrylic cap	0.991	0.90	8.57×10^{-3}
PTW normal, acrylic	0.994	1	8.51×10^{-3}
PTW transit, acrylic	0.994	1	8.51×10^{-3}
PTW micro, acrylic	0.988	1	8.46×10^{-3}
Shonka 0.1 cm³, acrylic	0.989	1	8.47×10^{-3}
Extradin T.E. (A-150)	0.983	1	8.28×10^{-3}
Extradin A.E. (C-552)	0.973	1	8.50×10^{-3}
Far West IC-18 (A-150)	0.989	1	8.33×10^{-3}
Capintec parallel plate, polystyrene	0.995	0	8.43×10^{-3}

These values were taken from Reference 21, in which W/e was taken to be 33.7 J/C and a wall correction factor, $\beta_{\text{wall}} = 1.005$. The wall correction factor β is the ratio of absorbed dose to the collision fraction kerma (22) in the chamber wall.

8.5 TRANSFER OF ABSORBED DOSE FROM ONE MEDIUM TO ANOTHER

Although water is the primary reference medium for dose calibrations, other media such as polystyrene and Lucite are frequently used for dose measurements. If a plastic phantom is used for calibration, the absorbed dose to the plastic should first be calculated and then transferred to absorbed dose to water. Further transfer of this dose to absorbed dose to tissue is considered as part of the treatment planning procedure and not of the basic calibration.

A. Photon Beams

The dose to any medium is related to dose to water by the following expression:

$$D_{\text{water}} = D_{\text{med}}\left(\frac{\bar{\mu}_{\text{en}}}{\rho}\right)_{\text{med}}^{\text{water}} \tag{8.49}$$

provided the spectral distribution and energy fluence of photons at the point of measurement in the medium is the same as at a comparable point in water. Due to the electron density (electrons per cm^3) differences between plastic phantoms and water, additional corrections for effective depth, geometry, and scatter are sometimes necessary. In the case of polystyrene, these corrections are insignificant, since the electron density of polystyrene is very close to that of water. However, the electron density of Lucite is significantly higher and therefore significant corrections are required when Lucite phantoms are used for dosimetry.

Suppose $D_{\text{plastic}}(d', r, \text{SSD})$ is the dose measured in a plastic phantom at the central axis of a beam where d' is the depth, r is the field size at the surface, and SSD is the source-surface distance. This dose can be transferred to dose in water by the following relationship:

$$D_{\text{water}}(d, r, \text{SSD}) = D_{\text{plastic}}(d', r, \text{SSD})$$

$$\cdot \left(\frac{\bar{\mu}_{\text{en}}}{\rho}\right)_{\text{plastic}}^{\text{water}} \cdot \left(\frac{\text{SSD} + d'}{\text{SSD} + d}\right)^2 \cdot \frac{\text{TAR}(r_d', d)}{\text{TAR}(r_d, d)} \tag{8.50}$$

where d is given by

$$d = d' \cdot \frac{\bar{\mu}_{\text{plastic}}}{\bar{\mu}_{\text{water}}} \tag{8.51}$$

$$r_d = r \cdot \frac{\text{SSD} + d}{\text{SSD}} \quad \text{and} \quad r_d' = \frac{r_d}{\rho_e}$$

$\bar{\mu}$ is the mean linear attenuation coefficient of the beam and ρ_e is the electron density of plastic relative to that of water. In the megavoltage range where

Compton effect is predominant, $\bar{\mu}_{\text{plastic}}/\bar{\mu}_{\text{water}}$ may be approximated by ρ_e. In the range of clinically used megavoltage beams, the ratio $\bar{\mu}_{\text{plastic}}/\bar{\mu}_{\text{water}}$ is close to 1.01 for polystyrene and 1.14 for Lucite.

The SSD correction in Equation 8.50 is necessitated by the shift of the point of measurement in the plastic phantom to the corresponding point in water. The term involving the ratio of TARs (or TMRs) corrects for differences in scatter between plastic and water for the same geometric field.

B. Electron Beams

If dose is measured in a plastic phantom at the depth of d_{max}, the dose to water is related to the dose to plastic by

$$D_{\text{water}} = D_{\text{plastic}} \cdot \left(\frac{\bar{S}}{\rho}\right)^{\text{water}}_{\text{plastic}} \cdot \phi^{\text{water}}_{\text{plastic}}$$

where $\dfrac{\bar{S}}{\rho}$ refers to the mean unrestricted stopping power of electrons at the point of measurement and $\phi^{\text{water}}_{\text{plastic}}$ is the ratio of the electron fluence at d_{max} in water to that in plastic. The fluence correction is necessitated by the fact that the fluence at d_{max} is a function of the mass angular scattering power of the phantom material. At the present time the data for $\phi^{\text{water}}_{\text{plastic}}$ are not available in the literature. Until the time these data are published, the user may determine these corrections by comparing absorbed dose measurements made in plastic phantom with those made in water. Preliminary data by Hogstrom and Almond (23) suggest that $\phi^{\text{water}}_{\text{polystyrene}}$ correction is significant especially for lower energies, e.g. about 1.03 for $\bar{E}_0 = 7$ MeV, decreasing down to about 1.01 for $\bar{E}_0 = 16$ MeV.

8.6 EXPOSURE FROM RADIOACTIVE SOURCES

Exposure rate from a radioactive source can be determined from the knowledge of its photon emission spectrum and the relevant mass energy absorption coefficients for air. A relationship between exposure, X, and energy fluence, Ψ, may be derived by comparing Equations 8.5 and 8.7, i.e.

$$D_{\text{air}} = X \cdot \frac{\bar{W}_{\text{air}}}{e} = \Psi \cdot \left(\frac{\mu_{\text{en}}}{\rho}\right)_{\text{air}}$$

Therefore,

$$X = \Psi \cdot \left(\frac{\mu_{\text{en}}}{\rho}\right)_{\text{air}} \cdot \frac{e}{\bar{W}_{\text{air}}} \tag{8.52}$$

Suppose a radioisotope emits N photons of different energy and with different probability per disintegration. Imagine a sphere of radius 1 m around this point source of activity 1 Ci. Since 1 Ci undergoes 3.7×10^{10} dps, and since area of a sphere of radius 1 m is 4π m^2 and since 1 h = 3600 sec, we have:

$$\text{Energy fluence/h at 1 m from 1-Ci source} = \frac{3.7 \times 10^{10} \times 3600}{4\pi}$$

$$\sum_{i=1}^{N} f_i E_i$$

where f_i is the number of photons emitted/decay of energy E_i. From Equation 8.52,

$$\text{Exposure/h at 1 m from 1-Ci source} = \dot{X} = \frac{3.7 \times 10^{10} \times 3600}{4\pi}$$

$$\sum_{i=1}^{N} f_i E_i \left(\frac{\mu_{en}}{\rho}\right)_{air,i} \cdot \frac{e}{\overline{W}_{air}}$$

where $\left(\dfrac{\mu_{en}}{\rho}\right)_{air,i}$ is the mass energy absorption coefficient in air for photon of energy E_i.

Substituting the values, $\dfrac{\overline{W}_{air}}{e} = 0.00873$ J/kg·R, 1 MeV = 1.602×10^{-19} J, and expressing mass energy absorption coefficient in m^2/kg, the above equation becomes:

$$\dot{X} = \frac{3.7 \times 10^{10} \times 3600}{4\pi \ (\text{m}^2)} \ (\text{h}^{-1}) \ \frac{1(\text{R})}{0.00873 \ (\text{J/kg})} \cdot 1.602 \times 10^{-19}\left(\frac{\text{J}}{\text{MeV}}\right)$$

$$\cdot \sum_{i=1}^{N} f_i E_i (\text{MeV}) \cdot \left(\frac{\bar{\mu}_{en}}{\rho}\right)_{air,i} \left(\frac{\text{m}^2}{\text{kg}}\right)$$

or

$$\dot{X} = 194.5 \sum_{i=1}^{N} f_i E_i \left(\frac{\mu_{en}}{\rho}\right)_{air,i} \ (\text{R h}^{-1}) \tag{8.53}$$

A quantity exposure rate constant Γ_δ has been defined by Reference 24 as

$$\Gamma_\delta = \frac{l^2}{A} \cdot (\dot{X})_\delta \tag{8.54}$$

where $\dot{X}_\delta$ is the exposure rate due to photons of energy greater than δ (a suitable cutoff for the energy spectrum) at a distance l from a point source of activity A. If $\dot{X}$ is in R/h, l is in m, and A is in Ci, the dimensions of Γ_δ become Rm^2 h^{-1} Ci^{-1}. It is also apparent that Γ_δ is numerically equal to $\dot{X}$ in Equation 8.53. Thus, the exposure rate constant may be written as:

$$\Gamma_\delta = 194.5 \sum_{i}^{N} f_i E_i \left(\frac{\mu_{en}}{\rho}\right)_{air,i} \ \text{Rm}^2 \ \text{h}^{-1} \ \text{Ci}^{-1} \tag{8.55}$$

where energy E_i is expressed in MeV and $\left(\dfrac{\mu_{en}}{\rho}\right)_{air,i}$ is in m^2/kg.

Example

Calculate the exposure rate constant for ^{60}Co. Determine the exposure rate in R/min from a 5000-Ci souce of ^{60}Co at a distance of 80 cm.

^{60}Co emits 2 γ-rays of energy 1.117 and 1.33 MeV per disintegration

f_i	E_i(MeV)	$\left(\dfrac{\mu_{en}}{\rho}\right)_{air,i}$ (m^2/kg)
1.00	1.17	0.00270
1.00	1.33	0.00261

$\Gamma_\delta = 194.5 \ (1.17 \times 0.00270 + 1.33 \times 0.00261) \ Rm^2 \ h^{-1} \ Ci^{-1}$

$= 1.29 \ Rm^2 \ h^{-1} \ Ci^{-1}$

Exposure rate from 5000-Ci ^{60}Co source at 1 meter $= 1.29 \times 5000$ R/h

$$= \frac{1.29 \times 5000}{60} \ R/min$$

$$= 107.5 \ R/min$$

Exposure rate at 80 cm $= 107.5 \times \left(\dfrac{100}{80}\right)^2$ R/min

$$= 168 \ R/min$$

The above calculation applies only very approximately to an actual cobalt teletherapy unit since exposure rate would depend not only on the source activity but also on the collimator scatter, source size, and self-absorption in the source.

8.7 MEASUREMENT OF ABSORBED DOSE

A. Calorimetry

Calorimetry is a basic method of determining absorbed dose in a medium. It is based on the principle that the energy absorbed in a medium from radiation appears ultimately as heat energy while a small amount may appear in the form of a chemical change. This results in a small increase in temperature of the absorbing medium which, if measured accurately, can be related to the energy absorbed per unit mass or the absorbed dose.

If a small volume of the medium is thermally isolated from the remainder, the absorbed dose D in this volume is given by

$$D = \frac{dE_h}{dm} + \frac{dE_s}{dm} \tag{8.56}$$

where dE_h is the energy appearing as heat in the absorber of mass d_m and dE_s is the energy absorbed or produced due to chemical change, called the heat defect (which may be positive or negative). Neglecting the latter for the moment, one can calculate the rise in temperature of water by the absorption of 1 Gy of dose:

$$1 \text{ Gy} = 1 \text{ J kg}^{-1} = \frac{1}{4.18} \text{ cal kg}^{-1}$$

where 4.18 is the mechanical equivalent of heat (4.18 J of energy = 1 cal of heat). Since the specific heat of water is 1 cal/g/°C or 10^3 cal/kg/°C, the rise in temperature, ΔT, produced by 1 Gy is

$$\Delta T = \frac{1}{4.18} \text{ (cal kg}^{-1}) \cdot \frac{1}{10^3} \text{ (kg cal}^{-1} \text{ °C)}$$

$$= 2.39 \times 10^{-4} \text{ °C}$$

In order to measure such a small temperature rise, thermistors are most commonly used. Thermistors are semiconductors which show a large change in electrical resistance with a small change in temperature (about 5% per 1°C). Thus, by measuring the change in resistance by an apparatus such as a Wheatstone bridge, one can calculate the absorbed dose.

Extensive literature exists on radiation calorimetry and the reader is referred to References 26 and 27 for detailed reviews. Most of these apparatuses are difficult to construct and, for various reasons, are considered impractical for clinical dosimetry. However, Domen (28) has recently described a simpler water calorimeter for absolute measurement of absorbed dose. Essential features of this calorimeter are briefly described below.

Figure 8.4 is a schematic drawing of Domen's calorimeter. An ultrasmall (0.25-mm diameter) bead thermistor is sandwiched between two 30-μm polyethylene films stretched on polystyrene rings. The thermistors are cemented to one of the films to increase thermal coupling. The films provide the necessary high and stable resistance ($>10^{11}$ Ω) between the thermistor leads and water.

The films held horizontally in a plastic frame are then immersed in an insulated tank of distilled water. Because of the low thermal diffusivity of water and imperviousness of polyethylene film to water, nearly negligible conductive heat transfer occurs at a point in the water medium. Therefore, a thermally isolated volume element of water is not necessary. This apparatus measures dose rates in water of about 4 Gy/min with a precision (for the reproducibility of measurements) of 0.5%.

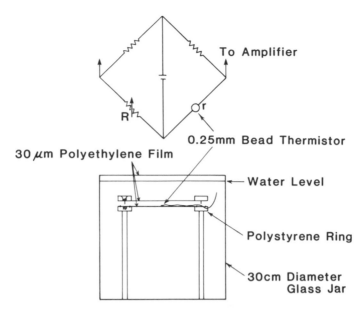

Figure 8.4. Schematic diagram of Domen's calorimeter. Redrawn from Ref. 28.

B. Chemical Dosimetry

The energy absorbed from ionizing radiation may produce a chemical change, and if this change can be determined, it can be used as a measure of absorbed dose. Many systems of chemical dosimetry have been proposed but the *ferrous sulfate* or the *Fricke dosimeter* is considered to be the most developed system for the precision measurement of absorbed dose. The use of this system has been fully discussed in References 13 and 29. A brief description will be provided here.

B.1. FERROUS SULFATE (FRICKE) DOSIMETER

The dosimeter consists of 1 mmol/liter ferrous sulfate (or ferrous ammonium sulfate), 1 mmol/liter NaCl, and 0.4 mol/liter sulfuric acid. The reason for NaCl in the solution is to counteract the effects of organic impurities present despite all the necessary precautions. When the solution is irradiated, the ferrous ions, Fe^{2+}, are oxidized by radiation to ferric ions, Fe^{3+}. The ferric ion concentration is determined by spectrophotometry of the dosimeter solution, which shows absorption peaks in the ultraviolet light at wavelengths of 224 and 304 nm.

B.2. G VALUE

The radiation chemical yield may be expressed in terms of the number of molecules produced per 100 eV of energy absorbed. This number is known as the G value. Thus, if the yield of ferric ions can be determined, the energy absorbed can be calculated when the G value is known.

Suppose a ΔM (moles/liter) concentration of ferric ions is produced by an absorbed dose of D grays.

$$D(\text{Gy}) = D(\text{J/kg}) = \frac{D}{1.602 \times 10^{-19}} \ (\text{eV/kg})$$

Molecules of ferric ions produced $= \Delta M \times 6.02 \times 10^{23}$ molecules/liter

$$\frac{\Delta M \times 6.02 \times 10^{23}}{\rho} \ \text{molecules/kg}$$

where ρ is the density of the solution in kg/liter.

No. of molecules produced per eV of energy absorbed

$$= \frac{\Delta M \times 6.02 \times 10^{23}}{\rho} \cdot \frac{1.602 \times 10^{-19}}{D}$$

$$= \frac{\Delta M}{\rho D} \cdot 9.64 \times 10^{4} \ \text{molecules/eV}$$

or

$$G = \frac{\Delta M}{\rho D} \cdot 9.64 \times 10^{4} \cdot 100 \ \text{molecules/100 eV}$$

$$= \frac{\Delta M}{\rho D} \cdot 9.64 \times 10^{6} \ \text{molecules/100 eV}$$

Thus

$$D = \frac{\Delta M}{\rho G} \cdot 9.64 \times 10^{6} \ (\text{Gy})$$

The G values for the Fricke dosimeter have been determined by many investigators. Table 8.6 gives the values recommended by Reference 13 for

Table 8.6.
Recommended (Reference 13) G values for the ferrous sulfate dosimeter (0.4 mol/liter H_2SO_4) for photon beams

Radiation	G Value (No./100 eV)
^{137}Cs	15.3 ± 0.3
2 MV	15.4 ± 0.3
^{60}Co	15.5 ± 0.2
4 MV	15.5 ± 0.3
5–10 MV	15.6 ± 0.4
11–30 MV	15.7 ± 0.6

photons from ^{137}Cs to 30 MV. A constant G value of 15.7 ± 0.6/100 eV is recommended for electrons in the energy range of 1 to 30 MeV for 0.4 mol/liter H_2SO_4 dosimeter solution (19).

C. Solid State Methods

There are several solid state systems available for the dosimetry of ionizing radiation. However, none of the systems is absolute, *i.e.* they need calibration in a known radiation field before they can be used for the determination of absorbed dose.

There are two types of solid state dosimeters: (a) integrating type dosimeters (thermoluminescent crystals, radiophotoluminescent glasses, optical density type dosimeters such as glass and film), and (b) electrical conductivity dosimeters (semiconductor junction detectors, induced conductivity in insulating materials). Of these, the most widely used systems for the measurement of absorbed dose are the thermoluminescent dosimeter (TLD) and film which are described below:

C.1. THERMOLUMINESCENCE DOSIMETRY

Many crystalline materials exhibit the phenomenon of thermoluminescence. When such a crystal is irradiated, a very minute fraction of the absorbed energy is stored in the crystal lattice. Some of this energy can be recovered later as visible light if the material is heated. This phenomenon of the release of visible photons by thermal means is known as thermoluminescence (TL).

The arrangement for measuring the TL output is shown schematically in Fig. 8.5. The irradiated material is placed in a heater cup or planchette where it is heated for a reproducible heating cycle. The emitted light is measured by

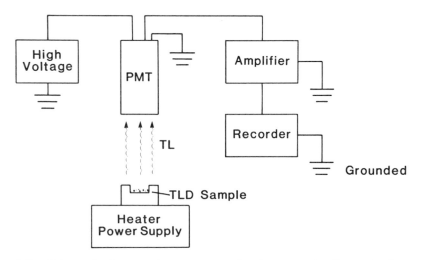

Figure 8.5. Schematic diagram showing apparatus for measuring thermoluminescence.

a photomultiplier tube (PMT) which converts light into an electrical current. The current is then amplified and measured by a recorder or a counter.

There are several TL phosphors available but the most noteworthy are lithium fluoride (LiF), lithium borate ($Li_2B_4O_7$), and calcium fluoride (CaF_2). Their dosimetric properties are listed in Table 8.7 (30). Of these phosphors, LiF is most extensively studied and most frequently used for clinical dosimetry. LiF in its purest form exhibits relatively little thermoluminescence. But the

Table 8.7.
Characteristics of various phosphors

Characteristic	LiF	Li_2B_{407}:Mn	CaF_2:Mn	CaF_2:nat	$CaSO_4$:Mn
Density (g/cc)	2.64	2.3	3.18	3.18	2.61
Effective Atomic No.	8.2	7.4	16.3	16.3	15.3
TL emission spectra (A)					
Range	3500–6000	5300–6300	4400–6000	3500–5000	4500–6000
Maximum	4000	6050	5000	3800	5000
Temperature of main TL glow peak	195°C	200°C	260°C	260°C	110°C
Efficiency at cobalt-60 (relative to LiF)	1.0	0.3	3	23	70
Energy response without added filter (30 keV/cobalt-60)	1.25	0.9	13	13	10
Useful range	mR–10^5 R	mR–10^6 R	mR–3 × 10^5 R	mR–10^4 R	R–10^4 R
Fading	Small, <5%/12 wk	10% in first month	10% in first month	No detectable fading	50–60% in the first 24 h
Light sensitivity	Essentially none	Essentially none	Essentially none	Yes	Yes
Physical form	Powder, extruded, Teflon-embedded, silicon-embedded, glass capillaries	Powder, Teflon-embedded	Powder, Teflon-embedded, hot-pressed chips, glass capillaries	Special dosimeters	Powder, Teflon-embedded

From Cameron *et al.* (30).

presence of a trace amount of impurities provides the radiation-induced TL. These impurities give rise to imperfections in the lattice structure of LiF and appear to be necessary for the appearance of the TL phenomenon.

C.2. SIMPLIFIED THEORY OF TLD

The chemical and physical theory of TLD is not exactly known, but simple models have been proposed to qualitatively explain the phenomenon. Figure 8.6 shows an energy-level diagram of an inorganic crystal exhibiting TL due to ionizing radiation.

In an individual atom, electrons occupy discrete energy levels. In a crystal lattice, on the other hand, electronic energy levels are perturbed by mutual interactions between atoms and give rise to energy bands: the "allowed" energy bands and the forbidden energy bands. In addition, the presence of impurities in the crystal creates energy traps in the forbidden region, providing metastable states for the electrons. When the material is irradiated, some of the electrons in the valence band (ground state) receive sufficient energy to be raised to the conduction band. The vacancy thus created in the valence band is called a positive hole. The electron and the hole move independently through their respective bands until they recombine (electron returning to the ground state) or until they fall into a trap (metastable state). If there is instantaneous emission of light due to these transitions, the phenomenon is called *fluorescence*. If an electron in the trap requires energy to get out of the trap and fall to the valence band, the emission of light in this case is called *phosphorescence* (delayed fluorescence). If phosphorescence at room temperature is very slow, but can be speeded up significantly with a moderate amount of heating (~300°C), the phenomenon is called *thermoluminescence*.

A plot of thermoluminescence against temperature is called a *glow curve* (Fig. 8.7). As the temperature of the TL material exposed to radiation is increased, the probability of releasing trapped electrons increases. The light emitted (TL) first increases, reaches a maximum value, and falls again to zero. Since most phosphors contain a number of traps at various energy levels in the forbidden band, the glow curve may consist of a number of glow peaks as

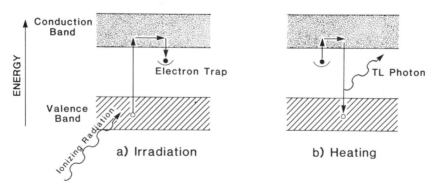

Figure 8.6.   A simplified energy-level diagram to illustrate thermoluminescence process.

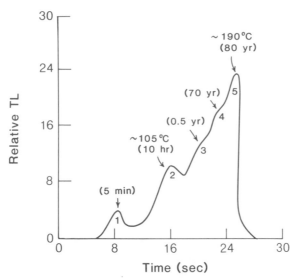

Figure 8.7. An example of glow curve of LiF (TLD-100) after phosphor has been annealed at 400°C for 1 h and read immediately after irradiation to 100 R. [Reprinted with permission from: Zimmerman *et al.* (34).]

shown in Fig. 8.7. The different peaks correspond to different "trapped" energy levels.

C.3. LITHIUM FLUORIDE

The TL characteristics of LiF have been studied extensively. For details, the reader is referred to the book by Cameron *et al.* (30).

Lithium fluoride has an effective atomic number of 8.2 compared to 7.4 for soft tissue. This makes this material very suitable for clinical dosimetry. Mass energy absorption coefficients for this material have been given by Greening *et al.* (31). The dose absorbed in LiF can be converted to dose in muscle by considerations similar to those discussed earlier. For example, under electronic equilibrium conditions, the ratio of absorbed doses in the two media will be the same as the ratio of their mass energy absorption coefficients. If the dimensions of the dosimeter are smaller than the ranges of the electrons crossing the dosimeter, then the Bragg-Gray relationship can also be used. The ratio of absorbed doses in the two media then will be the same as the ratio of mass stopping powers. The applicability of the Bragg-Gray cavity theory to TLD has been discussed by several authors (32, 33).

C.4. PRACTICAL CONSIDERATIONS

As stated earlier, the thermoluminescent dosimeter must be calibrated before it can be used for measuring an unknown dose. Since the response of the TLD materials is affected by their previous radiation history and thermal history, the material must be suitably annealed to remove residual effects. The

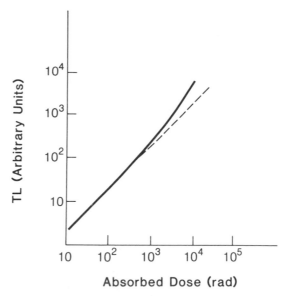

Figure 8.8. An example of TL *vs.* absorbed dose curve for TLD-100 powder (schematic).

standard pre-irradiation annealing procedure for LiF is 1 h of heating at 400°C and then 24 h at 80°C. The slow heating, namely 24 h at 80°C, removes peaks 1 and 2 of the glow curve (Fig. 8.7) by decreasing the "trapping efficiency." Peaks 1 and 2 can also be eliminated by postirradiation annealing for 10 min at 100°C. The need for eliminating peaks 1 and 2 arises from the fact that the magnitude of these peaks decreases relatively fast with time after irradiation. By removing these peaks by annealing, the glow curve becomes more stable and therefore predictable.

The dose response curve for TLD-100[3] is shown in Fig. 8.8. The curve is generally linear up to 10^3 rad but beyond this it becomes supralinear. The response curve, however, depends on many conditions which have to be standardized to achieve reasonable accuracy with TLD. The calibration should be done with the same TLD reader, in approximately the same quality beam and to approximately the same absorbed dose level.

The TLD response is defined as TL output per unit absorbed dose in the phosphor. Figure 8.9 gives the energy response curve for LiF (TLD-100) for photon energies below megavoltage range. The studies of energy response for photons above ^{60}Co and high energy electrons have yielded somewhat conflicting results. Whereas the data of Pinkerton *et al.* (35) and Crosby *et al.* (36) show some energy dependence, other studies (37) do not show this energy dependence.

---

[3] TLD-100, made by Harshaw Chemical Company, contains 7.5% ^{6}Li and 92.5% ^{7}Li.

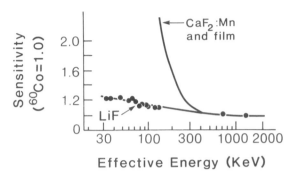

Figure 8.9. Energy response curve for LiF (TLD-100), CaF$_2$:Mn and a photographic film [Reprinted with permission from: Cameron *et al.* (30).]

When considerable care is used, precision of approximately 3% may be obtained using TLD powder or extruded material. Although not as precise as the ion chamber, TLD's main advantage is in measuring doses in regions where ion chamber cannot be used. For example, TLD is extremely useful for patient dosimetry by direct insertion into tissues or body cavities. Since TLD material is available in many forms and sizes, it can be used for special dosimetry situations such as for measuring dose distribution in the buildup region, around brachytherapy sources, and for personnel dose monitoring.

D. FILM DOSIMETRY

A radiographic film consists of a transparent film base (cellulose acetate or polyester resin) coated with an emulsion containing very small crystals of silver bromide. When the film is exposed to ionizing radiation or visible light, a chemical change takes place within the exposed crystals to form what is referred to as a *latent image*. When the film is developed, the affected crystals are reduced to small grains of metallic silver. The film is then *fixed*. The unaffected granules are removed by the fixing solution, leaving a clear film in their place. The metallic silver, which is not affected by the fixer, causes darkening of the film. Thus, the degree of blackening of an area of the film depends on the amount of free silver deposited and, consequently, on the radiation energy absorbed.

The degree of blackening of the film is measured by determining optical density with a densitometer. This instrument consists of a light source, a tiny aperture through which the light is directed and a light detector (photocell) to measure the light intensity transmitted through the film.

The optical density, OD, is defined as:

$$OD = \log \frac{I_0}{I_t} \tag{8.57}$$

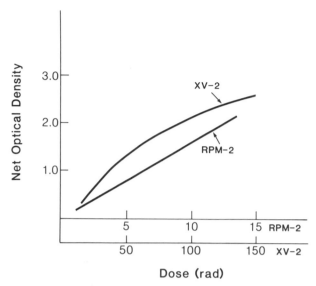

Figure 8.10.   Sensitometric curve of Kodak XV-2 film and Kodak RPM-2 (Type M) film.

where I_0 is the amount of light collected without film and I_t is the amount of light transmitted through the film. A densitometer gives a direct reading of optical density if it has been calibrated by a standard strip of film having regions of known optical density. In dosimetry, the quantity of interest is usually net optical density which is obtained by subtracting the reading for the base fog (OD of unexposed processed film) from the measured optical density.

A plot of net optical density as a function of radiation exposure or dose is termed the sensitometric curve or H-D curve.[4] Figure 8.10 shows examples of characteristic curves for two commonly used dosimetry films. Film speed and linearity of the sensitometric curve are the two main characteristics which are considered in selecting a film for dosimetry. If a film is exposed in the nonlinear region, corrections are necessary to convert optical density into dose.

Although, film is well established as a method of measuring electron beam distributions (Chapter 14), its usefulness in photon dosimetry is relatively limited. Because the photoelectric effect depends on the cube of the atomic number, the silver ($Z = 45$) in the film emulsion absorbs radiation below 150 keV very strongly by the photoelectric process. Since most clinical beams contain a scatter component of low energy photons, the correlation between optical density and dose becomes tenuous. In addition, film suffers from several potential errors such as changes in processing conditions, interfilm emulsion differences, and artifacts caused by air pockets adjacent to the film. For these

---

[4] The expression "H-D" is derived from the names of Hunter and Driffield, who in 1890 used such curves to characterize the response of photographic film to light.

reasons, absolute dosimetry with film is impractical. However, it is very useful for checking radiation fields, light-field coincidence, field flatness, and symmetry, and obtaining quick qualitative patterns of a radiation distribution.

In the megavoltage range of photon energies, however, film has been used to measure isodose curves with acceptable accuracy (±3%) (38–40). One of the techniques (40) consists of exposing the film packed tightly in a polystyrene phantom, parallel to the central axis of the beam. The film edge is carefully aligned with the phantom surface and air pockets between the film surface and the surrounding jacket are removed by punching holes near the corners. Optical densities are correlated with dose by using a depth-dependent sensitometric curve derived from known central axis depth dose data for a reference field such as 10 × 10 cm. The method is made practical by a computer-controlled densitometer and a computer program which performs the required isodensity-to-isodose curve conversion.

References

1. ICRU Report No. 33: *Radiation Quantities and Units*. Washington, DC, International Commission on Radiation Units and Measurements, 1980.
2. ICRU Report No. 31: *Average Energy Required to Produce an Ion Pair*. Washington, DC, International Commission on Radiation Units and Measurements, 1979.
3. Wyckoff HO: *Med Phys* 10:715, (communication) 1983.
4. Johns HE, Cunningham JR: *The Physics of Radiology*, 3rd ed. Springfield IL, Charles C Thomas, 1969.
5. Bragg WH: *Studies in Radioactivity*. New York, Macmillan, 1912.
6. Gray LH: An ionization method for the absolute measurement of gamma-ray energy. *Proc R Soc* A156:578, 1936.
7. Spencer LV, Attix FH: A theory of cavity ionization. *Radiat Res* 3:239, 1955.
8. Greening JR: An experimental examination of theories of cavity ionization. *Br J Radiol* 30:254, 1957.
9. Burlin TE: An experimental examination of theories relating the absorption of gamma-ray energy in medium to the ionization produced in a cavity. *Phys Med Biol* 6:33, 1961.
10. Burlin TE: Further examination of theories relating the absorption of gamma-ray energy in a medium to the ionization produced in a cavity. *Phys Med Biol* 11:255, 1966.
11. Berger MJ, Seltzer SM: *Tables of Energy Losses and Ranges of Electrons and Positrons, NASA SP-3012*. Washington, DC, National Aeronautics and Space Administration, 1964.
12. Berger MJ, Seltzer SM: *Additional Stopping Power and Range Tables for Protons, Mesons and Electrons, NASA SP-3036*. Washington, DC, National Aeronautics and Space Administration, 1966.
13. ICRU Report No. 14: *Radiation Dosimetry: X-rays and Gamma Rays with Maximum Photon Energies Between 0.6 and 50 MeV*. Washington, DC, International Commission on Radiation Units and Measurements, 1969.
14. Burlin TE: Cavity chamber theory. In Attix FH, Roesch WC (eds): *Radiation Dosimetry*, vol I, 2nd ed New York, Academic Press, 1969.
15. Almond PR, Svensson H: Ionization chamber dosimetry for photon and electron beams. *Acta Radiol* 16:177, 1977.
16. Lempert GD, Nath R, Schulz RJ: Fraction of ionization from electrons arising in the wall of an ionization chamber. *Med Phys* 10:1, 1983.
17. Greene D, Massey JB: The use of the Farmer-Baldwin and victrometer ionization chambers for dosimetry of high energy x-radiation. *Phys Med Biol* 13:287, 1968.
18. American Association of Physicists in Medicine (AAPM/SCRAD): Protocol for the dosimetry of x- and gamma-ray beams with maximum energies between 0.6 and 50 MeV. *Phys Med Biol* 16:379, 1971.
19. ICRU Report No. 21: *Radiation Dosimetry: Electrons with Initial Energies Between 1 and 50 MeV*. Washington, DC, International Commission on Radiation Units and Measurements, 1972.

20. Harder D: The effect of multiple electron scattering on ionization in gas-filled cavities. *Biophysik* 5:157, 1968.
21. American Association of Physicists in Medicine, RTC Task Group 21: A protocol for the determination of absorbed dose from high energy photon and electron beams. *Med Phys* 10:741, 1983.
22. Loevinger R: A formalism for calculation of absorbed dose to a medium from photon and electron beams. *Med Phys* 8:1 1981.
23. Hogstrom KR, Almond PR: The effect of electron multiple scattering on dose measured in non-water phantoms (presented at the Annual Meeting of the American Association of Physicists in Medicine, New Orleans). Abstract in *Med Phys* 9: 607 (abstr) 1982.
24. ICRU Report No. 19: *Radiation Quantities and Units.* Washington, DC, International Commission on Radiation Units and Measurements, 1971.
25. Hubbell JH: Photon mass attenuation and energy-absorption coefficients from 1 keV to 20 MeV. *Int J Appl Radiat Isotop* 33:1269, 1982.
26. Laughlin JS, Genna S: Calorimetry. In Attix FH, Roesch WC (eds): *Radiation Dosimetry*, vol II. New York, Academic Press, 1967, p 389.
27. Gunn SR: Radiometric calorimetry: a review. *Nucl Inst Methods* 29:1, 1964; 85:285, 1970; 135:251, 1976.
28. Domen SR: Absorbed dose water calorimeter. *Med Phys* 7:157, 1980.
29. ICRU Report No. 17: *Radiation Dosimetry: X-Rays Generated at Potentials of 5 to 150 kV.* Washington, DC, International Commission on Radiation Units and Measurements, 1970.
30. Cameron JR, Suntharalingam N, Kenney GN: *Thermoluminescent Dosimetry.* Madison, WI, The University of Wisconsin Press, 1968.
31. Greening JR, Law J, Redpath AT: Mass attenuation and mass energy absorption coefficients for LiF and $Li_2B_4O_7$ for photons from 1 to 150 keV. *Phys Med Biol* 17:585, 1972 (*Fundamentals of Radiation Dosimetry*. Bristol, Adam Hilger Ltd, 1981, p 128).
32. Paliwal BR, Almond PR: Application of cavity theories for electrons to LiF dosimeters. *Phys Med Biol* 20:547, 1975.
33. Holt JG, Edelstein GR, Clark TE: Energy dependence of the response of lithium fluoride TLD rods in high energy electron fields. *Phys Med Biol* 20:559, 1975.
34. Zimmerman DW, Rhyner CR, Cameron JR: Thermal annealing effects on the thermoluminescence of LiF. *Healthy Phys* 12:525, 1966.
35. Pinkerton A, Holt JG, Laughlin JS: Energy dependence of LiF dosimeters at high energies. *Phys Med Biol* 11:129, 1966.
36. Crosby EH, Almond PR, Shalek RJ: Energy dependence of LiF dosimeters at high energies. *Phys Med Biol* 11:131, 1966.
37. Suntharalingam N, Cameron JR: Thermoluminescent response of lithium fluoride to high-energy electrons (*High-Energy Radiation Therapy Dosimetry* issue). *Ann N Y Acad Sci* 161:77, 1969.
38. Jacobson A: 4 MeV x-ray film dosimetry. *Radiology* 103:703, 1972.
39. Patten L, Purdy J, Oliver G: Automated film dosimetry. *Med Phys* 1:110 (abstr) 1974.
40. Williamson JF, Khan FM, Sharma SC: Film dosimetry of megavoltage photon beams: a practical method of isodensity-to-isodose curve conversion. *Med Phys* 8: 94, 1981.
41. Day MJ, Greene D, Massey JB: Use of a Perspex sheath for ionization chamber measurements in a water phantom. *Phys Med Biol* 10:111, 1965.
42. ICRU Report 10b: *Physical Aspects of Irradiation, NBS Handbook 85.* Washington, DC, US Government Printing Office, 1962.

CHAPTER 9

Dose Distribution and Scatter Analysis

It is seldom possible to measure dose distribution directly in patients treated with radiation. Data on dose distribution are almost entirely derived from measurements in phantoms—tissue equivalent materials, usually large enough in volume to provide full scatter conditions for the given beam. These basic data are used in a dose calculation system devised to predict dose distribution in an actual patient. This chapter deals with various quantities and concepts which are useful for this purpose.

9.1 PHANTOMS

Basic dose distribution data are usually measured in a water phantom which closely approximates the radiation absorption and scattering properties of muscle and other soft tissues. Another reason for the choice of water as a phantom material is that it is universally available with reproducible radiation properties. A water phantom, however, poses some practical problems when using in conjunction with ion chambers and other detectors which are affected by water unless they are designed to be waterproof. In most cases, however, the detector is encased in a thin plastic (water equivalent) sleeve before immersion into the water phantom.

Since it is not always possible to put radiation detectors in water, solid dry phantoms have been developed as substitutes for water. Ideally, for a given material to be tissue or water equivalent, it must have the same effective atomic number, number of electrons per gram, and mass density. However, since the Compton effect is the most predominant mode of interaction for megavoltage photon beams in the clinical range, the necessary condition for water equivalence for such beams is the same electron density (number of electrons per cm^3) as that of water.

The electron density ρ_e of a material may be calculated from its mass density ρ_m and its atomic composition according to the formula:

$$\rho_e = \rho_m \cdot N_A \cdot \left(\frac{Z}{A}\right) \tag{9.1}$$

Table 9.1.
Physical properties of various phantom materials

Material	Chemical Composition	Mass Density (g/cm³)	Number of Electrons/g (×10²³)	Z_{eff}* (photoelectric)
Water	H_2O	1	3.34	7.42
Polystyrene	$(C_8H_8)_n$	1.03–1.05	3.24	5.69
Plexiglas (Perspex, Lucite)	$(C_5O_2H_8)_n$	1.16–1.20	3.24	6.48
Polyethylene	$(CH_2)_n$	0.92	3.44	6.16
Paraffin	C_nH_{2n+2}	0.87–0.91	3.44	5.42
Mix D	Paraffin: 60.8 Polyethylene: 30.4 MgO: 6.4 TiO_2: 2.4	0.99	3.41	7.05
M 3	Paraffin: 100 MgO: 29.06 $CaCO_3$: 0.94	1.06	3.34	7.35

Data are from Tubiana et al. (2) and Schulz and Nath (3).
* Z_{eff} for photoelectric effect is given by Equation 6.4.

where

$$\frac{Z}{A} = \sum_i a_i \cdot \left(\frac{Z_i}{A_i}\right) \qquad (9.2)$$

N_A is Avogadro's number and a_i is the fraction by weight of the ith element of atomic number Z_i and atomic weight A_i. Electron densities of various human tissues and body fluids have been calculated according to Equation 9.1 by Shrimpton (1). Values for some tissues of dosimetric interest are listed in Table 5.1.

Table 9.1 gives the properties of various phantoms which have been frequently used for radiation dosimetry. Of the commercially available phantom materials, Lucite and polystyrene are most frequently used as dosimetry phantoms. Although the mass density of these materials may vary depending upon a given sample, the atomic composition and the number of electrons per gram of these materials are sufficiently constant to warrant their use for high energy photon and electron dosimetry.

In addition to the homogeneous phantoms, anthropomorphic phantoms are frequently used for clinical dosimetry. One such commercially available system, known as Alderson Rando Phantom,[1] incorporates materials to simulate various body tissues—muscle, bone, lung, and air cavities. The phantom is shaped into a human torso (Fig. 9.1) and is sectioned transversely into slices for dosimetric applications.

---

[1] Alderson Research Laboratories, Inc., Stamford, Connecticut.

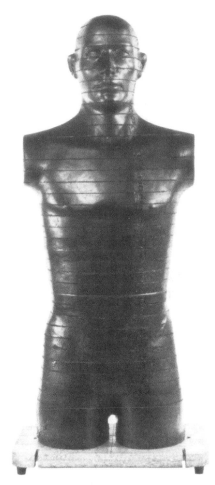

Figure 9.1. An anthropomorphic phantom (Alderson Rando Phantom) sectioned transversely for dosimetric studies.

White *et al.* (4) have developed extensive recipies for tissue substitutes. The method is based on adding particulate fillers to epoxy resins to form a mixture with radiation properties closely approximating that of a particular tissue. The most important radiation properties in this regard are the mass attenuation coefficient, the mass energy absorption coefficient, electron mass stopping, and angular scattering power ratios.

9.2 DEPTH DOSE DISTRIBUTION

As the beam is incident on a patient (or a phantom), the absorbed dose in the patient varies with depth. This variation depends on many conditions: beam energy, depth, field size, distance from source, and beam collimation system. Thus, the calculation of dose in the patient involves considerations with regard to these parameters and others as they affect depth dose distribution.

An essential step in the dose calculation system is to establish depth dose variation along the central axis of the beam. A number of quantities have been defined for this purpose, major among these being percentage depth dose (13), tissue-air ratios (5–8), tissue-phantom ratios (9–11), and tissue-maximum ratios (11, 12). These quantities are usually derived from measurements made in water phantoms using small ionization chambers. Although other dosimetry systems such as TLD, diodes, and film are occasionally used, ion chambers are preferred because of their better precision and smaller energy dependence.

9.3 PERCENTAGE DEPTH DOSE

One way of characterizing the central axis dose distribution is to normalize dose at depth with respect to dose at a reference depth. The quantity *percentage (or simply percent) depth dose* may be defined as the quotient, expressed as a percentage, of the absorbed dose at any depth d to the absorbed dose at a fixed reference depth d_0, along the central axis of the beam (Fig. 9.2). Percentage depth dose, P, is thus

$$P = \frac{D_d}{D_{d_0}} \times 100 \tag{9.3}$$

For orthovoltage (up to about 400 kVp) and lower energy x-rays, the reference

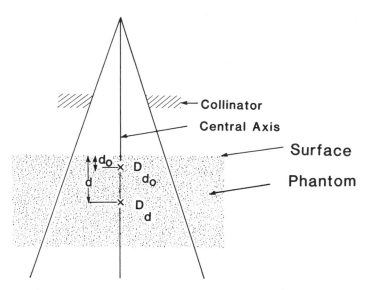

Figure 9.2. Percent depth dose is $(D_d/D_{d_0}) \times 100$, where d is any depth and d_0 is reference depth of maximum dose.

depth is usually the surface ($d_0 = 0$). For higher energies the reference depth is taken at the position of the *peak absorbed dose* ($d_0 = d_m$).

In clinical practice, the peak absorbed dose on the central axis is sometimes called the *maximum dose*, the *dose maximum*, the *given dose* or simply the D_{max}. Thus.

$$D_{\max} = \frac{D_d}{P} \times 100 \qquad (9.4)$$

A number of parameters affect the central axis depth dose distribution. These include beam quality or energy, depth, field size and shape, source to surface distance, and beam collimation. A discussion of these parameters will now be presented.

A. Dependence on Beam Quality and Depth

The percentage depth dose (beyond the depth of maximum dose) increases with beam energy. Higher energy beams have greater penetrating power and thus deliver higher percent depth dose (Fig. 9.3). If the effects of inverse square law and scattering are not considered, the percentage depth dose variation with depth is governed approximately by exponential attenuation. Thus, the beam quality affects the percentage depth dose by virtue of the average attenuation coefficent $\bar{\mu}$.[2] As the $\bar{\mu}$ decreases, the more penetrating

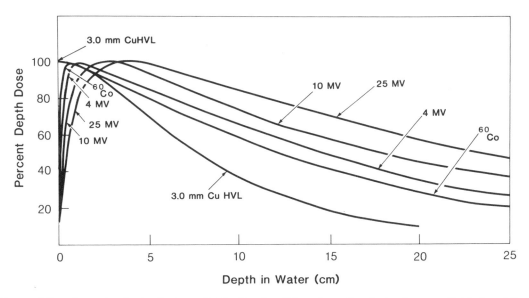

Figure 9.3. Central axis depth dose distribution for different quality photon beams. Field size, 10 × 10 cm; SSD = 100 cm for all beams except for 3.0 mm Cu HVL, SSD = 50 cm. Data are from Reference 13 and the Appendix.

the beam becomes, resulting in a higher percentage depth dose at any given depth beyond the build-up region.

A.1. INITIAL DOSE BUILD-UP

As seen in Fig. 9.3, the percent depth dose decreases with depth beyond the depth of maximum dose. However, there is an initial build-up of dose which becomes more and more pronounced as the energy is increased. In the case of the orthovoltage or lower energy x-rays, the dose builds up to a maximum on or very close to the surface. But for higher energy beams, the point of maximum dose lies deeper into the tissue or phantom. The region between the surface and the point of maximum dose is called the *dose build-up region*.

The dose build-up effect of the higher energy beams gives rise to what is clinically known as the *skin-sparing effect*. For megavoltage beams such as cobalt-60 and higher energies, the surface dose is much smaller than the D_{max}. This offers a distinct advantage over the lower energy beams where the D_{max} occurs at the skin surface. Thus, in the case of the higher energy photon beams, higher doses can be delivered to the deep-seated tumors without exceeding the tolerance of the skin. This, of course, is possible both because of the higher percent depth dose at the tumor and the lower surface dose at the skin. This topic is discussed in greater detail in Chapter 13.

The physics of dose build-up may be explained as follows. 1) As the high energy photon beam enters the patient or the phantom, high speed electrons are ejected from the surface and the subsequent layers. 2) These electrons deposit their energy a significant distance away from their site of origin. 3) Because of 1 and 2 above, the electron fluence and hence the absorbed dose increases with depth until it reaches a maximum. However, the photon energy fluence continuously decreases with depth and, as a result, the production of secondary electrons also decreases with depth. The net effect is that beyond a certain depth the dose eventually begins to decrease with depth.

It may be instructive to explain the build-up phenomenon in terms of absorbed dose and a quantity known as *kerma*. The kerma, K (<u>K</u>inetic <u>E</u>nergy <u>R</u>eleased in the <u>M</u>edium) may be defined (14) as "the quotient of dE_{tr} by dm, where dE_{tr} is the sum of the initial kinetic energies of all the charged ionizing particles (electrons) liberated by uncharged ionizing particles (photons) in a material of mass dm."

$$K = \frac{dE_{tr}}{dm}$$

The unit for kerma is the same as for the dose, *i.e.* J/kg. The name for the unit is gray (Gy). Also the special unit is rad which may be used temporarily.

Since kerma represents the energy transferred from photons to directly

---

[2] $\bar{\mu}$ is the average attenuation coefficient for the heterogeneous beam.

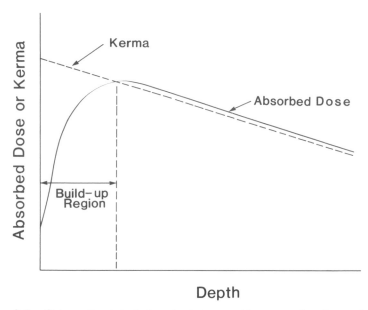

Figure 9.4. Schematic plot of absorbed dose and kerma as functions of depth.

ionizing electrons, the kerma is maximum at the surface and decreases with depth due to the decrease in the photon energy fluence (Fig. 9.4). The absorbed dose, on the other hand, first increases with depth as the high speed electrons ejected at various depths travel downstream. As a result, there is an electronic build-up with depth. However, the dose, as it depends on the electron fluence, reaches a maximum at a depth approximately equal to the range of electrons in the medium. Beyond this depth, the dose decreases as kerma continues to decrease, resulting in a decrease in secondary electron production and hence a net decrease in electron fluence. As seen in Fig. 9.4, the kerma curve is initially higher than the dose curve but falls below the dose curve beyond the build-up region. This effect is explained by the fact that the areas under the two curves taken to infinity must be the same.

B. Effect of Field Size and Shape

Field size may be specified either geometrically or dosimetrically. The *geometrical field size* is defined (15) as "the projection, on a plane perpendicular to the beam axis, of the distal end of the collimator as seen from the front center of the source." This definition usually corresponds to the field defined by the light localizer, arranged as if a point source of light is located at the center of the front surface of the radiation source. The *dosimetric* or the *physical* field size is the distance intercepted by a given isodose curve (usually 50% isodose) on a plane perpendicular to the beam axis at a stated distance from the source.

Unless stated otherwise, the term field size in this book will denote geometric field size. In addition, the field size will be defined at a predetermined distance such as the *SSD* (*source-surface distance*) or the *SAD* (*source-axis distance*). The latter term is the distance from the source to axis of gantry rotation known as the *isocenter*.

For an infinitesimally small field or a 0 × 0 field, the depth dose at a point is effectively due to the primary radiation, *i.e.* the photons which have traversed the overlying medium without interacting. The contribution of the scattered photons to the depth dose in this case is negligibly small or zero. But as the field size is increased, the contribution of the scattered radiation to the absorbed dose increases. Since this increase in scattered dose is greater at larger depths than at the depth of $D_{\max}$, the percent depth dose increases with increasing field size.

The increase in percent depth dose due to increase in field size is dependent on beam quality. Since the scattering probability or cross section decreases with energy increase and the higher energy photons are scattered more predominantly in the forward direction, the field size dependence of percent depth dose is less pronounced for the higher energy beams than for the lower energy beams.

Percent depth dose data for radiotherapy beams are usually tabulated for square fields. Since the majority of the treatments encountered in clinical practice require rectangular and irregularly shaped (blocked) fields, a system of equating square fields to different field shapes is required. Semi-empirical methods have been developed to relate central axis depth dose data for square, rectangular, circular, and irregularly shaped fields. Although general methods (based on Clarkson's principle—to be discussed later in this chapter) are available, simpler methods have been developed specifically for interrelating square, rectangular, and circular field data.

Day (16) and others (17, 18) have shown that, for central axis depth dose distribution, a rectangular field may be approximated by an equivalent square or by an equivalent circle. Data for equivalent squares, taken from Reference 13, are given in Table 9.2. As an example, consider a 10 × 20 cm field. From Table 9.2, the equivalent square is 13.0 × 13.0 cm. Thus, the percent depth dose data for a 13 × 13 cm field (obtained from standard tables) may be applied as an approximation to the given 10 × 20 cm field.

A simple rule of thumb method has been developed by Sterling *et al.* (28) for equating rectangular and square fields. According to this rule, a rectangular field is equivalent to a square field if they have the same area/perimeter (A/P). For example, the 10 × 20 cm field has an A/P of 3.33. The square field which has the same A/P is 13.3 × 13.3 cm, a value very close to that given in Table 9.2.

The following formulae are useful for quick calculation of the equivalent field parameters: For rectangular fields

$$A/P = \frac{a \times b}{2(a + b)} \tag{9.5}$$

Table 9.2.
Equivalent squares of rectangular fields

Long Axis (cm)	2	4	6	8	10	12	14	16	18	20	22	24	26	28	30
2	2.0														
4	2.7	4.0													
6	3.1	4.8	6.0												
8	3.4	5.4	6.9	8.0											
10	3.6	5.8	7.5	8.9	10.0										
12	3.7	6.1	8.0	9.6	10.9	12.0									
14	3.8	6.3	8.4	10.1	11.6	12.9	14.0								
16	3.9	6.5	8.6	10.5	12.2	13.7	14.9	16.0							
18	4.0	6.6	8.9	10.8	12.7	14.3	15.7	16.9	18.0						
20	4.0	6.7	9.0	11.1	13.0	14.7	16.3	17.7	18.9	20.0					
22	4.0	6.8	9.1	11.3	13.3	15.1	16.8	18.3	19.7	20.9	22.0				
24	4.1	6.8	9.2	11.5	13.5	15.4	17.2	18.8	20.3	21.7	22.9	24.0			
26	4.1	6.9	9.3	11.6	13.7	15.7	17.5	19.2	20.9	22.4	23.7	24.9	26.0		
28	4.1	6.9	9.4	11.7	13.8	15.9	17.8	19.6	21.3	22.9	24.4	25.7	27.0	28.0	
30	4.1	6.9	9.4	11.7	13.9	16.0	18.0	19.9	21.7	23.3	24.9	26.4	27.7	29.0	30.0

Taken from Reference 13.

where a is field width and b is field length. For square fields, since $a = b$,

$$A/P = \frac{a}{4} \qquad (9.6)$$

where a is the side of the square. From Equations 9.5 and 9.6, it is evident that the side of an equivalent square of a rectangular field is $4 \times A/P$. For example, 10×15 cm field has an A/P of 3.0. Its equivalent square is 12×12 cm. This agrees closely with the value of 11.9 given in Table 9.2.

Although the concept of A/P is not based on sound physical principles, it is widely used in clinical practice and has been extended as a field parameter to apply to other quantities such as backscatter factors, tissue-air ratios, and even beam output in air or in phantom. The reader may, however, be cautioned against an indiscriminate use of A/P. For example, the A/P parameter, as such, does not apply to circular or irregularly shaped fields, although radii of equivalent circles may be obtained by the relationship:

$$r = \frac{4}{\sqrt{\pi}} \cdot A/P \qquad (9.7)$$

The above equation can be derived by assuming that the equivalent circle is the one that has the same area as the equivalent square. Validity of this approximation has been verified from the table of equivalent circles given in Reference 13.

C. Dependence on Source-Surface Distance (SSD)

Photon fluence emitted by a point source of radiation varies inversely as a square of the distance from the source. Although the clinical source (isotopic source or focal spot) for external beam therapy has a finite size, the source-surface distance is usually chosen to be large (≥80 cm) so that the source dimensions become unimportant in relation to the variation of photon fluence with distance. In other words, the source can be considered as a point at large source-surface distances. Thus, the exposure rate or "dose rate in free space" (Chapter 8) from such a source varies inversely as the square of the distance. Of course, the inverse square law dependence of dose rate assumes that we are dealing with a primary beam, without scatter. In a given clinical situation, however, collimation or other scattering material in the beam may cause deviation from the inverse square law.

Percent depth dose increases with SSD due to the effects of the inverse square law. Although the actual dose rate at a point decreases with increase in distance from the source, the percent depth dose, which is a relative dose with respect to a reference point, increases with SSD. This is illustrated in Fig. 9.5 in which relative dose rate from a point source of radiation is plotted

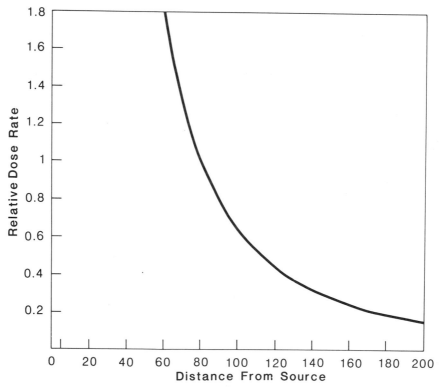

Figure 9.5.   Plot of relative dose rate as inverse square law function of distance from a point source. Reference distance = 80 cm.

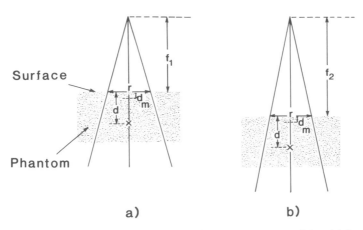

Figure 9.6. Change of percent depth dose with SSD. Irradiation condition (a) has SSD = f_1 and condition (b) has SSD = f_2. For both conditions, field size on the phantom surface, $r \times r$, and depth d are the same.

as a function of distance from the source, following the inverse square law. The plot shows that the drop in dose rate between two points is much greater at smaller distances from the source than at large distances. This means that the percent depth dose, which represents depth dose relative to a reference point, decreases more rapidly near the source than far away from the source.

In clinical radiotherapy, SSD is a very important parameter. Since percent depth dose determines how much dose can be delivered at depth relative to the surface dose or D_{max}, the SSD needs to be as large as possible. However, since dose rate decreases with distance, the SSD, in practice, is set at a distance which provides a compromise between dose rate and percent depth dose. For the treatment of deep seated lesions with megavoltage beams, the minimum recommended SSD is 80 cm.

Tables of percent depth dose for clinical use are usually measured at a standard SSD (80 or 100 cm for megavoltage units). In a given clinical situation, however, the SSD set on a patient may be different from the standard SSD. For example, larger SSDs are required for treatment techniques that involve field sizes larger than the ones available at the standard SSDs. Thus, the percent depth doses for a standard SSD must be converted to those applicable to the actual treatment SSD. Although more accurate methods are available (to be discussed later in this chapter), we discuss an approximate method in this section: the *Mayneord F Factor* (19). This method is based on a strict application of the inverse square law, without considering changes in scattering, as the SSD is changed.

Figure 9.6 shows two irradiation conditions, which differ only with regard to SSD. Let $P(d,r,f)$ be the percent depth dose at depth d for SSD = f and a field size r (*e.g.* a square field of dimensions $r \times r$). Since the variation in dose with depth is governed by three effects, namely, inverse square law, exponential attenuation, and scattering,

$$P(d,r,f_1) = 100 \cdot \left(\frac{f_1 + d_m}{f_1 + d}\right)^2 \cdot e^{-\mu(d-d_m)} \cdot K_s \qquad (9.8)$$

where μ is the linear attenuation coefficient for the primary and K_s is a function which accounts for the change in scattered dose. Ignoring the change in the value of K_s from one SSD to another,

$$P(d,r,f_2) = 100 \cdot \left(\frac{f_2 + d_m}{f_2 + d}\right)^2 \cdot e^{-\mu(d-d_m)} \cdot K_s \qquad (9.9)$$

Dividing Equation 9.9 by 9.8, we have

$$\frac{P(d,r,f_2)}{P(d,r,f_1)} = \left(\frac{f_2 + d_m}{f_1 + d_m}\right)^2 \cdot \left(\frac{f_1 + d}{f_2 + d}\right)^2 \qquad (9.10)$$

The terms on the right-hand side of Equation 9.10 are called the Mayneord F factor. Thus,

$$F = \left(\frac{f_2 + d_m}{f_1 + d_m}\right)^2 \cdot \left(\frac{f_1 + d}{f_2 + d}\right)^2 \qquad (9.11)$$

It can be shown that the F factor is greater than 1 for $f_2 > f_1$ and less than 1 for $f_2 < f_1$. Thus, it may be restated that the percent depth dose increases with increase in SSD.

EXAMPLE 1

The percent depth dose for a 15×15 field size, 10-cm depth, and 80-cm SSD is 58.4 (^{60}Co beam). Find the percent depth dose for the same field size and depth for 100-cm SSD.

From Equation 9.11, assuming $d_m = 0.5$ cm for ^{60}Co γ rays

$$F = \left(\frac{100 + 0.5}{80 + 0.5}\right)^2 \left(\frac{80 + 10}{100 + 10}\right)^2$$

$$= 1.043$$

From Equation 9.10,

$$\frac{P(10,15,100)}{P(10,15,80)} = 1.043$$

Thus, the desired percent depth dose is

$$P(10,15,100) = P(10,15,80) \times 1.043$$

$$= 58.4 \times 1.043$$

$$= 60.9$$

More accurate methods which take scattering change into account would yield a value close to 60.6.

The Mayneord F factor method works reasonably well for small fields since the scattering is minimal under these conditions. However, the method can give rise to significant errors under extreme conditions such as lower energy, large field, large depth, and large SSD change. For example, the error in dose at 20 cm depth for a 30 × 30 cm field and 160-cm SSD (^{60}Co beam) will be about 3% if the percent depth dose is calculated from the 80-cm SSD tables.

In general, the Mayneord F factor overestimates the increase in percent depth dose with increase in SSD. For example, for large fields and lower energy radiation where the proportion of scattered radiation is relatively greater, the factor $\dfrac{1 + F}{2}$ applies more accurately. Factors intermediate between F and $\dfrac{1 + F}{2}$ have also been used for certain conditions (19).

9.4 TISSUE-AIR RATIO

Tissue-air ratio was first introduced by Harold Johns (5) in 1953 and was originally called "tumor-air ratio." At that time, this quantity was intended specifically for rotation therapy calculations. In rotation therapy, the radiation source moves in a circle around the axis of rotation which is usually placed in the tumor. Although the source-surface distance (SSD) may vary depending upon the shape of the surface contour, the source-axis distance remains constant.

Since the percent depth dose depends on the SSD (Section 9.3C), the SSD correction to the percent depth dose will have to be applied to correct for the varying SSD—a procedure which becomes cumbersome to apply routinely in clinical practice. A simpler quantity, namely, the tissue-air ratio (TAR) has been defined to remove the SSD dependence. Since the time of its introduction, the concept of TAR has been refined to facilitate calculations not only for rotation therapy but also for stationary isocentric techniques as well as irregular fields.

Tissue-air ratio may be defined as the ratio of the dose (D_d) at a given point in the phantom to the dose in free space (D_{fs}) at the same point. This is illustrated in Fig. 9.7. For a given quality beam, TAR depends on depth d and field size r_d at that depth,

$$\mathrm{TAR}(d, r_d) = \frac{D_d}{D_{fs}} \tag{9.12}$$

A. Effect of Distance

One of the most important properties attributed to TAR is that it is independent of the distance from the source. This, however, is an approximation which is usually valid to an accuracy of better than 2% over the range of distances used clinically. This useful result can be deduced as follows:

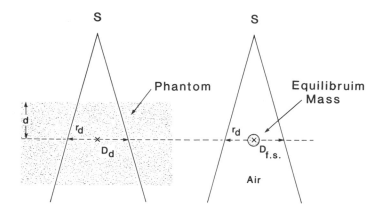

Figure 9.7. Illustration of the definition of tissue-air ratio. TAR $(d, r_d) = D_d/D_{fs}$.

Since TAR is the ratio of the two doses, D_d and D_{fs}, at the same point, the distance dependence of the photon fluence is removed. Thus, the TAR represents modification of the dose at a point due only to attenuation and scattering of the beam in the phantom compared to the dose at the same point in the miniphantom (or equilibrium phantom) placed in free air. Since the primary beam is attenuated exponentially with depth, the TAR for the primary beam is only a function of depth, not of SSD. The case of the scatter component, however, is not obvious. Nevertheless, Johns *et al.* (20) have shown that the fractional scatter contribution to the depth dose is almost independent of the divergence of the beam and depends only on the depth and the field size at that depth. Hence the tissue-air ratio which involves both the primary and scatter component of the depth dose is independent of the source distance.

B. Variation with Energy, Depth, and Field Size

Tissue-air ratio varies with energy, depth, and field size very much like the percent depth dose. For the megavoltage beams, the tissue-air ratio builds up to a maximum at the depth of maximum dose (d_m) and then decreases with depth more or less exponentially. For a narrow beam or a 0×0 field size in which scatter contribution to the dose can be neglected, the TAR beyond d_m varies approximately exponentially with depth

$$\text{TAR}(d, 0) = e^{-\bar{\mu}(d-d_m)} \tag{9.13}$$

where $\bar{\mu}$ is the average attenuation coefficient of the beam for the given phantom. As the field size is increased, the scattered component of the dose increases and the variation of TAR with depth becomes more complex. However, for high energy megavoltage beams, where the scatter is minimal and is directed more or less in the forward direction, the TAR variation with depth can still be approximated by an exponential function, provided an effective attenuation coefficient (μ_{eff}) for the given field size is used.

B.1. BACKSCATTER FACTOR (BSF)

The term backscatter factor is simply the tissue-air ratio at the depth of maximum dose on central axis of the beam. It may be defined as the ratio of the dose on central axis at the depth of maximum dose to the dose at the same point in free space. Mathematically,

$$\text{BSF} = \frac{D_{\max}}{D_{fs}} \tag{9.14}$$

or

$$\text{BSF} = \text{TAR}(d_m, r_{d_m}) \tag{9.15}$$

where r_{d_m} is the field size at the depth d_m of maximum dose.

The backscatter factor, like the tissue-air ratio, is independent of distance from the source and depends only on the beam quality and field size. Figure 9.8 shows backscatter factors for various quality beams and field areas. Whereas BSF increases with field size, its maximum value occurs for beams having a half-value layer between 0.6 and 0.8 mm Cu, depending upon field size. Thus, for the orthovoltage beams with usual filtration, the backscatter factor can be as high as 1.5 for large field sizes. This amounts to a 50% increase in dose near the surface compared to the dose in free space or, in terms of exposure, 50% increase in exposure on the skin compared to the exposure in air.

For megavoltage beams (^{60}Co and higher energies), the backscatter factor is much smaller. For example, BSF for a 10×10 cm field for ^{60}Co is 1.036. This means that the $D_{\max}$ will be 3.6% higher than the dose in free space. This increase in dose is due to the radiation scatter reaching the point of $D_{\max}$ from the overlying and underlying tissues. As the beam energy is increased, the scatter is further reduced and so is the backscatter factor. Above about 8 MV, the scatter at the depth of $D_{\max}$ becomes negligibly small and the backscatter factor approaches its minimum value, namely unity.

C. Relationship between TAR and Percent Depth Dose

Tissue-air ratio and percent depth dose are interrelated. The relationship can be derived as follows: Considering Fig. 9.9a, let $\text{TAR}(d, r_d)$ be the tissue-air ratio at point Q for a field size r_d at depth d. Let r be the field size at the surface, f be the SSD, and d_m be the reference depth of maximum dose at point P. Let $D_{fs}(P)$ and $D_{fs}(Q)$ be the doses in free space at points P and Q, respectively (Fig. 9b and c). $D_{fs}(P)$ and $D_{fs}(Q)$ are related by inverse square law.

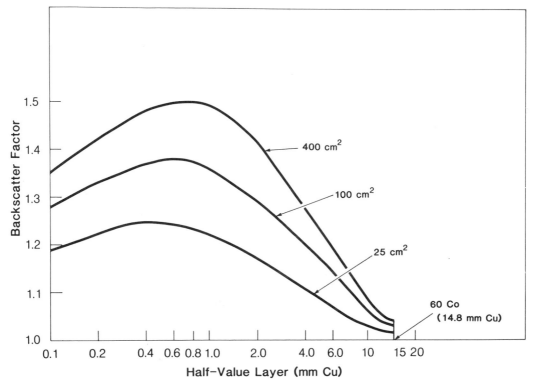

Figure 9.8. Variation of backscatter factors with beam quality (half-value layer). Data are for circular fields (13, 21).

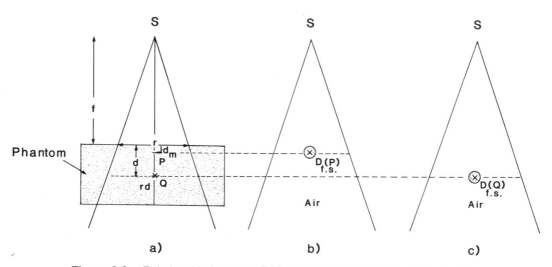

Figure 9.9. Relationship between TAR and percent depth dose. See text.

$$\frac{D_{fs}(Q)}{D_{fs}(P)} = \left(\frac{f + d_m}{f + d}\right)^2 \tag{9.16}$$

The field sizes r and r_d are related by:

$$r_d = r \cdot \frac{f + d}{f} \tag{9.17}$$

By definition of TAR,

$$\text{TAR}(d,r_d) = \frac{D_d(Q)}{D_{fs}(Q)} \tag{9.18}$$

or

$$D_d(Q) = \text{TAR}(d,r_d) \cdot D_{fs}(Q) \tag{9.19}$$

Since

$$D_{\max}(P) = D_{fs}(P) \cdot \text{BSF}(r) \tag{9.20}$$

and, by definition, the percent depth dose $P(d,r,f)$ is given by

$$P(d,r,f) = \frac{D_d(Q)}{D_{\max}(P)} \tag{9.21}$$

we have, from Equations 9.19, 9.20, and 9.21,

$$P(d,r,f) = \text{TAR}(d,r_d) \cdot \frac{1}{\text{BSF}(r)} \cdot \frac{D_{fs}(Q)}{D_{fs}(P)} \tag{9.22}$$

From Equations 9.16 and 9.22,

$$P(d,r,f) = \text{TAR}(d,r_d) \cdot \frac{1}{\text{BSF}(r)} \cdot \left(\frac{f + d_m}{f + d}\right)^2 \tag{9.23}$$

C.1. CONVERSION OF PERCENT DEPTH DOSE FROM ONE SSD TC ANOTHER—THE TAR METHOD

In Section 9.3C, we discussed a method of converting percent depth dose from one SSD to another. That method used the Mayneord F factor which is derived solely from inverse square law considerations. A more accurate method is based on the interrelationship between percent depth dose and TAR. This TAR method can be derived from Equation 9.23 as follows.

Suppose f_1 is the SSD for which the percent depth dose is known and f_2 is the SSD for which the percent depth dose is to be determined. Let r be the field size at the surface and d be the depth, for both cases. Referring to Fig. 9.6, let r_{d,f_1} and r_{d,f_2} be the field sizes projected at depth d in Fig. 9.6, a and b, respectively.

$$r_{d,f_1} = r \cdot \frac{f_1 + d}{f_1} \qquad (9.24)$$

$$r_{d,f_2} = r \cdot \frac{f_2 + d}{f_2} \qquad (9.25)$$

From Equation 9.23,

$$P(d,r,f_1) = \text{TAR}(d,r_{d,f_1}) \cdot \frac{1}{\text{BSF}(r)} \cdot \left(\frac{f_1 + d_m}{f_1 + d} \right)^2 \qquad (9.26)$$

and

$$P(d,r,f_2) = \text{TAR}(d,r_{d,f_2}) \cdot \frac{1}{\text{BSF}(r)} \cdot \left(\frac{f_2 + d_m}{f_2 + d} \right)^2 \qquad (9.27)$$

From Equations 9.26 and 9.27, the conversion factor is given by

$$\frac{P(d,r,f_2)}{P(d,r,f_1)} = \frac{\text{TAR}(d,r_{d,f_2})}{\text{TAR}(d,r_{d,f_1})} \cdot \left[\left(\frac{f_1 + d}{f_2 + d} \right)^2 \cdot \left(\frac{f_2 + d_m}{f_1 + d_m} \right)^2 \right] \qquad (9.28)$$

The last term in the brackets is the Mayneord factor. Thus, the TAR method corrects the Mayneord F factor by the ratio of TARs for the fields projected at depth for the two SSDs.

Burns (22) has developed the following equation to convert percent depth dose from one SSD to another

$$P(d,r,f_2) = P\left(d, \frac{r}{\sqrt{F}}, f_1 \right) \cdot \frac{\text{BSF}(r/\sqrt{F})}{\text{BSF}(r)} \cdot F \qquad (9.29)$$

where F is the Mayneord F factor given by $\left(\frac{f_1 + d}{f_2 + d} \right)^2 \cdot \left(\frac{f_2 + d_m}{f_1 + d_m} \right)^2$. The above equation is based on the concept that TARs are independent of the source distance. Burns' equation may be used in a situation where TARs are not available but instead a percent depth dose table is available at a standard SSD along with the backscatter factors for various field sizes.

As mentioned earlier, for high energy x-rays, *i.e.* above 8 MV, the variation of percent depth dose with field size is small and the backscatter factor is negligible. Equations 9.28 and 9.29 then simplify to a use of Mayneord F factor.

PRACTICAL EXAMPLES

In this section, we will present examples of typical treatment calculations using the concepts of percent depth dose, backscatter factor, and tissue-air ratio. Although a more general system of dosimetric calculations will be presented in the next chapter, these examples are presented here to illustrate the concepts presented thus far.

EXAMPLE 2

A patient is to be treated with an orthovoltage beam having a half-value layer of 3 mm Cu. Supposing that the machine is calibrated in terms of exposure rate in air, find the time required to deliver 200 cGy (rad) at 5 cm depth, given the following data: exposure rate = 100 R/min at 50 cm, field size = 8 × 8 cm, SSD = 50 cm, percent depth dose = 64.8, backscatter factor = 1.20, and rad/R = 0.95 (check these data in Reference 13).

$$\text{Dose rate in free space} = \text{exposure rate} \times \text{rad/R factor} \times A_{eq}$$

$$= 100 \times 0.95 \times 1.00$$

$$= 95 \text{ cGy/min}$$

$$D_{max} \text{ rate} = \text{dose rate free space} \times \text{BSF}$$

$$= 95 \times 1.20$$

$$= 114 \text{ cGy/min}$$

Tumor dose to be delivered = 200 cGy

$$D_{max} \text{ to be delivered} = \frac{\text{tumor dose}}{\text{percent depth dose}} \times 100$$

$$= \frac{200}{64.8} \times 100$$

$$= 308.6 \text{ cGy}$$

$$\text{Treatment time} = \frac{D_{max} \text{ to be delivered}}{D_{max} \text{ rate}}$$

$$= \frac{308.6}{114}$$

$$= 2.71 \text{ min}$$

EXAMPLE 3

A patient is to be treated with ^{60}Co radiation. Supposing that the machine is calibrated in air in terms of dose rate free space, find the treatment time to deliver 200 cGy (rad) at a depth of 8 cm, given the following data: dose rate free space = 150 cGy/min at 80.5 cm for a field size of 10 × 10 cm, SSD = 80 cm, percent depth dose = 64.1, and backscatter factor = 1.036.

$$D_{max} \text{ rate} = 150 \times 1.036 = 155.4 \text{ cGy/min}$$

$$D_{max} = \frac{200}{64.1} \times 100 = 312 \text{ cGy}$$

$$\text{Treatment time} = \frac{312}{155.4} = 2.01 \text{ min}$$

EXAMPLE 4

Determine the time required to deliver 200 cGy (rad) with a ^{60}Co γ ray beam at the *isocenter* (a point of intersection of the collimator axis and the gantry axis of rotation) which is placed at 10 cm depth in a patient. Given the following data: SAD = 80 cm, field size = 6 $\times$ 12 cm (at the isocenter), dose rate free space at the SAD for this field = 120 cGy/min and TAR = 0.681.

$$A/P \text{ for } 6 \times 12 \text{ cm field} = \frac{6 \times 12}{2(6 \times 12)} = 2$$

Side of equivalent square field = $4 \times A/P = 8$ cm

TAR(10,8 $\times$ 8) = 0.681 (given)

$D_d = 200$ cGy (given)

Since $\text{TAR} = \dfrac{D_d}{D_{fs}}$

$$D_{fs} = \frac{200}{0.681} = 293.7 \text{ cGy}$$

$$D_{fs} \text{ rate} = 120 \text{ cGy/min (given)}$$

$$\text{Treatment time} = \frac{293.7}{120} = 2.45 \text{ min}$$

D. Calculation of Dose in Rotation Therapy

The concept of tissue-air ratios is most useful for calculations involving isocentric techniques of irradiation. Rotation or arc therapy is a type of isocentric irradiation in which the source moves continuously around the axis of rotation.

The calculation of depth dose in rotation therapy involves the determination of average TAR at the isocenter. The contour of the patient is drawn in a plane containing the axis of rotation. The isocenter is then placed within the contour (usually in the middle of the tumor or a few centimeters beyond it) and radii are drawn from this point at selected angular intervals (*e.g.* 20°) (Fig. 9.10). Each radius represents a depth for which TAR can be obtained from the TAR table, for the given beam energy and field size defined at the isocenter. The TARs are then summed and averaged to determine $\overline{\text{TAR}}$, as illustrated in Table 9.3.

EXAMPLE 5

For the data given in Table 9.3, determine the treatment time to deliver 200 cGy (rad) at the center of rotation, given the data: dose rate free space for 6 × 6 cm field at the SAD is 86.5 cGy/min.

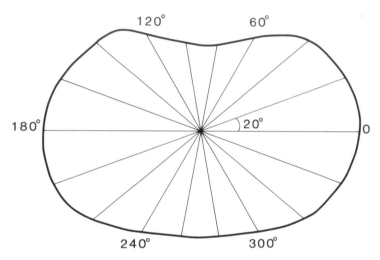

Figure 9.10. Contour of patient with radii drawn from the isocenter of rotation at 20° intervals. Length of each radius represents a depth for which TAR is determined for the field size at the isocenter. (See Table 9.3.)

Table 9.3.
Determination of average *TAR* at the center of rotation. ^{60}Co beam, field size at the isocenter = 6 × 6 cm

Angle	Depth along Radius	TAR	Angle	Depth along Radius	TAR
0	16.6	0.444	180	16.2	0.450
20	16.0	0.456	200	16.2	0.450
40	14.6	0.499	220	14.6	0.499
60	11.0	0.614	240	12.4	0.563
80	9.0	0.691	260	11.2	0.606
100	9.4	0.681	280	11.0	0.614
120	11.4	0.597	300	12.0	0.580
140	14.0	0.515	320	14.2	0.507
160	15.6	0.470	340	16.0	0.456

Average tissue-air ratio ($\overline{\text{TAR}}$) = 9.692/18 = 0.538.

$\overline{\text{TAR}}$ = 0.538 (as calculated in Table 9.3)

Dose to be delivered at isocenter = 200 cGy (given)

Dose free space to be delivered at isocenter $= \dfrac{200}{0.538} = 371.8$ cGy

Dose rate free space at isocenter = 86.5 cGy/min (given)

Treatment time $= \dfrac{371.8}{86.5} = 4.30$ min

9.5 SCATTER-AIR RATIO (SAR)

Scatter-air ratios are used for the purpose of calculating scattered dose in the medium. The computation of the primary and the scattered dose separately is particularly useful in the dosimetry of irregular fields.

Scatter-air ratio may be defined as the ratio of the scattered dose at a given point in the phantom to the dose in free space at the same point. The scatter-air ratio like the tissue-air ratio is independent of the source-surface distance but depends on the beam energy, depth, and field size.

Since the scattered dose at a point in the phantom is equal to the total dose minus the primary dose at that point, scatter-air ratio is mathematically given by the difference between the TAR for the given field and the TAR for the 0 × 0 field.

$$\text{SAR}(d,r_d) = \text{TAR}(d,r_d) - \text{TAR}(d,0) \qquad (9.30)$$

Hence, TAR(d,0) represents the primary component of the beam since for a beam of 0 × 0 field size no scattered radiation is produced in the phantom.

Since SARs are primarily used in calculating scatter in a field of any shape, SARs are tabulated as functions of depth and radius of a circular field at that depth. Also, since SAR data are derived from TAR data for rectangular or square fields, radii of equivalent circles may be obtained from the table in Reference 13 or by Equation 9.7.

A. Dose Calculation in Irregular Fields—Clarkson's Method

Any field other than the rectangular, square, or circular field may be termed irregular. Irregularly shaped fields are encountered in radiotherapy when radiation sensitive structures are shielded from the primary beam or when the field extends beyond the irregularly shaped patient body contour. Examples of such fields are the mantle and inverted Y fields employed for the treatment of Hodgkin's disease. Since the basic data [percent depth dose, tissue-air ratios, or tissue-maximum ratios (to be discussed later)] are available usually for rectangular fields, methods are required to use these data for general cases of irregularly shaped fields. One such method, originally proposed by Clarkson (23) and later developed by Cunningham (24, 25), has proved to be the most general in its application.

Clarkson's method is based on the principle that the scattered component of the depth dose, which depends on the field size and shape, can be calculated separately from the primary component which is independent of the field size and shape. A special quantity, SAR, is used to calculate the scattered dose. This method has been discussed in detail in the literature (26, 27) and only a brief discussion will be presented here.

Let us consider an irregularly shaped field as shown in Fig. 9.11. Assume this field cross section to be at depth d and perpendicular to the beam axis. Let Q be the point of calculation in the plane of the field cross section. Radii are drawn from Q to divide the field into elementary sectors. Each sector is characterized by its radius and can be considered as part of a circular field of that radius. If we suppose the sector angle is 10°, then the scatter contribution from this sector will be $10°/360° = \frac{1}{36}$ of that contributed by a circular field

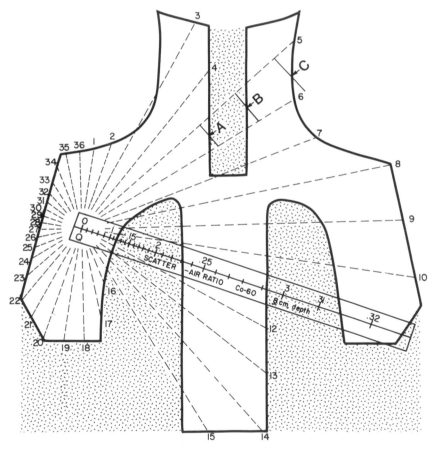

Figure 9.11. Outline of mantle field in a plane perpendicular to the beam axis and at a specified depth. Radii are drawn from point Q, the point of calculation. Sector angle = 10°. Redrawn from Reference 26.

of that radius and centered at Q. Thus, the scatter contribution from all the sectors can be calculated and summed by considering each sector to be a part of its own circle whose scatter-air ratio is already known and tabulated.

Using an SAR table for circular fields, the SAR values for the sectors are calculated and then summed to give the average scatter-air ratio $\overline{\text{SAR}}$ for the irregular field at point Q. For sectors passing through a blocked area, the net SAR is determined by subtracting the scatter contribution by the blocked part of sector. For example, net $(\text{SAR})_{QC} = (\text{SAR})_{QC} - (\text{SAR})_{QB} + (\text{SAR})_{QA}$.

The computed $\overline{\text{SAR}}$ is converted to average tissue-air ratio $(\overline{\text{TAR}})$ by the equation

$$\overline{\text{TAR}} = \text{TAR}(0) + \overline{\text{SAR}} \tag{9.30}$$

where $\text{TAR}(0)$ is the tissue-air ratio for 0×0 field, *i.e.* $\text{TAR}(0) = e^{-\bar{\mu}(d-d_m)}$, where $\bar{\mu}$ is the average linear attenuation coefficient for the beam and d is the depth of point Q.

The percent depth dose $(\%DD)$ at Q may be calculated relative to D_{max} on the central axis using Equation 9.23.

$$\%DD = 100 \times \overline{\text{TAR}} \times \left(\frac{f + d_m}{f + d}\right)^2 \bigg/ \text{BSF} \tag{9.31}$$

where BSF is the backscatter factor for the irregular field and can be calculated by Clarkson's method. This involves determining $\overline{\text{TAR}}$ at the depth d_m on the central axis, using the field contour or radii projected at the depth d_m.

In clinical practice, additional corrections are usually necessary such as for the variation of SSD within the field and the primary beam profile. The details of these corrections will be discussed in the next chapter.

References

1. Shrimpton PC: Electron density values of various human tissues: *in vitro* Compton scatter measurements and calculated ranges. *Phys Med Biol* 26:907, 1981.
2. Tubiana M, Dutreix J, Dutreix A, Jocky P: *Bases Physiques de la Radiotherapie et de la Radiobiologie.* Masson ET Cie, Éditeurs, Paris, 1963, p 458.
3. Schulz RJ, Nath R: On the constancy in composition in polystyrene and polymethylmethacrylate plastics. *Med Phys* 6:153, 1979.
4. White DR, Martin RJ, Darlison R: Epoxy resin based tissue substitutes. *Br J Radiol* 50:814, 1977.
5. Johns HE, Whitmore GF, Watson TA, Umberg FH: A system of dosimetry for rotation therapy with typical rotation distributions. *J Can Assn Radiol* 4:1, 1953.
6. Johns HE: Physical aspects of rotation therapy. *Am J Roentgenol* 79:373, 1958.
7. Cunningham JR, Johns HE, Gupta SK: An examination of the definition and the magnitude of back-scatter factor for cobalt 60 gamma rays. *Br J Radiol* 38:637, 1965.
8. Gupta SK, Cunningham JR: Measurement of tissue-air ratios and scatter functions for large field sizes for cobalt 60 gamma radiation. *Br J Radiol* 39:7, 1966.
9. Karzmark CJ, Dewbert A, Loevinger R: Tissue-phantom ratios—an aid to treatment planning. *Br J Radiol* 38:158, 1965.
10. Saunders JE, Price RH, Horsley RJ: Central axis depth doses for a constant source-tumor distance. *Br J Radiol* 41:464, 1968.

11. Holt JG, Laughlin JS, Moroney JP: Extension of concept of tissue-air ratios (TAR) to high energy x-ray beams. *Radiology* 96:437, 1970.
12. Khan FM, Sewchand W, Lee J, Williamson JF: Revision of tissue-maximum ratio and scatter-maximum ratio concepts for cobalt 60 and higher energy x-ray beams. *Med Phys* 7:230, 1980.
13. Hospital Physicists' Association: Central axis depth dose data for use in radiotherapy. *Br J Radiol* (Suppl 11), 1978.
14. International Commission on Radiation Units and Measurements (ICRU): *Report 33, Radiation Quantities and Units.* Washington, DC, United States National Bureau of Standards, 1980.
15. International Commission on Radiation Units and Measurements (ICRU): *Report 24, Determination of Absorbed Dose in a Patient Irradiated by Beams of X or Gamma Rays in Radiotherapy Procedures.* Washington, DC, United States National Bureau of Standards, 1976.
16. Day MJ: A note on the calculation of dose in x-ray fields. *Br J Radiol* 23:368, 1950.
17. Jones DEA: A note on back-scatter and depth doses for elongated rectangular x-ray fields. *Br J Radiol* 22:342, 1949.
18. Batho HF, Theimer O, Theimer R: A consideration of equivalent circle method of calculating depth doses for rectangular x-ray fields. *J Can Assn Radiol* 7:51, 1956.
19. Mayneord WV, Lamerton LF: A survey of depth dose data. *Br J Radiol* 14:255, 1944.
20. Johns HE, Bruce WR, Reid WB: The dependence of depth dose on focal skin distance. *Br J Radiol* 31:254, 1958.
21. Johns HE, Hunt JW, Fedoruk SO: Surface back-scatter in the 100 kV to 400 kV range. *Br J Radiol* 27:443, 1954.
22. Burns JE: Conversion of depth doses from one FSD to another. *Br J Radiol* 31:643, 1958.
23. Clarkson JR: A note on depth doses in fields of irregular shape. *Br J Radiol* 14:265, 1941.
24. Johns HE, Cunningham JR: *The Physics of Radiology*, 3rd ed. Springfield, IL, Charles C Thomas, 1969.
25. Cunningham JR: Scatter-air ratios. *Phys Med Biol* 17:42, 1972.
26. American Association of Physicists in Medicine: *Dosimetry Workshop: Hodgkin's Disease*, Chicago, IL. M. D. Anderson Hospital, Houston, TX, Radiological Physics Center, 1970.
27. Khan FM, Levitt SH, Moore VC, Jones TK: Computer and approximation methods of calculating depth dose in irregularly shaped fields. *Radiology* 106:433, 1973.
28. Sterling TD, Perry H, Katz L: Derivation of a mathematical expression for the percent depth dose surface of cobalt 60 beams and visualization of multiple field dose distributions. *Br J Radiol* 37:544, 1964.

CHAPTER 10

A System of Dosimetric Calculations

Several methods are available for calculating absorbed dose in a patient. Two of these methods using percent depth doses and tissue-air ratios (TAR) were discussed in Chapter 9. However, there are some limitations to these methods. For example, the dependence of percent depth dose on source-surface distance (SSD) makes this quantity unsuitable for isocentric techniques. Although TARs and SARs eliminate that problem, their application to beams of energy higher than those of ^{60}Co has been seriously questioned (1–3) as they require measurement of dose in free space. As the beam energy increases, the size of the chamber buildup cap for in-air measurements has to be increased and it becomes increasingly difficult to calculate the dose in free space from such measurements. In addition, the material of the buildup cap is usually different from that of the phantom and this introduces a bias or uncertainty in the TAR measurements.

In order to overcome the limitations of the TAR, Karzmark *et al.* (1) introduced the concept of tissue-phantom ratio (TPR). This quantity retains the properties of the TAR but limits the measurements to the phantom rather than in air. A few years later, Holt *et al.* (18) introduced yet another quantity, tissue-maximum ratio (TMR), which also limits the measurements to the phantom.

In this chapter we develop a dosimetric system based on the TMR concept, although a similar system can also be derived from the TPR concept (4).

10.1 DOSE CALCULATION PARAMETERS

The dose to a point in a medium may be analyzed into primary and scattered components. The primary dose is contributed by the initial or original photons emitted from the source and the scattered dose is due to the scattered photons. The scattered dose can be further analyzed into collimator and phantom components since the two can be varied independently by blocking. For example, blocking a portion of the field does not significantly change the output or exposure in the open portion of the beam (5, 6) but may substantially reduce the phantom scatter.

The above analysis presents one practical difficulty, namely, the determination of primary dose in a phantom which excludes both the collimator and phantom scatter. However, for megavoltage photon beams, it is reasonably accurate to consider collimator scatter as part of the primary beam so that the phantom scatter could be calculated separately. We, therefore, define an *effective primary dose* as the dose due to the primary photons as well as those scattered from the collimating system. The effective primary in a phantom may be thought of as the dose at depth minus the phantom scatter. Alternatively, the effective primary dose may be defined as the depth dose expected in the field when scattering volume is reduced to zero while keeping the collimator opening constant.

A. Collimator Scatter Correction Factor (S_c)

The beam output (exposure rate, dose rate in free space or energy fluence rate) measured in air depends on the field size. As the field size is increased, the output increases because of the increased collimator scatter which is added to the primary beam. This increase in scatter is due to the increase in the surface area of the collimator as the collimator opens to a larger size.

The collimator scatter correction factor (S_c) is commonly called the *output factor* and may be defined as the ratio of the output in air for a given field to that for a reference field (*e.g.* 10 × 10 cm). S_c may be measured with an ion chamber with a buildup cap of size large enough to provide maximum dose buildup for the given energy beam. The measurement setup is shown in Fig. 10.1A. Readings are plotted against field size [side of equivalent square or

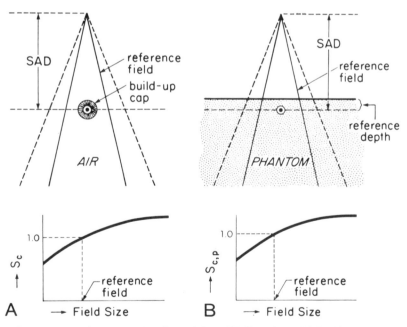

Figure 10.1. Arrangement for measuring S_c and $S_{c,p}$. (A) Chamber with buildup cap in air to measure output relative to a reference field, for determining S_c *vs.* field size. (B) Measurements in a phantom at a fixed depth for determining $S_{c,p}$ *vs.* field size. [Reprinted with permission from: Khan *et al.* (4).]

area/perimeter (A/P)] and the values are normalized to the reference field, 10 × 10 cm.

In the measurement of S_c factors, the field must fully cover the buildup cap for all field sizes if measurements are to reflect relative photon fluences. For small fields, one may take the measurements at large distances from the source so that the smallest field covers buildup cap. Normally, the collimator scatter correction factors are measured at the SAD. However, larger distances can be used provided the field sizes are all defined at the SAD.

B. Phantom Scatter Correction Factor (S_p)

The phantom scatter correction factor takes into account the change in scatter radiation originating in the phantom at a reference depth as the field size is changed. S_p may be defined as the ratio of the dose rate for a given field at a reference depth (e.g. depth of maximum dose) to the dose rate at the same depth for the reference field size (e.g. 10 × 10 cm), with the same collimator opening. In this definition, it should be noted that S_p is related to the changes in the area of the phantom irradiated for a fixed collimator opening. Thus, one could determine S_p, at least in concept, by using a large field incident on phantoms of various cross-sectional sizes.

For photon beams for which backscatter factors can be accurately measured (e.g. ^{60}Co and 4 MV), S_p factor at the depth of maximum dose may be defined simply as the ratio of backscatter factor (BSF) for the given field to that for the reference field (see Appendix A). Mathematically,

$$S_p(r) = \frac{\text{BSF}(r)}{\text{BSF}(r_0)} \tag{10.1}$$

where r_0 is the reference field size (10 × 10 cm).

A more practical method of measuring S_p, which can be used for all beam energies, consists of indirect determination from the following equation (for derivation, see Appendix A):

$$S_p(r) = \frac{S_{c,p}(r)}{S_c(r)} \tag{10.2}$$

where $S_{c,p}(r)$ is the total scatter correction factor defined as the dose rate at a reference depth for a given field r divided by the dose rate at the same point and depth for the reference field size (10 × 10 cm) (Fig. 10.1B). Thus, $S_{c,p}(r)$ contains both the collimator and phantom scatter and when divided by $S_c(r)$ yields $S_p(r)$.

C. Tissue-Phantom and Tissue-Maximum Ratios

The tissue-phantom ratio (TPR) is defined as the ratio of the dose at a given point in phantom to the dose at the same point at a fixed reference depth, usually 5 cm. This is illustrated in Fig. 10.2. The corresponding quantity for the scattered dose calculation is called the scatter-phantom ratio (SPR),

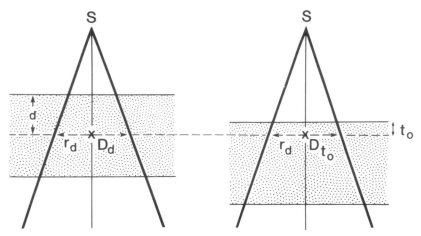

Figure 10.2. Diagram illustrating the definitions of tissue-phantom ratio (TPR) and tissue-maximum ratio (TMR). $\text{TPR}(d, r_d) = \dfrac{D_d}{D_{t_0}}$, where t_0 is a reference depth. If t_0 is the reference depth of maximum dose, then $\text{TMR}(d, r_d) = \text{TPR}(d, r_d)$.

which is analogous in use to the scatter-air ratio discussed in the previous chapter. Details of the TPR and SPR concepts have been discussed in the literature (1, 3, 4).

TPR is a general function which may be normalized to any reference depth. But there is no general agreement concerning the depth to be used for this quantity, although 5-cm depth is the usual choice for most beam energies. On the other hand, the point of central axis $D_{\max}$ has a simplicity that is very desirable in dose computations. If adopted as a fixed reference depth, the quantity TPR gives rise to the *tissue-maximum ratio* (TMR). Thus, TMR is a special case of TPR and may be defined as the ratio of the dose at a given point in phantom to the dose at the same point at the reference depth of maximum dose (see Fig. 10.2).

For megavoltage beams in the range of 20–45 MV, the depth of maximum dose (d_m) has been found to depend significantly on field size (7, 8) as well as on SSD (9, 10). In order that the calculative functions be independent of machine parameters, they should not involve measurements in the buildup region. Therefore, the reference depth must be equal to or greater than the largest d_m. Since d_m tends to decrease with field size (7) and increase with SSD (9), one should choose d_m for the smallest field and the largest SSD. In practice, one may plot $[(\%DD) \times (SSD + d)^2]$ as a function of depth d to find d_m (10). This eliminates dependence on SSD. The maximum d_m can then be obtained by plotting d_m as a function of field size and extrapolating to 0×0 field size.

The *reference depth of maximum dose* (t_0), as determined above, should be used for percent depth dose, TMR, and S_p factors, irrespective of field size and SSD.

C.1. PROPERTIES OF TMR

The concept of tissue-maximum ratio is based on the assumption that the fractional scatter contribution to the depth dose at a point is independent of the divergence of the beam and depends only on the field size at the point and the depth of the overlying tissue. This has been shown to be essentially true by Johns *et al.* (11). This principle which also underlies TAR and TPR makes all these functions practically independent of source-surface distance. Thus, a single table of TMRs can be used for all SSDs for each radiation quality.

Figure 10.3 shows TMR data for for 10-MV x-ray beams as an example.

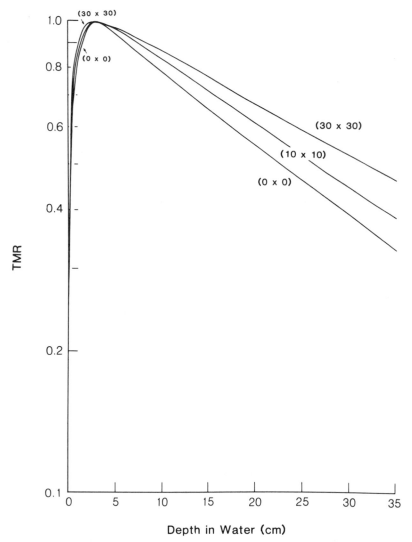

Figure 10.3.   Plot of TMR for 10-MV x-rays as a function of depth for a selection of field sizes.

The curve for 0×0 field size shows the steepest drop with depth and is due entirely to the primary beam. For megavoltage beams, the primary beam attenuation can be approximately represented by

$$\text{TMR}(d, 0) = e^{-\mu(d-t_0)} \tag{10.3}$$

where μ is the effective linear attenuation coefficient and t_0 is the reference depth of maximum dose. μ can be determined from TMR data by plotting μ as a function of field size (side of equivalent square) and extrapolating it back to 0×0 field.

TMR and percent depth dose P are interrelated by the following equation (see Appendix B for derivation).

$$\text{TMR}(d, r_d) = \left(\frac{P(d, r, f)}{100}\right)\left(\frac{f + d}{f + t_0}\right)^2 \left(\frac{S_p(r_{t_0})}{S_p(r_d)}\right) \tag{10.4}$$

where

$$f = \text{SSD}, \ r_d = r \cdot \left(\frac{f + d}{f}\right)$$

$$r_{t_0} = r \cdot \left(\frac{f + t_0}{f}\right)$$

Here the percent depth dose is referenced against the dose at depth t_0 so that $P(t_0, r, f) = 100$ for all field sizes and SSDs.

Although TMRs can be measured directly, they can also be calculated from percent depth doses, as shown by Equation 10.4. For ^{60}Co, Equations 10.2 and 10.4 can be used to calculate TMRs. In addition, TMRs can be derived from TAR data in those cases, such as ^{60}Co, where TARs are accurately known:

$$\text{TMR}(d, r_d) = \frac{\text{TAR}(d, r_d)}{\text{BSF}(r_d)} \tag{10.5}$$

D. Scatter-Maximum Ratio (SMR)

SMR, like the SAR, is a quantity designed specifically for the calculation of scattered dose in a medium. It may be defined (4) as the ratio of the scattered dose at a given point in phantom to the effective primary dose at the same point at the reference depth of maximum dose. Mathematically,

$$\text{SMR}(d, r_d) = \text{TMR}(d, r_d)\left(\frac{S_p(r_d)}{S_p(0)}\right) - \text{TMR}(d, 0) \tag{10.6}$$

For derivation of the above equation, see Appendix C.

From Equations 10.1, 10.5, and 10.6, it can be shown that for ^{60}Co γ rays, SMRs are the same as SARs. However, for higher energies, SMRs should be calculated from TMRs by using Equations 9.7 and 10.6.

Another interesting relationship can be obtained at the reference depth of maximum dose (t_0). Since TMR at depth t_0 is unity by definition, Equation 10.6 becomes:

$$\text{SMR}(t_0, r_{t_0}) = \frac{S_p(r_{t_0})}{S_p(0)} - 1 \tag{10.7}$$

This equation will be used later in Section 10.2C.

10.2 PRACTICAL APPLICATIONS

Radiotherapy institutions vary in their treatment techniques and calibration practices. For example, some rely exclusively on the SSD or the SAD (isocentric) type techniques while others use both. Accordingly, units are calibrated in air or in phantom at a suitable reference depth. In addition, clinical fields, although basically rectangular or square, are often shaped irregularly to protect critical or normal regions of the body. Thus, a calculation system must be generally applicable to the above practices, with acceptable accuracy and simplicity for routine use.

A. Accelerator Calculations

A.1. SSD TECHNIQUE

Percent depth dose is a suitable quantity for calculations involving SSD techniques. Machines are usually calibrated to deliver 1 rad (10^{-2} Gy) per monitor unit (MU) at the reference depth t_0, for a reference field size 10×10 cm and a source-to-calibration point distance of SCD. Assuming that the S_c factors relate to collimator field sizes defined at the SAD, the monitor units necessary to deliver a certain tumor dose (TD) at depth d for a field size r at the surface at any SSD are given by

$$\text{MU} = \frac{\text{TD} \times 100}{(\%\text{DD})_d \times S_c(r_c) \times S_p(r) \times (\text{SSD factor})} \tag{10.8}$$

where r_c is the collimator field size, given by $r_c = r \cdot \dfrac{\text{SAD}}{\text{SSD}}$ and

$$\text{SSD factor} = \left(\frac{\text{SCD}}{\text{SSD} + t_0}\right)^2$$

It must be remembered that, whereas the field size for the S_c factor is defined at the SAD, the S_p factors relate to the field irradiating the patient.

Example 1. A 4-MV linear accelerator is calibrated to give 1 rad (10^{-2} Gy) per MU in phantom at a reference depth of maximum dose of 1 cm, 100-cm SSD, and 10×10 cm field size. Determine the MU values to deliver 200 rads to a patient at 100-cm SSD, 10-cm depth, and 15×15 cm field size, given

$S_c(15 \times 15) = 1.020$, $S_p(15 \times 15) = 1.010$, %DD = 65.1. From Equation 10.8

$$MU = \frac{200 \times 100}{65.1 \times 1.020 \times 1.010 \times 1} = 298$$

A form for treatment calculations is shown in Fig. 10.4 with the above calculations filled in.

Example 2. Determine the MU for the treatment conditions given in Example 1 except that the treatment SSD is 120 cm, given $S_c(12.5 \times 12.5) = 1.010$ and percent depth dose for the new SSD is 66.7.

Field size projected at SAD(= 100 cm) $= 15 \times \dfrac{100}{120} = 12.5$ cm

$S_c(12.5 \times 12.5)$ is given as 1.010 and $S_p(15 \times 15) = 1.010$

$$\text{SSD factor} = \left(\frac{100 + 1}{120 + 1}\right)^2 = 0.697$$

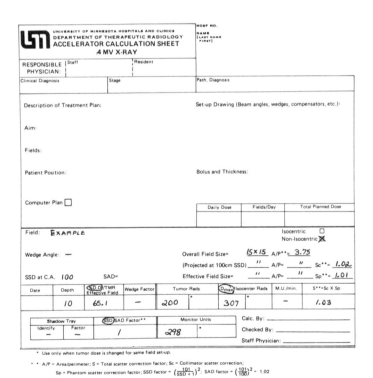

Figure 10.4. Accelerator calculation sheet.

From Equation 10.8,

$$MU = \frac{200 \times 100}{66.7 \times 1.010 \times 1.010 \times 0.697} = 442$$

A.2. ISOCENTRIC TECHNIQUE

TMR is the quantity of choice for dosimetric calculations involving isocentric techniques. Since the unit is calibrated to give 1 rad (10^{-2} Gy)/MU at the reference depth t_0, calibration distance SCD and for the reference field (10 × 10 cm), then the monitor units necessary to deliver isocenter dose (ID) at depth d are given by:

$$MU = \frac{ID}{TMR(d,\ r_d) \times S_c(r_c) \times S_p(r_d) \times SAD\ factor} \qquad (10.9)$$

where

$$SAD\ factor = \left(\frac{SCD}{SAD}\right)^2$$

Example 3. A tumor dose of 200 rads is to be delivered at the isocenter which is located at a depth of 8 cm, given 4-MV x-ray beam, field size at the isocenter = 6 × 6 cm, $S_c(6 \times 6) = 0.970$, $S_p(6 \times 6) = 0.990$, machine calibrated at SCD = 100 cm, TMR(8, 6 × 6) = 0.787. Since the calibration point is at the SAD, SAD factor = 1. Thus, using Equation 10.9,

$$MU = \frac{200}{0.787 \times 0.970 \times 0.990 \times 1} = 265$$

Example 4. Calculate MU values for the case in Example 3, if the unit is calibrated nonisocentrically, *i.e.* source to calibration point distance = 101 cm.

$$SAD\ factor = \left(\frac{101}{100}\right)^2 = 1.020$$

Thus,

$$MU = \frac{200}{0.787 \times 0.970 \times 0.99 \times 1.02} = 260$$

B. Cobalt-60 Calculations

The above calculation system is sufficiently general that it can be applied to any radiation generator including ^{60}Co. In the latter case, the machine can be calibrated either in air or in phantom provided the following information is available: 1) dose rate $\dot{D}_0(t_0, r_0, f_0)$ in phantom at depth t_0 of maximum dose for a reference field r_0 and standard SSD f_0; 2) S_c factors; 3) S_p factors; 4) percent depth doses; and 5) TMR values. If universal depth dose data for ^{60}Co (Reference 11) are used, then the S_p factors and TMRs can be obtained by using Equations 10.1 and 10.5. In addition, the SSD used in these calculations should be confined to a range for which the output in air obeys an inverse square law for a constant collimator opening.

A form for cobalt calculations is presented in Fig. 10.5.

Example 5. A tumor dose of 200 rads is to be delivered at 8-cm depth, using 15 × 15 cm field size, 100-cm SSD, and penumbra trimmers up. The unit is calibrated to give 130 rads/min in phantom at 0.5 cm depth for a 10 × 10 cm field with trimmers up and SSD = 80 cm. Determine the time of irradiation, given $S_c(12 \times 12) = 1.012$, $S_p(15 \times 15) = 1.014$, and %DD (8, 15 × 15, 100) = 68.7.

$$\text{Field size projected at SAD (= 80 cm)} = 15 \times \frac{80}{100} = 12 \text{ cm} \times 12 \text{ cm}$$

$$\text{SSD factor} = \left(\frac{80 + 0.5}{100 + 0.5}\right)^2 = 0.642$$

$$\text{Time} = (\text{TD} \times 100)/[\dot{D}_0(0.5, 10 \times 10, 80) \times \%DD(8, 15 \times 15, 100)$$

$$\times S_c(12 \times 12) \times S_p(15 \times 15) \times \text{SSD factor}]$$

$$= \frac{200 \times 100}{130 \times 68.7 \times 1.012 \times 1.014 \times 0.642}$$

$$= 3.40 \text{ min}$$

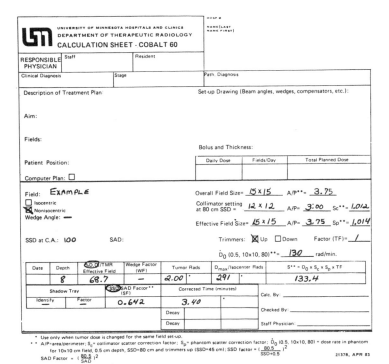

Figure 10.5. Calculation sheet—cobalt-60.

C. Irregular Fields

Dosimetry of irregular fields using TMRs and SMRs is analogous to the method using TARs and SARs (Section 9.5). Since the mathematical rationale of the method has been discussed in detail in the literature (4), only a brief outline will be presented here to illustrate the procedure.

An irregular field at depth d may be divided into n elementary sectors with radii emanating from point Q of calculation (see Fig. 9.10, Chap. 9). A Clarkson type integration (Section 9.5) may be performed to give averaged scatter-maximum ratio $(\overline{SMR}(d, r_d))$ for the irregular field r_d:

$$\overline{SMR}(d, r_d) = \frac{1}{n} \sum_{i=1}^{n} SMR(d, r_i) \tag{10.10}$$

where r_i is the radius of the ith sector at depth d and n is the total number of sectors ($n = 2\pi/\Delta\theta$, where $\Delta\theta$ is the sector angle).

The computed $\overline{SMR}(d, r_d)$ is then converted to $\overline{TMR}(d, r_d)$ by using Equation 10.6.

$$\overline{TMR}(d, r_d) = [TMR(d, 0) + \overline{SMR}(d, r_d)] \times \frac{S_p(0)}{\overline{S}_p(r_d)} \tag{10.11}$$

where $\overline{S}_p(r_d)$ is the averaged S_p for the irregular field r_d and $S_p(0)$ is the S_p for the 0×0 area field. The above equation is strictly valid only for points along the central axis of a beam that is normally incident on an infinite phantom with flat surface. For off-axis points in a beam with nonuniform primary dose profile, one should write:

$$\overline{TMR}(d, r_d) = [K_p \cdot TMR(d, 0) + \overline{SMR}(d, r_d)] \times \frac{S_p(0)}{\overline{S}_p(r_d)} \tag{10.12}$$

where K_p is the off-axis ratio representing primary dose at point Q relative to that at the central axis.

$\overline{TMR}(d, r_d)$ may be converted into percent depth dose $P(d, r, f)$ by using Equation 10.4.

$$P(d, r, f) = 100[K_p \cdot TMR(d, 0) + \overline{SMR}(d, r_d)]$$
$$\times \frac{S_p(0)}{\overline{S}_p(r_d)} \times \frac{\overline{S}_p(r_d)}{\overline{S}_p(r_{t_0})} \times \left(\frac{f + t_0}{f + d}\right)^2 \tag{10.13}$$

From Equations 10.7 and 10.13 we get the final expression:

$$P(d, r, f) = 100[K_p \cdot TMR(d, 0) + \overline{SMR}(d, r_d)]$$
$$\times \frac{1}{1 + \overline{SMR}(t_0, r_{t_0})} \times \left(\frac{f + t_0}{f + d}\right)^2 \tag{10.14}$$

Thus, the calculation of percent depth dose for an irregular field requires a

Clarkson integration over the function SMR both at the point of calulation Q as well as at the reference depth (t_0) at central axis.

C.1. SSD VARIATION WITHIN THE FIELD

The percent depth dose at Q is normalized with respect to the $D_{\max}$ on the central axis at depth t_0. Let f_0 be the nominal SSD along the central axis, g be the vertical gap distance, $i.e.$ "gap" between skin surface over Q and the nominal SSD plane, and d be the depth of Q from skin surface. The percent depth dose is then given by

$$\%DD = 100 \times [K_p \cdot TMR(d, 0) + \overline{SMR}(d, r_d)]$$

$$\times \frac{1}{1 + \overline{SMR}(t_0, r_{t_0})} \times \left(\frac{f + t_0}{f + g + d}\right)^2 \quad (10.15)$$

The sign of g should be set positive or negative depending upon the SSD over Q being larger or smaller than the nominal SSD.

C.2. COMPUTER PROGRAM

A computer algorithm embodying Clarkson's principle and scatter-air ratios was developed by Cunningham $et\ al.$ (17) at the Princess Margaret Hospital, Toronto and was published in 1970. Another program, based on the same principle, was developed by the author at the University of Minnesota. It was originally written for the CDC-3300 computer using SARs (12) and later rewritten for the Artronix PC-12 and PDP 11/34 computers. The latter versions use SMRs instead of SARs.

The following data are permanently stored in this computer program: (a) a table of SMRs as functions of radii of circular fields; and (b) the off-axis ratios K_p, measured in air, using an appropriate buildup cap. For energies ≥ 8 MV, K_p values may be measured in phantom at the depth of $D_{\max}$. These data are then stored in the form of a table of K_p as a function of l/L where l is the lateral distance of a point from the central axis and L is the distance along the same line to the geometric edge of the beam. Usually large fields are used for these measurements.

The following data are provided for a particular patient. (a) Contour points: the outline of the irregular field can be drawn from the port (field) film with actual blocks or markers in place to define the field. The field contour is then digitized and the coordinates stored in the computer.

(b) The coordinates (x, y) of the points of calculation are also entered, including the reference point, usually on the central axis, against which the percent depth doses are calculated.

(c) Patient measurements: patient thickness at various points of interest, SSDs, and source to film distance are measured and recorded as shown in Fig. 10.6 for a mantle field as an example.

Figure 10.7 shows a daily dose table calculated by the computer for a typical

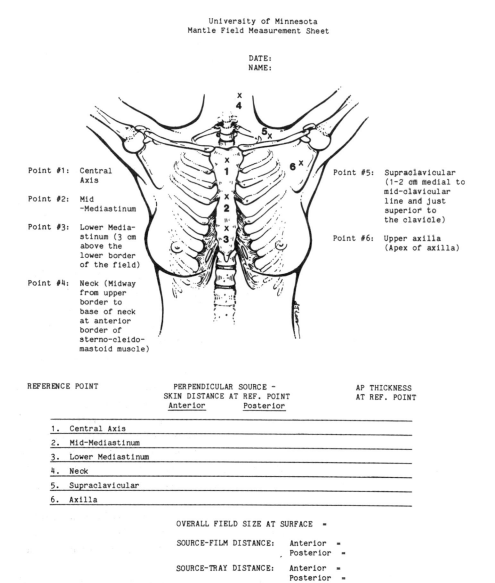

University of Minnesota
Mantle Field Measurement Sheet

DATE:
NAME:

Point #1: Central Axis

Point #2: Mid -Mediastinum

Point #3: Lower Mediastinum (3 cm above the lower border of the field)

Point #4: Neck (Midway from upper border to base of neck at anterior border of sterno-cleido-mastoid muscle)

Point #5: Supraclavicular (1-2 cm medial to mid-clavicular line and just superior to the clavicle)

Point #6: Upper axilla (Apex of axilla)

REFERENCE POINT	PERPENDICULAR SOURCE - SKIN DISTANCE AT REF. POINT		AP THICKNESS AT REF. POINT
	Anterior	Posterior	
1. Central Axis			
2. Mid-Mediastinum			
3. Lower Mediastinum			
4. Neck			
5. Supraclavicular			
6. Axilla			

OVERALL FIELD SIZE AT SURFACE =

SOURCE-FILM DISTANCE: Anterior =
                        Posterior =

SOURCE-TRAY DISTANCE: Anterior =
                        Posterior =

Figure 10.6. Form for recording patient and dosimetric data for mantle field. Note that the measurement points are standardized by anatomical landmarks.

TREATMENT NO.	DMAX ANT	DMAX POST	CA 1	M MED 2	MID 3	WEEK 4	S CLAV 5	U AX 6	L AX 7
1	157		150	147	142	169	173	157	157
2		187	300	294	284	338	346	314	314
3	374		450	442	426	537	519	470	471
4		374	600	589	568	676	692	627	629
5	562		750	736	710	845	865	784	786
6		562	900	883	851	1014	1038	941	943
7	749		1350	1030	993	1183	1211	1098	1100
8		749	1200	1177	1135	1352	1385	1254	1257
9	936		1350	1325	1277	1520	1558	1411	1414
10		936	1500	1472	1419	1689	1731	1568	1571
11	1123		1650	1619	1561	1858	1904	1725	1729
12		1123	1800	1766	1703	2027	2077	1881	1886
13	1310		1950	1913	1845	2196	2250	2038	2043
14		1310	2100	2060	1987	2365	2423	2195	2200
15	1498		2250	2208	2129	2534	2596	2352	2357
16		1498	2400	2355	2271	2703	2769	2509	2514
17	1685		2550	2502	2412	2872	2942	2665	2671
18		1685	2700	2649	2554	3041	3115	2822	2829
19	1872		2850	2796	2696	3210	3288	2979	2986
20		1872	3000	2943	2838	3379	3461	3136	3143
21	2059		3150	3091	2980	3548	3634	3293	3300
22		2059	3300	3238	3122	3717	3807	3449	3457
23	2247		3450	3385	3264	3886	3981	3606	3614
24		2247	3600	3532	3406	4055	4154	3763	3771
25	2434		3750	3679	3548	4224	4327	3920	3928
26		2434	3900	3826	3690	4392	4500	4077	4086 Rt
27	2621		4050	3974	3832	4561	4673	4233	4243
28		2621	4200	4121	3974	4730	4846	4390	4400
29	2808		4350	4268	4115	4899	5019	4547	4557 Lt
30		2808	4500	4415	4257	5068	5192	4704	4714
31	2995		4650	4562	4399	5237	5365	4860	4871
32		2995	4800	4709	4541	5406	5538	5017	5028
33	3183		4950	4857	4683	5575	5711	5174	5186
34		3183	5100	5004	4825	5744	5884	5331	5343
35	3370		5250	5151	4967	5913	6057	5488	5500

Figure 10.7. Computer output sheet showing cumulative midthickness doses for a mantle field. Total dose to various points is programmed by a line drawn through the table. As soon as a given area reaches its prescribed dose, it is shielded during subsequent treatments. It is not necessary to recalculate the table with this change in blocking since only a few treatments are affected.

mantle field. Such a table is useful in programming treatments so that the dose to various regions of the field can be adjusted. The areas that receive the prescribed dose after a certain number of treatments are shielded for the remaining sessions.

10.3 OTHER PRACTICAL METHODS OF CALCULATING DEPTH DOSE DISTRIBUTION

A. Irregular Fields

Clarkson's technique is a general method of calculating depth dose distribution in an irregularly shaped field but it is not practical for routine manual calculations. Even when computerized, it is time consuming since a considerable amount of input data is required by the computer program. However, with the exception of mantle, inverted Y, and a few other complex fields, reasonably accurate calculations can be made for most blocked fields using an approximate method (12) discussed below.

Figure 10.8 shows a number of blocked fields encountered in radiotherapy. Approximate rectangles may be drawn containing the point of calculation so as to include most of the irradiated area surrounding the point and exclude only those areas that are remote to the point. In so doing, a blocked area may

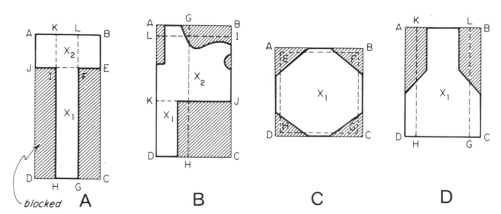

Figure 10.8. Examples of irregularly shaped fields. Equivalent rectangles for dose at points of interest are shown by dashed lines. Points *vs.* equivalent rectangles are: (A) 1, *GHKL*; 2, *ABEJ*; (B) 1, *AGHD*; 2, *LIJK*; (C) 1, *EFGH*; (D) 1, *KLGH*. (Reprinted with permission from: Levitt SH, Tapley N (eds): *Technological Basis of Radiation Therapy: Practical Clinical Applications.* Philadelphia, Lea and Febiger, in press, 1983.

be included in the rectangle provided this area is small and is remotely located relative to that point. The rectangle thus formed may be called the *effective field* while the unblocked field, defined by the collimator, may be called the *collimator field.*

Once the effective field has been determined, one may proceed with the usual calculations as discussed in Section 10.2. However, it is important to remember that, whereas the S_c factors are related to the collimator field, the percent depth dose, TMR, or S_p corresponds to the effective field.

B. Point Off-Axis

It is possible to calculate depth dose distributions at any point within the field or outside the field using Clarkson's technique. However, as stated earlier, it is not practical for manual calculations. Day (13) has proposed a particularly simple calculation method for rectangular fields. In this method, percent depth dose can be calculated at any point within the medium using the central axis data.

In order to calculate dose at any point Q, the field is imagined to be divided into four sections (Fig. 10.9) and their contribution is computed separately. Thus, the dose at depth d along the axis through Q is given by ¼(sum of central axis dose at depth d for fields $2a \times 2b$, $2a \times 2c$, $2d \times 2b$, and $2d \times 2c$).

Suppose the dose in free space on the central axis through P at SSD + d_m is 100 cGy (rad) and its value at a corresponding point over Q is $K_Q \times 100$,

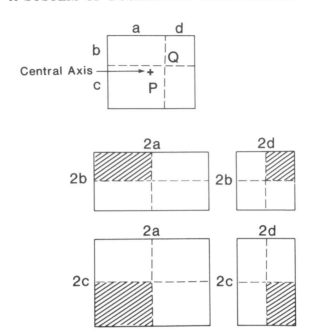

Figure 10.9. Day's method of calculating dose at any point Q in a rectangular field. See text.

where K_Q is the off-axis ratio determined in air from the primary beam profile. If the BSF and central axis %DD for rectangular fields are available, the dose at depth d along the axis through Q will be given by

$$\frac{K_Q \times 100}{4} \text{ (sum of BSF} \times \text{\%DD at depth } d \text{ for fields}$$

$$2a \times 2b, 2a \times 2c, 2d \times 2b, \text{ and } 2d \times 2c)$$

Since the $D_{\max}$ at P is $100 \times \text{BSF}[(a + d) \times (b + c)]$, the percent depth dose at depth d along the axis through Q, relative to $D_{\max}$ at P, will be given by

$$\frac{K_Q}{4 \times \text{BSF}[(a + d) \times (b + c)]} \text{ (sum of BSF} \times \text{\%DD at depth } d \text{ for fields}$$

$$2a \times 2b, 2a \times 2c, 2d \times 2b, \text{ and } 2d \times 2c)$$

EXAMPLE 6

Suppose in Fig. 10.9 that the overall field size is 15×15 cm. Find the percent depth dose at point Q at 10 cm depth, given $a = 10$, $b = 5$, $c = 10$, and $d = 5$. Assume ^{60}Co beam with $K_Q = 0.98$ and SSD = 80 cm.

Using the above procedure and consulting Table A.9.1 in the Appendix at the end of the book, the required percent depth dose is given by

$$\frac{K_Q}{4 \times \text{BSF}(15 \times 15)} [\text{BSF}(20 \times 10) \times \%DD(20 \\ \times 10) + BSF(20 \times 20) \times \%DD(20 \times 20) \\ + \text{BSF}(10 \times 10) \times \%DD(10 \times 10) + \text{BSF}(10 \times 20) \times \%DD(10 \times 20)]$$

or

$$\frac{0.98}{4 \times 1.052} [(1.043 \times 56.3) + (1.061 \times 60.2) \\ + (1.036 \times 55.6) + (1.043 \times 56.3)] = 55.8$$

In the above example, if the primary beam profile was flat, *i.e.* $K_Q = 1$, the percent depth dose at Q would be 56.9 which is still less than 58.4, the percent depth dose at P. This off-axis decrease in dose is due to the reduced scatter at point Q compared to point P. Similarly, it can be shown that the magnitude of the reduction in scatter depends on the distance of Q from P as well as depth. Thus, the depth dose profile across the field is a function not only of the beam flatness in air but also the depth in the phantom.

For higher energy beams (≥ 8 MV), the above procedure may be further simplified by assuming BSF = 1 for all field sizes. Also Day's procedure can be adopted using S_p values instead of BSF since the two quantities are related by Equation 10.1.

C. Point Outside the Field

Day's method can be extended also to the case of determining dose distribution at points outside the field limits. In Fig. 10.10, a rectangular field of dimensions $a \times b$ is shown with the central axis passing through P. Suppose Q is a point outside the field at a distance c from the field border. Imagine a rectangle adjacent to the field such that it contains point Q and has dimensions $2c \times b$. Place another rectangle of dimensions $a \times b$ on the other side of Q such that the field on the right side of Q is a mirror image of the field on the left, as shown in the figure. The dose at point Q at depth d is then given by subtracting the depth dose at Q for field $2c \times b$ from that for field $(2a + 2c) \times b$ and dividing by 2. The procedure is illustrated by the following example.

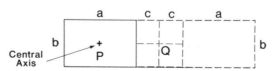

Figure 10.10. Calculation of depth dose outside a rectangular field. See text.

EXAMPLE 7

Suppose it is required to determine percent depth dose at Q (relative to D_{max} at P) outside a 15×10 cm field at a distance of 5 cm from the field border. In Fig. 10.10, then, $a = 15$, $b = 10$, and $c = 5$. Suppose Q is at the center of the middle rectangle of dimensions $2c \times b$. Then, the dose D_Q at 10-cm depth is given by

$$\tfrac{1}{2}[D_Q(40 \times 10) - D_Q(10 \times 10)]$$

If D_Q is normalized to D_{max} at P, one gets the percent depth dose at Q or $\% D_Q$.

$$\% D_Q = \frac{1}{BSF(15 \times 15)} \cdot \tfrac{1}{2}[BSF(40 \times 10) \times \% DD(40$$

$$\times 10) - BSF(10 \times 10) \times \% DD(10 \times 10)]$$

Thus for a ^{60}Co beam at SSD = 80 cm,

$$\% D_Q = \frac{1}{1.052} \cdot \tfrac{1}{2}[1.054 \times 58.8 - 1.036 \times 55.6] = 2.1$$

Again for higher energy beams, the above procedure is simplified by assuming BSF = 1. Also, if S_p values are known instead of BSF, the above calculation can be performed by substituting S_p for BSF.

D. Point under the Block

As discussed earlier, the dose distribution in a blocked field is best determined by Clarkson's method of irregular field dosimetry. However, if the blocked portion of the field is approximated to a rectangle, a simpler method known as negative field method may be used. The concept of negative field has been described in the literature (14, 15). In this method, the dose at any point is equal to the dose from the overall (unblocked) field minus the dose expected if the entire field were blocked, leaving the shielded volume open. In other words, the blocked portion of the field is considered a negative field and its contribution is subtracted from the overall field dose distribution.

A computerized negative field method is not only a fast method of calculating isodose distribution in blocked fields, it is very convenient for manual point dose calculation. Its practical usefulness will be illustrated by the example discussed below.

EXAMPLE 8

A patient is treated with a split field of overall size 15×15 cm, blocked in the middle to shield a region of size 4×15 cm on the surface (Fig. 10.11). Calculate (a) the treatment time to deliver 200 cGy (rad) at 10 cm depth at point P in the open portion of the field and (b) what percentage of that dose is received at point Q in the middle of the blocked area, given ^{60}Co beam, SSD

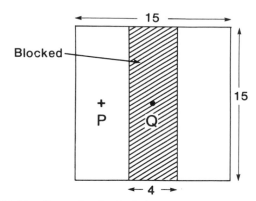

Figure 10.11.   Example of calculating depth dose under a block.

= 80 cm, dose rate free space for 15 × 15 cm field at 80.5 cm = 120 rads/min, lead block thickness = 5 cm with primary beam transmission of 5%, and shadow tray (or block tray) transmission = 0.97.

(a) Approximate equivalent field at point $P \simeq 5.5 \times 15$, assuming negligible scatter contribution to P from the other open portion of the field across the blocked area.

$A/P(5.5 \times 15) = 2.01$

Equivalent square = $4 \times A/P = 8 \times 8$ cm

$\%DD(10, 8 \times 8, 80) = 54.0$

BSF = 1.029

$$\text{Treatment time} = \frac{200 \times 100}{120 \times 1.029 \times 54.0 \times 0.97}$$

$$= 3.09 \text{ min}$$

(b) $D_Q = D_Q(15 \times 15) - D_Q(4 \times 15) \times (1 - T)$ where T is the transmission factor for the lead block.

$D_Q(15 \times 15)$ = (dose rate free space × time) × BSF × %DD

$$= 120 \times 3.09 \times 1.052 \times \frac{58.4}{100}$$

$$= 227.8 \text{ cGy}$$

$$D_Q(4 \times 15) = 120 \times 3.09 \times 1.023 \times \frac{52.3}{100} \quad [A/P(4 \times 15) = 1.58.$$
$$\text{Equivalent square} = 6.3 \times 6.3 \text{ cm}]$$

$$= 198.4 \text{ cGy}$$

Thus

$$D_Q = 227.8 - 198.4(1 - 0.05)$$

$$= 39.3 \text{ cGy}$$

Since $D_p = 200$ cGy (given)

$$D_Q \text{ as a percentage of } D_p = \frac{D_Q}{D_p} \times 100 = \frac{39.3}{200} \times 100$$

$$= 20\%$$

Alternative. Let us project all fields at depth = 10 cm.

$$\text{Magnification} = \frac{80 + 10}{80} = 1.125$$

Projected fields.

(15×15) cm $\times 1.125 = 17 \times 17$ cm

(4×15) cm $\times 1.125 = 4.5 \times 17$ cm $= 7 \times 7$ cm eq square

(5.5×15) cm $\times 1.125 = 6.2 \times 17$ cm $= 9 \times 9$ cm eq square

$$\frac{D_Q}{D_p} = \frac{\text{TAR}(10, 17 \times 17) - [\text{TAR}(10, 7 \times 7)](1 - T)}{\text{TAR}(10, 9 \times 9)}$$

$$= \frac{0.771 - 0.667(1 - 0.05)}{0.694}$$

$$= 0.20 \text{ or } 20\%$$

Alternative. Since $\text{TAR}(d, r_d) = \text{TMR}(d, r_d) \cdot S_p(r_d)$ (from Equation 10.5)

$$\frac{D_Q}{D_p} = \frac{\text{TMR}(10, 17 \times 17) \cdot S_p(17 \times 17) - \text{TMR}(10, 7 \times 7) \cdot S_p(7 \times 7)(1 - T)}{\text{TMR}(10, 9 \times 9) \cdot S_p(9 \times 9)}$$

Substituting values from Table A.9.2 in the Appendix at the end of the book

$$\frac{D_Q}{D_p} = \frac{0.733 \times 1.02 - 0.651 \times 0.989(1 - 0.05)}{0.672 \times 0.997}$$

$$= 0.20 \text{ or } 20\%$$

Note that although the primary transmission through the lead block is only 5%, the dose at 10-cm depth under the block in the middle is about 20% of the dose in the open portion. This increase in dose is due to the internal scatter contributed by the open areas of the field to point Q. Of course, the dose under the block depends on the extent of the blocked area, overall field size, block thickness, depth, and location of point Q.

APPENDIX

A. Derivation of S_p

$S_p(r)$, as defined in Section 10.1B, is the ratio of dose rate for the given field (r) at a reference depth to the dose rate at the same point for the reference field (r_0), with the same collimator opening. This is illustrated in Fig. 10.12. The given field in diagram A is blocked down to the size of the reference field in diagram B without changing the collimator opening. Thus, both arrangements have the same collimator scatter factor, $S_c(r)$, but different phantom scatter. Let D_{fs} and D_{max} be the free space dose rate and D_{max} dose rate, respectively. Then, at the reference depth of maximum dose,

$$S_p(r) = \frac{D_{max} \text{ in arrangement A}}{D_{max} \text{ in arrangement B}}$$

$$= \frac{D_{fs}(r_0) \cdot S_c(r) \cdot \text{BSF}(r)}{D_{fs}(r_0) \cdot S_c(r) \cdot \text{BSF}(r_0)} \tag{A1}$$

$$= \frac{\text{BSF}(r)}{BSF(r_0)} \tag{A2}$$

which is the same as Equation 10.1.

Equation A1 can also be written as:

$$S_p(r) = \frac{D_{fs}(r) \cdot \text{BSF}(r)}{D_{fs}(r_0) \cdot \text{BSF}(r_0) \cdot S_c(r)}$$

$$= \frac{D_{max}(r)}{D_{max}(r_0) \cdot S_c(r)}$$

$$= \frac{S_{c,p}(r)}{S_c(r)} \tag{A3}$$

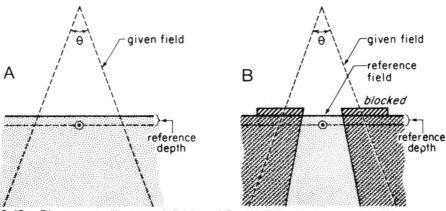

Figure 10.12. Diagrams to illustrate definition of S_p. (A) Dose in phantom at reference depth for a given field. (B) Dose at the same point for a reference field with the same collimator opening. [Reprinted with permission from: Khan *et al.* (4).]

where $S_{c,p}(r)$ is the total scatter correction factor defined as the ratio of D_{max} dose rate for a given field to the D_{max} dose rate for the reference field (see Fig. 10.1B).

B. Derivation of TMR

In Fig. 10.2, let D_1 and D_2 be the doses at depths d and t_0 (reference depth of maximum dose), respectively. Let r, r_{t_0}, and r_d be the field sizes at distances f, $f + t_0$, and $f + d$ from the source, respectively. Then, by definition

$$\text{TMR}(d, r_d) = \frac{D_1}{D_2} \qquad (A4)$$

and

$$\frac{D_1}{D(t_0, r_{t_0}, f)} = \frac{P(d, r, f)}{100} \qquad (A5)$$

where $D(t_0, r_{t_0}, f)$ is the dose at depth t_0, field size r_{t_0} and SSD $= f$.

$$\frac{D_2}{D(t_0, r_{t_0}, f)} = \frac{S_p(r_d)}{S_p(r_{t_0})} \cdot \left(\frac{f + t_0}{f + d}\right)^2 \qquad (A6)$$

Combining Equations A4, A5, and A6,

$$\text{TMR}(d, r_d) = \frac{P(d, r, f)}{100} \left(\frac{f + d}{f + t_0}\right)^2 \left(\frac{S_p(r_{t_0})}{S_p(r_d)}\right) \qquad (A7)$$

C. Derivation of SMR

Referring to Fig. 10.2, let $D_1(d, r_d)$ be the dose at point 1 and $D_2(t_0, r_d)$ be the dose at point 2 for field size r_d. Let $D_1(d, 0)$ and $D_2(t_0, 0)$ be the corresponding doses for 0×0 field with the same collimator opening. Then,

$$\text{SMR}(d, r_d) = \frac{D_1(d, r_d) - D_1(d, 0)}{D_2(t_0, 0)} \qquad (A8)$$

or

$$\text{SMR}(d, r_d) = \frac{D_1(d, r_d)}{D_2(t_0, r_d)} \times \frac{D_2(t_0, r_d)}{D_2(t_0, r_0)} \times \frac{D_2(t_0, r_0)}{D_2(t_0, 0)} - \frac{D_1(d, 0)}{D_2(t_0, 0)} \qquad (A9)$$

where r_0 is the reference field (10×10 cm) for normalizing S_p factors. Since

$$\text{TMR}(d, r_d) = \frac{D_1(d, r_d)}{D_2(t_0, r_d)}$$

$$\text{TMR}(d, 0) = \frac{D_1(d, 0)}{D_2(t_0, 0)}$$

$$S_p(r_d) = \frac{D_2(t_0, r_d)}{D_2(t_0, r_0)}$$

and

$$S_p(0) = \frac{D_2(t_0, 0)}{D_2(t_0, r_0)}$$

Equation A9 becomes

$$\text{SMR}(d, r_d) = \text{TMR}(d, r_d) \cdot \frac{S_p(r_d)}{S_p(0)} - \text{TMR}(d, 0) \qquad \text{(A10)}$$

References

1. Karzmark CJ, Deubert A, Loevinger R: Tissue-phantom ratios—an aid to treatment planning. *Br J Radiol* 38:158, 1965.
2. Holt JG: Letter to the editor. *Am Assoc Phys Med Q Bull* 6:127, 1972.
3. Saunders JE, Price RH, Horsley RJ: Central axis depth doses for a constant source-tumor distance. *Br J Radiol* 41:464, 1968.
4. Khan FM, Sewchand W, Lee J, Williamson JF: Revision of tissue-maximum ratio and scatter-maximum ratio concepts for cobalt 60 and higher energy x-ray beams. *Med Phys* 7:230, 1980.
5. Khan FM: Dose distribution problems in cobalt teletherapy. Thesis, University of Minnesota, p 106, 1969.
6. Cundiff JH, Cunningham JR, Golden R, Holt G, Lanzl M, Meurk L, Ovadia J, Page V, Pope RA, Sampiere VA, Saylor WL, Shalek RJ, Suntharalingam N: In *Dosimetry Workshop on Hodgkin's Disease* compiled by RPC/AAPM. Houston, MD Anderson Hospital, 1970.
7. Almond P, Roosenbeek EV, Browne R, Milcamp J, Williams CB: Variation in the position of the central axis maximum build-up point with field size for high-energy photon beams (Letter to the Editor). *Br J Radiol* 43:911, 1970.
8. Dawson DJ: Percentage depth doses for high energy x-rays. *Phys Med Biol* 21:226, 1976.
9. Bagne F: Physical aspects of supervoltage x-ray therapy. *Med Phys* 1:266, 1974.
10. Suntharalingam N, Steben DJ: Physical characterization of 45-MV photon beams for use in treatment planning. *Med Phys* 4:134, 1977.
11. Johns HE, Bruce WR, Reid WB: The dependence of depth dose on focal skin distance. *Br J Radiol* 31:254, 1958.
12. Khan FM, Levitt SH, Moore VC, Jones TK: Computer and approximation methods of calculating depth dose in irregularly shaped fields. *Radiology* 106:433, 1973.
13. Day MJ: A note on the calculation of dose in x-ray fields. *Br J Radiol* 23:368, 1950.
14. Sundbom L: Method of dose planning on application of shielding filters in cobalt 60 teletherapy. *Acta Radiol Ther Phys Biol* 3:210, 1965.
15. Khan FM: Computer dosimetry of partially blocked fields in cobalt teletherapy. *Radiology* 97:405, 1970.
16. Hospital Physicists' Association: Central axis depth dose data for use in radiotherapy. *Br J Radiol* Suppl 11, 1978.
17. Cunningham JR, Shrivastava PN, Wilkinson JM: Computer calculation of dose within an irregularly shaped beam. In *Dosimetry Workshop on Hodgkin's Disease*, compiled by RPC/AAPM. Houston, MD Anderson Hospital, 1970.
18. Holt JG, Laughlin JS, Moroney JP: The extension of the concept of tissue-air ratios (TAR) to high energy x-ray beams. *Radiology* 96:437, 1970.

CHAPTER 11

Treatment Planning I: Isodose Distributions

The central axis depth dose distribution by itself is not sufficient to characterize a radiation beam which produces a dose distribution in a three-dimensional volume. In order to represent volumetric or planar variation in absorbed dose, distributions are depicted by means of *isodose curves* which are lines passing through points of equal dose. The curves are usually drawn at regular intervals of absorbed dose and expressed as a percentage of the dose at a reference point. Thus, the isodose curves represent levels of absorbed dose in the same manner that isotherms are used for heat and isobars for pressure.

11.1 ISODOSE CHART

An *isodose chart* for a given beam consists of a family of isodose curves usually drawn at equal increments of percent depth dose, representing the variation in dose as a function of depth and transverse distance from the central axis. The depth dose values of the curves are normalized either at the point of maximum dose on the central axis or at a fixed distance along the central axis in the irradiated medium. The charts in the first category are applicable when the patient is treated at a constant SSD irrespective of beam direction. In the second category, the isodose curves are normalized at a certain depth beyond the depth of maximum dose, corresponding to the axis of rotation of an isocentric therapy unit. This type of representation is especially useful in rotation therapy but can also be used for stationary isocentric treatments. Figure 11.1, A and B, shows both types of isodose charts for a ^{60}Co γ ray beam.

Examination of the isodose charts in Fig. 11.1 reveals some general properties of x- and γ-ray dose distributions.

1) The dose at any depth is greatest on the central axis of the beam and gradually decreases toward the edges of the beam, with the exception of some beams which exhibit areas of high dose or "horns" near the surface in the periphery of the field. These horns are created by the flattening filter which is usually designed to overcompensate near the surface in order to obtain flat isodose curves at greater depths.

2) Near the edges of the beam (the penumbra region), the dose rate decreases rapidly as a function of lateral distance from the beam axis. As discussed in Section 4.7, the width of geometric penumbra, which exists both

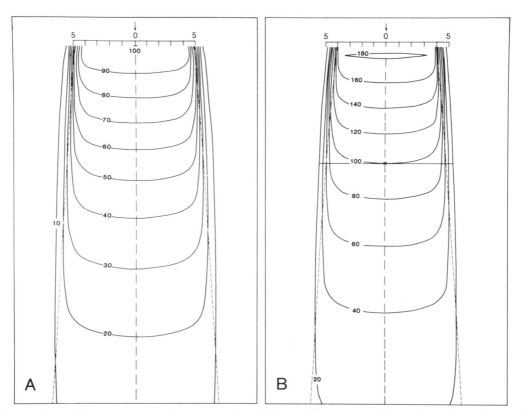

Figure 11.1. Example of an isodose chart. A, SSD type, ^{60}Co beam, SSD = 80 cm, field size = 10 × 10 cm at surface. B, SAD type, ^{60}Co beam, SAD = 100 cm, depth of isocenter = 10 cm, field size at isocenter = 10 × 10 cm. (Data from University of Minnesota Hospitals, Eldorado 8 Cobalt Unit, source size = 2 cm.)

inside and outside the geometrical boundaries of the beam, depends on source size, distance from the source, and source-to-diaphragm distance.

3) Near the beam edge, falloff of the beam is due not only to the geometric penumbra but also to the reduced side scatter. Therefore, the geometric penumbra is not the best measure of beam sharpness near the edges. Instead the term *physical penumbra* may be used. The *physical penumbra* width is defined as the lateral distance between two specified isodose curves at a specified depth (*e.g.* lateral distance between 90% and 20% isodose lines at the depth of D_{max}).

4) Outside the geometric limits of the beam and the penumbra, the dose variation is due to side scatter from the field and both leakage and scatter from the collimator system. Beyond this collimator zone, the dose distribution is governed by the lateral scatter from the medium and leakage from the head of the machine (often called *therapeutic housing* or *source housing*).

Figure 11.2 shows the dose variation across the field at a specified depth.

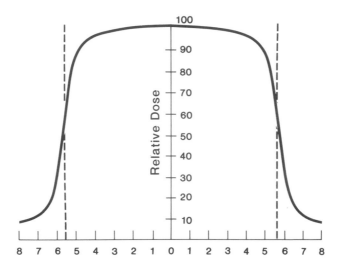

Figure 11.2. Depth dose profile showing variation of dose across the field. ^{60}Co beam, SSD = 80 cm, depth = 10 cm, field size at surface = 10 × 10 cm. Dotted line indicates geometric field boundary at 10-cm depth.

Such a representation of the beam is known as the *beam profile*. It may be noted that the field size is defined as the lateral distance between the 50% isodose lines at a reference depth. This definition is practically achieved by a procedure called the beam *alignment* in which the field-defining light is made to coincide with the 50% isodose lines of the radiation beam projected on a plane perpendicular to the beam axis and at the standard SSD or SAD.

Another way of depicting the dose variation across the field is to plot isodose curves in a plane perpendicular to the central axis of the beam (Fig. 11.3). Such a representation is useful for treatment planning in which the field sizes are determined on the basis of an isodose curve (*e.g.* 90%) that adequately covers the target volume.

11.2 MEASUREMENT OF ISODOSE CURVES

Isodose charts can be measured by means of ion chambers, solid state detectors, or radiographic films (Chapter 8). Of these, the ion chamber is the most reliable method, mainly because of its relatively flat energy response and precision. Although any of the phantoms described in Section 9.1 may be used for isodose measurements, water is the medium of choice for ionometric measurements. The chamber can be made waterproof by a thin plastic sleeve which covers the chamber as well as the portion of the cable immersed in the water.

As measurement of isodose charts has been discussed in some detail in ICRU Report 23 (see Reference 1), only a few important points will be discussed here. The ionization chamber used for isodose measurements should

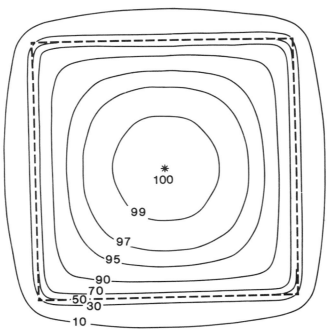

Figure 11.3.   Cross sectional isodose distribution in a plane perpendicular to the central axis of the beam. Isodose values are normalized to 100% at the center of the field.

be small so that measurements can be made in regions of high dose gradient, such as that near the edges of the beam. It is recommended that the sensitive volume of the chamber be less than 15 mm long and have an inside diameter of 5 mm or less. Energy independence of the chamber is another important requirement. Since the x-ray beam spectrum changes with position in the phantom due to scatter, the energy response of the chamber should be as flat as possible. This can be checked by obtaining the exposure calibration of the chamber for orthovoltage (1–4 mm Cu) and ^{60}Co beams. A variation of about 5% in response throughout this energy range is acceptable.

Automatic devices for measuring isodose curves have been developed for rapid mapping of the isodose curves. These systems are designed to be either stand-alone or computer-driven. Basically, the apparatus (Fig. 11.4) consists of two ionization chambers, referred to as the detector A (or probe) and the monitor B. Whereas the probe is arranged to move in the tank of water to sample the dose rate at various points, the monitor is fixed at some point in the field to monitor the beam intensity with time. The ratio of the detector to the monitor response (A/B) is recorded as the probe is moved in the phantom. Thus, the final response A/B is independent of fluctuations in output. In the stand-alone system, the probe searches for points at which A/B is equal to a preset percentage value of A/B measured at a reference depth or the depth of maximum dose. The motion of the probe is transmitted to the plotter which records its path, the isodose curve.

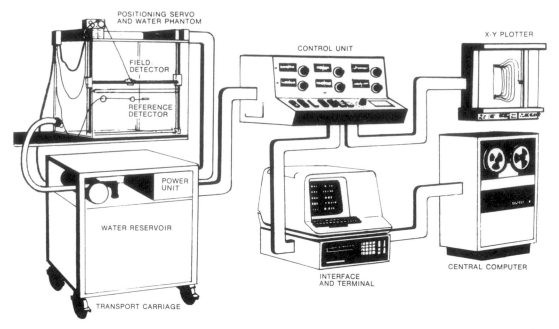

Figure 11.4. Schematic diagram of an automatic isodose plotter system, "Therados RFA-3." (Reprinted with permission from: Instrument AB Therados, Uppsala, Sweden.)

In the computer-driven models, the chamber movement of the probe is controlled by a computer program. The probe to monitor ratio is sampled as the probe moves across the field at preset increments. These beam profiles are measured at a number of depths, determined by computer program. The data thus measured are stored in the computer in the form of a matrix which can then be transformed into isodose curves or other formats allowed by the computer program.

A. Sources of Isodose Charts

Acquisition of isodose charts is discussed in ICRU Report 23 (1). Atlases of premeasured isodose charts for a wide range of radiotherapy equipment are available from the sources listed in References 2, 3, and 4. In addition, isodose distributions may also be obtained from manufacturers of radiation generators or from other institutions having the same unit. However, the user is cautioned against accepting isodose charts from any source and using them as basis for patient treatment without adequate verification. The first and most important check to be performed is to verify that the central axis depth dose data corresponds with percent depth dose data measured independently in a water phantom. A deviation of 2% or less in local dose is acceptable up to depths of 20 cm. The edges of the distribution should be checked by measuring beam profiles for selected field sizes and depths. An agreement within 2 mm in the penumbra region is acceptable.

Besides direct measurements, isodose charts can also be generated by calculations using various algorithms for treatment planning (5–9). Some of these programs are commercially available with treatment planning computers. Again, the applicability of the computer-generated isodose curves to the user's machine must be carefully checked.

11.3 PARAMETERS OF ISODOSE CURVES

Among the parameters that affect the single beam isodose distribution are beam quality, source size, beam collimation, field size, source-surface distance (SSD), and the source-diaphragm distance (SDD). A discussion of these parameters will be presented in the context of treatment planning.

A. Beam Quality

As discussed earlier, the central axis depth dose distribution depends on the beam energy. As a result, the depth of a given isodose curve increases with beam quality. Beam energy also influences isodose curve shape near the field borders. Greater lateral scatter associated with lower energy beams causes the isodose curves outside the field to bulge out. In other words, the absorbed dose in the medium outside the primary beam is greater for low energy beams than for those of higher energy.

Physical penumbra depends on beam quality as illustrated in Fig. 11.5. As expected, the isodose curves outside the primary beam (*e.g.* 10% and 5%) are greatly distended in the case of orthovoltage radiation. Thus, one disadvantage of the orthovoltage beams is the increased scattered dose to tissue outside the treatment region. For megavoltage beams, on the other hand, the scatter outside the field is minimized due to predominantly forward scattering and becomes more a function of collimation than energy.

B. Source Size, SSD, and SDD—the Penumbra Effect

These three parameters affect the shape of isodose curves by virtue of the geometric penumbra, discussed in Section 4.7. In addition, the SSD affects the percent depth dose and therefore the depth of the isodose curves.

As discussed earlier, the dose variation across the field border is a complex function of geometric penumbra, lateral scatter, and collimation. Therefore, the field sharpness at depth is not simply determined by the source or focal spot size. For example, by using penumbra trimmers or secondary blocking, the isodose sharpness at depth for ^{60}Co beams with a source size less than 2 cm in diameter can be made comparable to higher energy linac beams although the focal spot size of these beams is usually less than 2 mm. Comparison of isodose curves for ^{60}Co, 4 and 10 MV in Fig. 11.5, illustrates the point that the physical penumbra width for these beams is more or less similar.

C. Collimation and Flattening Filter

The term collimation is used here to designate not only the collimator blocks that give shape and size to the beam but also the flattening filter and

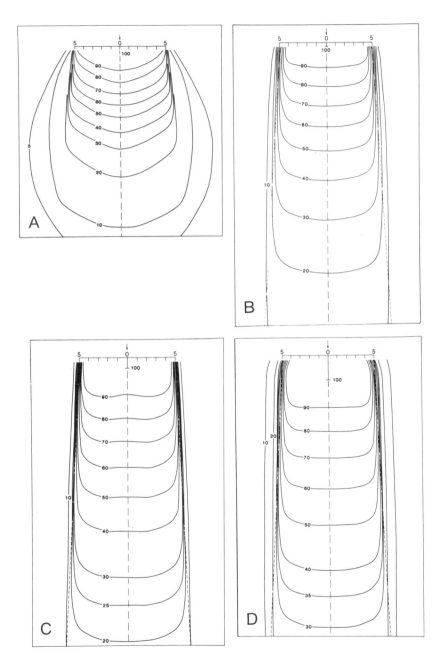

Figure 11.5. Isodose distributions for different quality radiations. A, 200 kVp, SSD = 50 cm, HVL = 1 mm Cu, field size = 10 × 10 cm. B, ^{60}Co, SSD = 80 cm, field size = 10 × 10 cm. C, 4-MV x-rays, SSD = 100 cm, field size = 10 × 10 cm. D, 10-MV x-rays, SSD = 100 cm, field size = 10 × 10 cm.

other absorbers or scatterers in the beam between the target and the patient. Of these, the flattening filter which is used for megavoltage x-ray beams has the greatest influence in determining the shape of the isodose curves. Without this filter, the isodose curves will be conical in shape showing markedly increased x-ray intensity along the central axis and a rapid reduction transversely. The function of the flattening filter is to make the beam intensity distribution relatively uniform across the field (*i.e.* "flat"). Therefore, the filter is thickest in the middle and tapers off toward the edges.

The cross sectional variation of the filter thickness also causes variation in the photon spectrum or beam quality across the field due to selective hardening of the beam by the filter. In general, the average energy of the beam is somewhat lower for the peripheral areas compared to the central part of the beam. This change in quality across the beam causes the flatness to change with depth. However, the change in flatness with depth is not only caused by the selective hardening of the beam across the field but also the changes in the distribution of radiation scatter as the depth increases.

Beam flatness is usually specified at 10-cm depth with the maximum limits set at the depth of maximum dose. By careful design of the filter and accurate placement in the beam, it is possible to achieve flatness to within ±3% of the central axis dose value at 10-cm depth. This degree of flatness should extend over the central area bounded by at least 80% of the field dimensions at the specified depth or 1 cm from the edge of field. The above specification is satisfactory for the precision required in radiotherapy.

In order to obtain acceptable flatness at 10-cm depth, an area of high dose near the surface may have to be accepted. Although the extent of the high dose regions or "horns" varies with the design of the filter, lower energy beams exhibit a larger variation than higher energy beams. In practice, it is acceptable to have these "superflat" isodose curves near the surface provided no point in any plane parallel to the surface receives dose greater than 107% of the central axis value (10).

D. Field Size

Field size is one of the most important parameters in treatment planning. Adequate dosimetric coverage of the tumor requires a determination of appropriate field size. This determination must always be made dosimetrically rather than geometrically. In other words, a certain isodose curve (*e.g.* 90%) enclosing the treatment volume should be the guide in choosing a field size rather than the geometric dimensions of the field.

Great caution should also be exercised in using field sizes smaller than 6 cm in which a relatively large part of the field is in the penumbra region. Depending upon the source size, collimation, and design of the flattening filter, the isodose curves for small field sizes, in general, tend to be bell-shaped. Thus, treatment planning with isodose curves should be mandatory for small field sizes.

The isodose curvature for ^{60}Co increases as the field size becomes overly large unless the beam is flattened by a flattening filter. The reason for this effect is the progressive reduction of scattered radiation with increasing distance from the central axis as well as the obliquity of the primary rays. The effect becomes particularly severe with elongated fields such as cranial spinal fields used in the treatment of medulloblastoma. In these cases, one needs to calculate doses at several off-axis points or use a beam-flattening compensator.

11.4 WEDGE FILTERS

Frequently, special filters or absorbing blocks are placed in the path of a beam to modify its isodose distribution. The most commonly used beam-modifying device is the *wedge filter*. This is a wedge-shaped absorber which causes a progressive decrease in the intensity across the beam, resulting in a tilt of the isodose curves from their normal positions. As shown in Fig. 11.6 the isodose curves are tilted toward the thin end, the degree of tilt being dependent on the slope of the wedge filter. In actual wedge filter design, the sloping surface is made either straight or sigmoid in shape, the latter design being used to produce straighter isodose curves.

The wedge is usually made of a dense material, such as lead or copper, and is mounted on a transparent plastic tray which can be inserted in the beam at a specified distance from the source (Fig. 11.7). This distance is arranged such that the wedge tray is always at a distance of at least 15 cm from the skin

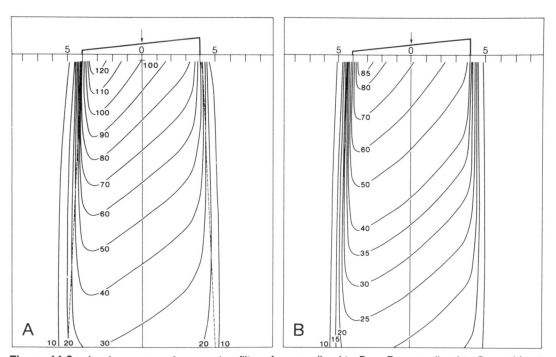

Figure 11.6. Isodose curves for a wedge filter. A, normalized to D_{max}. B, normalized to D_{max} without the wedge. ^{60}Co, wedge angle = 45° field size = 8 × 10 cm, SSD = 80 cm.

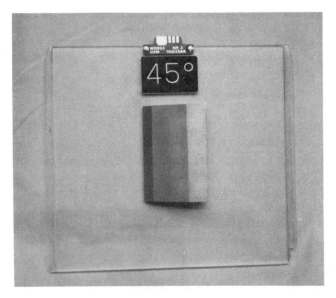

Figure 11.7.   Photograph of a 45° wedge filter for a 4-MV x-ray linac (ATC 400).

surface, so as to avoid destroying the skin-sparing effect of the megavoltage beam.

A. Wedge Isodose Angle

The term *wedge isodose angle* (or simply *wedge angle*) refers to "the angle through which an isodose curve is titled at the central ray of a beam at a specified depth" (11). In this definition, one should note that the wedge angle is the angle between the isodose curve and the normal to the central axis, as shown in Fig. 11.6. In addition, the specification of depth is important since, in general, the presence of scattered radiation causes the angle of isodose tilt to decrease with increasing depth in the phantom. However, there is no general agreement as to the choice of reference depth. Some choose depth as a function of field size (*e.g.* ½ or ⅔ of the beam width) while others define wedge angle as the angle between the 50% isodose curve and the normal to the central axis. The latter choice, however, becomes impractical when higher energy beams are used. For example, the central axis depth of the 50% isodose curve for a 10-MV beam lies at about 18 cm for a 10 × 10 cm field and 100-cm SSD. This depth is too large in the context of wedge filter application. As will be discussed in Section 11.7, the wedge filters are mostly used for treating superficial tumors, *e.g.* not more than 10 cm deep. Therefore, the current recommendation is to use a single reference depth of 10 cm for wedge angle specification (11).

B. Wedge Transmission Factor

The presence of a wedge filter decreases the output of the machine which must be taken into account in treatment calculations. This effect is characterized by the *wedge transmission factor* (or simply *wedge factor*), defined as the ratio of outputs with and without the wedge, at a point along the central axis of the beam. This factor can be measured either in air or in phantom at the depth of maximum dose.

The wedge factor is sometimes incorporated into the isodose curves, as shown in Fig. 11.6B. In this case, the depth dose distribution is normalized relative to the D_{max} without the wedge. For example, the isodose curve at depth of D_{max} is 72%, indicating that the wedge factor is already taken into account in the isodose distribution. If such a chart is used for isodose planning, no further correction should be applied to the output. In other words, the machine output corresponding to the open beam should be used.

A more common approach is to normalize the isodose curves relative to the central axis D_{max} with the wedge in the beam. As seen in Fig. 11.6A, the 100% dose is indicated at the depth of D_{max}. With this approach, the output of the beam must be corrected using the wedge factor.

C. Wedge Systems

Wedge filters are of two main types. The first may be called the *individualized wedge system* which requires a separate wedge for each beam width, optimally designed to minimize the loss of beam output. A mechanism is provided to align the thin end of the wedge with the border of the light field (Fig. 11.8A). The second system uses a *"universal wedge,"* i.e. a single wedge serves for all beam widths. Such a filter is fixed centrally in the beam while the field can be opened to any size. As illustrated in Fig. 11.8B, only a small part of this wedge, i.e. ABC, is effective in producing the given wedge angle. The rest ($ACDE$), being unwedged, does not contribute to the isodose tilt but unnecessarily reduces the beam intensity. Since the individualized system economizes on the beam output, it is preferred for use in cobalt teletherapy. The universal wedge, on the other hand, is useful for linear accelerator beams where the output is plentiful. From the setup and treatment planning point of view, the universal wedge is simpler to use than the individualized filter.

D. Effect on Beam Quality

In general, the wedge filter alters the beam quality by preferentially attenuating the lower energy photons (beam hardening) and, to a lesser extent, by Compton scattering which results in energy degradation (beam softening). For ^{60}Co beam, because the primary beam is essentially monoenergetic, the presence of the wedge filter does not significantly alter the central axis percent depth dose distribution. For x-rays, on the other hand, there can be some beam hardening (12) and, consequenty, the depth dose distribution can be somewhat altered, especially at large depths.

Although the wedge filters produce some change in beam quality, as noted above, the effect is not large enough to alter other calculation parameters such as the backscatter factor or the equivalent square which may be assumed to be the same as for the corresponding open beams. Even central axis percent

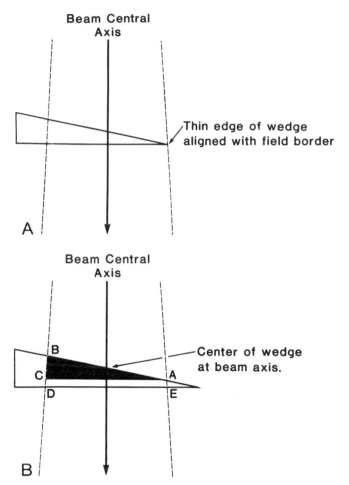

Figure 11.8. Schematic representation of (A) individualized wedge for a specific field width in which the thin end of wedge is always aligned with the field border; and (B) universal wedge is which the center of wedge filter is fixed at beam axis and field can be opened to any width.

depth doses, TARs or TMRs may be assumed unchanged for small depths (*e.g.* less than 10 cm).

E. Design of Wedge Filters

The design of wedge filters for megavoltage beams has been described by many authors (13–16). Here we will briefly present the design of a universal wedge filter following the technique of Aron and Scapicchio (16). The principle of this method is to determine the ratio of percent depth doses at various points for wedged and nonwedged fields. The thickness of the wedge filter material at these points is then determined from these ratios and the knowledge of the half-value layer or the attenuation coefficient of the given beam for the filter material.

Figure 11.9 illustrates the design of a wedge filter. A line is drawn at a selected depth across the nonwedged field at right angles to the central axis. This depth should correspond to the reference depth used for the wedge angle definition. Fan lines, representing rays from the source, are drawn at fixed intervals (*e.g.* 1 cm) on both sides of the central axis. A series of parallel lines is drawn making angle with the central axis equal to the complement of the given wedge angle and intersecting the central axis at the same points of intersection as the nonwedged isodose lines. A table is constructed which includes the percentage depth doses at the points of intersection of the fan lines and the reference depth line, for the nonwedged isodose curves and the wedged isodose lines (sloping lines). The ratio of the wedged to nonwedged values is calculated as shown in Table 11.1. These ratios are normalized to the highest value within the field (excluding the penumbra region) to give the relative transmission ratio along the designated fan lines. A wedge filter of a given material can then be designed to provide these transmission ratios.

11.5 COMBINATION OF RADIATION FIELDS

Treatment by a single photon beam is seldom used except in some cases where the tumor is superficial. The following criteria of acceptability may be used for a single field treatment: (a) the dose distribution within the tumor

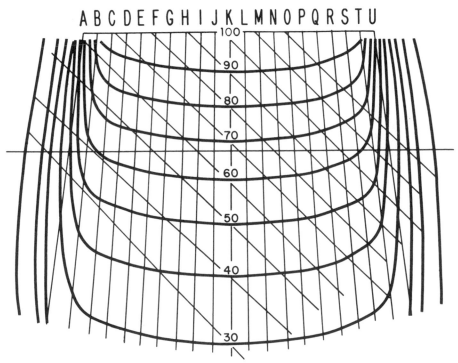

Figure 11.9. New 45° lines constructed parallel to one another, intersecting central axis at same points of intersection as nonwedge isodose lines. Redrawn from Aron and Scapicchio (16).

Table 11.1
Transmission ratios for the construction of wedge filter

	A	B	C	E	G	I	K	M	O	Q	S	T	U
Nonwedge iso-dose	40	55	62	65	67	68	68	68	67	65	62	55	40
Wedge iso-dose	35	39	41	47	53	60	68	76	86	95	105	110	115
Ratio Wedge/nonwedge	0.875	0.710	0.660	0.720	0.790	0.880	1.00	1.12	1.28	1.46	1.70	1.20	2.88
Transmission ratio			0.387	0.425	0.462	0.515	0.59	0.66	0.75	0.86	1.0		
mm Pb			15.2	13.6	12.2	10.5	8.3	6.5	4.5	2.3	0		

From Reference 16.

volume is reasonably uniform (*e.g.* within ±5%); (b) the maximum dose to the tissues in the beam is not excessive (*e.g.* not more than 110% of the prescribed dose); and (c) normal critical structures in the beam do not receive doses near or beyond tolerance. Whereas single fields of superficial x-rays are routinely used for treating skin cancers which are confined to a depth of a few millimeters, single megavoltage beams are used only in rare cases where a combination of beams is either technically difficult or results in unnecessary or excessive irradiation of the normal tissues. Examples of a few treatments which use single megavoltage beams are the supraclavicular region, internal mammary nodes (anterior field), and the spinal cord (posterior field). Although the dose distribution is not ideal, the single field technique in these cases results in simplicity of setup without violating the above criteria of acceptability.

For treatment of most tumors, however, a combination of two or more beams is required for an acceptable distribution of dose within the tumor and the surrounding normal tissues. Although radiation fields may be combined in many ways, the discussion here will be confined to the basic principles which are useful in treating tumors involving different sites.

A. Parallel Opposed Fields

The simplest combination of two fields is a pair of fields directed along the same axis from opposite sides of the treatment volume. The advantages of the parallel opposed fields are the simplicity and reproducibility of setup, homogeneous dose to the tumor, and less chances of geometrical miss (compared to angled beams), provided the field size is large enough to provide adequate lateral coverage of the tumor volume. A disadvantage is the excessive dose to normal tissues and critical organs above and below the tumor.

A composite isodose distribution for a pair of parallel opposed fields may be obtained by adding the depth dose contribution of each field (Fig. 11.10). The manual procedure consists of joining the points of intersection of isodose curves for the individual fields which sum to the same total dose value. The

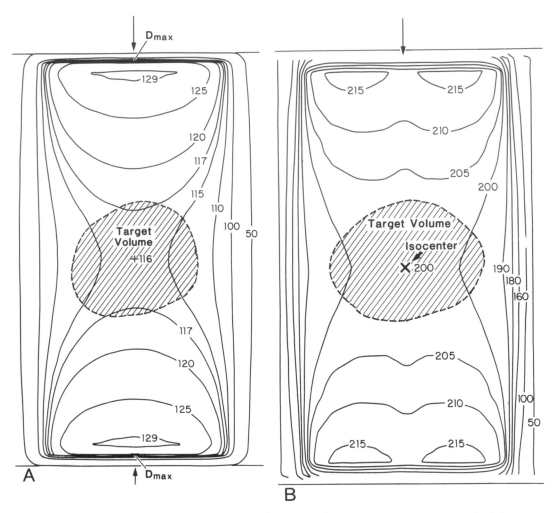

Figure 11.10. Composite isodose distribution for a pair of parallel opposed fields. A, Each beam is given a weight of 100 at the depth of D_{max}. B, Isocentric plan with each beam weighted 100 at the isocenter.

resultant distribution shows the combined isodose distribution normalized to the individual beam weights. The beams are usually weighted in dose units of 100 at the depth of D_{max} in the case of SSD techniqus or at the isocenter for the isocentric techniques. For the example shown in Fig. 11.10A, the minimum percent isodose surrounding the tumor is 110. This means that the minimum dose to the tumor (with a generous margin) is 110 rads if 100 rads are delivered at the depth of D_{max} by each field. Thus, if the tumor dose were to be specified at this isodose level, one could calculate the D_{max} dose and the treatment time for each field. For the isocentric plan shown in Fig. 11.10B, the beam weights refer to doses delivered to the isocenter. Thus, the 190% isodose curve represents the specified minimum dosage level if each beam delivered 100 rads to its isocenter. Once the isocenter dose is calculated, one can determine the treatment time or monitor units as described in Section 10.2.

A.1. PATIENT THICKNESS *VS.* DOSE UNIFORMITY

One advantage of equally weighted parallel opposed beams is that the dose distribution within the irradiated volume can be made uniform. However, the uniformity of distribution depends on the patient thickness, beam energy, and beam flatness. In general, as the patient thickness increases or the beam energy decreases, the central axis maximum dose near the surface increases relative to the midpoint dose. This effect is shown in Fig. 11.11 in which two opposing beams are placed 25 cm apart with the midpoint dose normalized to 100. The curves for cobalt-60 and 4 MV show that for a patient of this thickness parallel opposed beams would give rise to an excessively higher dose to the subcutaneous tissues compared to the tumor dose at the midpoint. As the energy is increased to 10 MV, the distribution becomes almost uniform and at 25 MV it shows significant sparing of the superficial tissues relative to the midline structures.

The ratio of maximum *peripheral dose* to midpoint dose is plotted in Fig. 11.12 as a function of patient thickness for a number of beam energies. Such data are useful in choosing the appropriate beam energy for a given patient thickness when using parallel opposed fields. For example, acceptable uniformity of dose, *i.e.* within ±5%, is achievable with ^{60}Co or 4–6-MV beams for

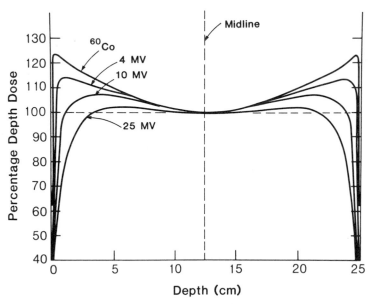

Figure 11.11. Depth dose curves for parallel opposed field normalized to midpoint value. Patient thickness = 25 cm, field size = 10 × 10 cm, SSD = 100 cm.

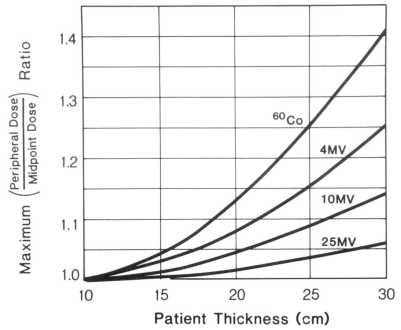

Figure 11.12. Ratio of maximum peripheral dose to the midpoint dose plotted as a function of patient thickness for different beam qualities. Parallel opposed fields, field size = 10 × 10 cm, SSD = 100 cm.

thicknesses of about 15 cm or less (*e.g.* head, neck, and extremities). However, for thicknesses of 20 cm or greater (*e.g.* thorax, abdomen, and pelvis), 10 MV or higher energies must be used in order to spare the normal subcutaneous tissues.

A.2. EDGE EFFECT (LATERAL TISSUE DAMAGE)

When treating with multiple beams, the question arises: should one treat one field per day or all fields per day? Wilson and Hall (17) have discussed this problem in terms of cell survival curves and Ellis's time-dose-fractionation formula (18, 19). For parallel opposed beams, they have shown that treating with one field per day produces greater biological damage to normal subcutaneous tissue than treating with two fields per day despite the fact that the total dose is the same. Apparently, the biological effect in the normal tissue is greater if it receives alternating high and low dose fractions compared to the equal but medium size dose fractions resulting from treating both fields daily. This phenomenon has been called "*the edge effect*" or "the tissue lateral damage" (20). The problem becomes more severe when larger thicknesses (*e.g.* ≥20 cm) are treated with one field per day using a lower energy beam (*e.g.* ≤6 MV). In such cases, the dose per fraction to the subcutaneous tissues, although delivered on alternate days, becomes prohibitively high.

A.3. INTEGRAL DOSE

One way of comparing dose distributions for different quality beams is to calculate the *integral dose* for a given tumor dose. Integral dose is a measure of the total energy absorbed in the treated volume. If a mass of tissue receives a uniform dose, then the integral dose is simply the product of mass and dose. However, in practice, the absorbed dose in the tissue is nonuniform so rather complex mathematical formulas are required to calculate it.

For a single beam of x- or γ radiation, Mayneord (21) formulated the following expression:

$$\Sigma = 1.44 \, D_0 A d_{1/2}(1 - e^{-0.693d/d_{1/2}})\left(1 + \frac{2.88d_{1/2}}{\text{SSD}}\right) \tag{11.1}$$

where Σ is the integral dose, D_0 is the peak dose along the central axis, A is the geometric area of the field, d is the total thickness of patient in the path of the beam, $d_{1/2}$ is the half-value depth or the depth of 50% depth dose and SSD is the source-surface distance. The term $\left(1 + \dfrac{2.88d_{1/2}}{\text{SSD}}\right)$ is a correction for geometric divergence of the beam.

Since integral dose is basically the product of mass and dose, its unit is the gram-rad or kilogram-gray or simply joule (since 1 gray = 1 joule/kg). Figure 11.13 shows the integral dose as a function of the energy of radiation, for a tumor dose of the 100 rads (1 rad = 10^{-2} Gy) at a depth of 12.5 cm in the patient of 25-cm thickness treated with parallel opposed beams (22). The curve shows a useful result, namely the higher the photon energy the lower the integral dose.

Although it is generally believed that the probability of damage to normal tissue increases with the increase in the integral dose, this quantity is seldom

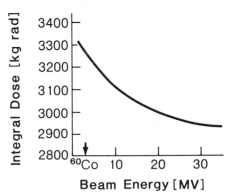

Figure 11.13. Integral dose as a function of photon beam energy, when 100 rads are delivered at a midpoint of a 25-cm-thick patient. Field size, 10 cm diameter at an SSD of 100 cm. Redrawn from Podgorsak *et al.* (22).

used clinically to plan dosages or predict treatment outcome. However, it does provide qualitative guidelines for treatment planning for selecting beam energy, field sizes, and multiplicity of fields. As a general rule, one should keep the integral dose to a minimum provided the adequacy of tumor irradiation and the sparing of critical organs are not compromised.

B. Multiple Fields

One of the most important objectives of treatment planning is to deliver maximum dose to the tumor and minimum dose to the surrounding tissues. In addition, dose uniformity within the tumor volume and sparing of critical organs are important considerations in judging a plan. Some of the strategies useful in achieving these goals are: (a) using fields of appropriate size; (b) increasing the number of fields or *portals*; (c) selecting appropriate beam directions; (d) adjusting beam weights (dose contribution from individual fields); (e) using appropriate beam energy; and (f) using beam modifiers such as wedge filters and compensators. Although obtaining a combination of these parameters which yields an optimal plan is time consuming if done manually, treatment-planning computers are now available that can do the job quickly and accurately. Some of these systems are highly interactive so that the user can almost instantly modify, calculate, and examine various plans to select one that is clinically superior.

In Section 11.5A, we discussed the case of two parallel opposed fields. Although the technique results in uniform irradiation of the tumor, there is little sparing of the surrounding normal tissue. In fact, the dose to the peripheral tissues can be significantly higher than the midline dose. Reduction of dose to subcutaneous tissue and normal tissue surrounding the tumor can be achieved by using a combination of three or more fields. Figure 11.14 illustrates various multiple field arrangements in which the beam enters the patient from various directions, always directed at the tumor. Thus, by using multiple fields, the ratio of the tumor dose to the normal tissue dose is increased. Figure 11.15, A and B, shows typical examples of multiple fields, one used for the treatment of the esophagus and the other for the prostate. Fig. 11.15C illustrates a fixed SSD-type technique in which the beam weights are delivered to D_{max} points. In actual practice, one may use a combination of parallel opposed fields and multiple fields to achieve the desired dose distribution.

Although multiple fields can provide good distribution, there are some clinical and technical limitations to these techniques. For example, certain beam angles are prohibited because of the presence of critical organs in those directions. Also, the setup accuracy of a treatment may be better with parallel opposed than with the multiple angled beam arrangement. It is, therefore, important to realize that the acceptability of a treatment plan depends not only on the dose distribution on paper but also on the practical feasibility, setup accuracy, and reproducibility of the treatment technique.

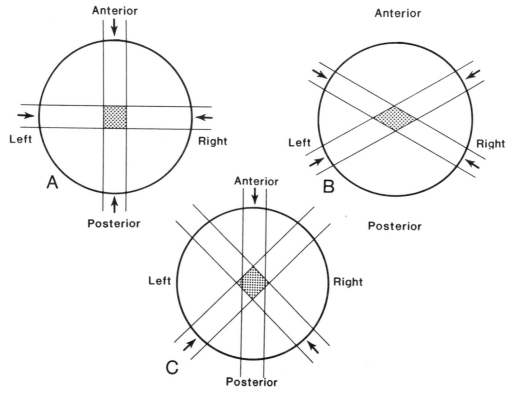

Figure 11.14. Schematic diagram showing examples of multiple fields. A, Two opposing pairs at right angles. B, Two opposing pairs at 120°. C, Three fields: one anterior and two posterior oblique, at 45° with the vertical.

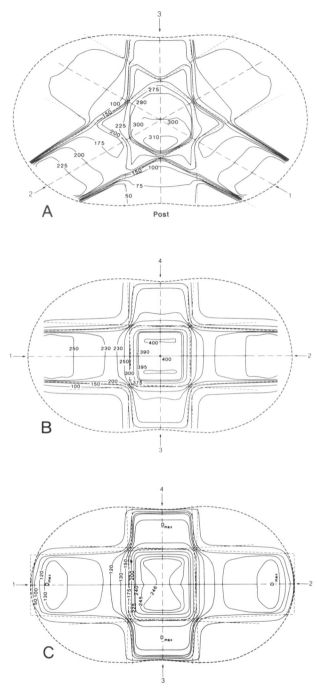

Figure 11.15. Examples of multiple field plans. A, Three-field isocentric technique. Each beam delivers 100 units of dose at the isocenter. 4 MV, field size = 8 × 8 cm at isocenter, SAD = 100 cm. B, Four-field isocentric technique. Ech beam delivers 100 units of dose at the isocenter. 10 MV, field size = 8 × 8 cm at isocenter, SAD = 100 cm. C, Four-field SSD technique in which all beams are weighted 100 units at their respective points of D_{max}; 10 MV, field size = 8 × 8 cm at surface, SSD = 100 cm.

225

11.6 ISOCENTRIC TECHNIQUES

Most modern machines are constructed so that the source of radiation can rotate about a horizontal axis. The gantry of the machine is capable of rotating through 360° with the collimator axis moving in a vertical plane. The *isocenter* is the point of intersection of the collimator axis and the gantry axis.

A. Stationary Beams

The isocentric technique of irradiation consists of placing the isocenter of the machine at a depth within the patient and directing the beams from different directions. The distance of the source from the isocenter or the SAD remains constant irrespective of the beam direction. However, the SSD in this case may change depending on the beam direction and the shape of the patient contour. For any beam direction, the following relationship holds:

$$SSD = SAD - d \qquad (11.2)$$

where d is the depth of the isocenter. Knowing the depth and position of isocenter from one direction such as the anterior-posterior, the SSD can be calculated according to Equation 11.2 and set up from that direction. Then the positioning of subsequent fields simply requires moving the gantry and not the patient.

Although all techniques for which SSD ≤ SAD can be carried out isocentrically, the major advantage of this method is the ease with which multiple field setups (three or more) can be treated when all fields are treated the same day. Not only does this technique dispense with the setting up of SSD for each beam direction, it relies primarily on the accuracy of machine isocentricity and not on the skin marks which are unreliable points of reference in most cases.

The treatment calculations for isocentric treatments have been presented in Section 10.2A.2. Figure 11.15, A and B, shows examples of isodose distribution for isocentric techniques.

B. Rotation Therapy

Rotation therapy is a special case of the isocentric technique in which the beam moves continuously about the patient, or the patient is rotated while the beam is held fixed. Although this technique has been used for treating tumors of the esophagus, bladder, prostate, cervix, and brain, the technique offers little advantage over the isocentric technique using multiple stationary beams. For example, the esophagus can be treated equally well with three fields, the prostate and bladder with four fields (sometimes combined with parallel opposed fields), and brain with two or three fields or with wedges depending upon the size and location of the tumor. Many times it is a matter of individual preference, although one technique may offer particular advantages over the other with regard to patient positioning, blocking, and the size of volume to be irradiated. Especially when intricate blocking is required, rotation therapy should not be attempted.

Rotation therapy is best suited for small deep seated tumors. If the tumor is confined within a region extending not more than halfway from the center of the contour cross section, rotation therapy may be a proper choice. However, rotation therapy is not indicated if 1) volume to be irradiated is too large, 2) the external surface differs markedly from a cylinder, and 3) the tumor is too far off-center.

Calculation for rotation therapy can be made in the same way as for the stationary isocentric beams except that a reasonably large number of beams should be positioned around the patient contour at fixed angular intervals. The dose rate at the isocenter is given by:

$$\dot{D}_{iso} = \dot{D}_{ref} \times \bar{T} \tag{11.3}$$

where $\dot{D}_{ref}$ is the reference dose rate related to the quantity $\bar{T}$ which may be average tissue-air ratio or tissue-maximum ratio (averaged over all depths at the selected angles). In the case of tissue-air ratios, $\dot{D}_{ref}$ is the dose rate in free space for the given field at the isocenter. A method of manual calculations based on this system has been discussed in Section 9.4D. If the tissue maximum ratios (TMR) are used, $\dot{D}_{ref}$ is the D_{max} dose rate for the given field at the SAD. Using the TMR system discussed in Chapter 10,

$$\dot{D}_{iso} = \dot{D}_0 \times S_c \times S_p \times \overline{TMR} \tag{11.4}$$

where $\dot{D}_0$ is the D_{max} dose rate for a 10×10 cm field at the SAD, and S_c and S_p are the collimator and phantom scatter correction factors for the given field size at the isocenter. In the case of a linear accelerator, $\dot{D}_0$ is the monitor unit (MU) rate (assuming 1 MU = 1 rad (cGy) at the isocenter for a depth of D_{max} for a 10×10 cm field.

EXAMPLE

A patient is to receive 250 rads at the isocenter by rotation therapy, using 4-MX x-rays, 6×10 cm field at the isocenter, and SAD of 100 cm. If $\overline{TMR}$ calculated according to the procedure in Section 9.4D is 0.756, calculate the number of monitor units to be set on the machine, if the machine output is set at 200 MU/min, and given S_c (6×10) = 0.98 and S_p (6×10) = 0.99. From Equation 11.4,

$$\dot{D}_{iso} = \dot{D}_0 \times S_c \times S_p \times \overline{TMR}$$

or

$$\dot{D}_{iso} = 200 \times 0.98 \times 0.99 \times 0.746$$

$$= 144.8 \text{ rad/min}$$

$$\text{Treatment time} = \frac{250 \text{ rad}}{144.8 \text{ rad/min}} = 1.73 \text{ min}$$

$$\text{Total MU to be set} = 200 \text{ (MU/min)} \times 1.73 \text{ min}$$

$$= 345 \text{ MU}$$

Gantry rotation speed is set so that 345 MU are delivered at the conclusion of the rotation. Some machines perform only one rotation while others can perform a specified number of arcs or rotations in a pendulum manner. Most modern machines allow for automatic adjustment of rotation speed to deliver a preset number of monitor units by the end of a single rotation.

The determination of complete isodose curves for rotation therapy by manual means is very time consuming. It is essentially the same procedure as used in multiple fixed beams, but with a large number of beams. The isocentric isodose chart (Fig. 11.1B) in which isodoses are normalized to a point at depth on central axis is used with the isocenter placed at the point of normalization. By summing the isodose values at selected points while the chart is placed at different angles, the dose distribution can be determined relative to the isocenter. Because of the tedium involved in the procedure, this task is ideally suited for computer application. Such programs are available with commercial treatment planning computers.

Figure 11.16 shows three examples of isodose distribution for rotation therapy: (a) 100° arc rotation; (b) 180° arc rotation; and (c) full 360° rotation. It should be noted that whereas the maximum dose for the 360° rotation occurs at the isocenter, for the partial arcs it is displaced toward the irradiated sector. This illustrates an important principle that in arc therapy or when oblique fields are directed through one side of a patient, they should be aimed a suitable distance beyond the tumor area. This is sometimes referred to as "past pointing." The extent of past pointing required to bring the maximum dose to the tumor site depends on the arc angle and should be determined for an individual case by actual isodose planning.

11.7 WEDGE FIELD TECHNIQUES

Relatively superficial tumors, extending from the surface to a depth of several centimeters, can be irradiated by two "wedged" beams directed from the same side of the patient. Figure 11.17A shows isodose distribution of two angled beams with no wedge in the beams. It is seen that in the region of overlap of the beams, the dose distribution is quite nonuniform. The dose is highest in the superficial or proximal region of overlap and falls off to lower values toward the deeper areas. By inserting appropriate wedge filters in the beam and positioning them with the thick ends adjacent to each other, the angled field distribution can be made fairly uniform (Fig. 11.17B). Each wedged beam in this case has a reduced dose in the superficial region relative to the deeper region so that the dose gradient in the overlap region is minimized. The dose falls off rapidly beyond the region of overlap or the "plateau" region, which is clinically a desirable feature.

There are three parameters that affect the plateau region in terms of its depth, shape, and dose distribution: θ, ϕ, and S, where θ is the wedge angle (Section 11.4A), ϕ is the hinge angle, and S is the separation. These parameters are illustrated in Fig. 11.18. The hinge angle is the angle between the central axes of the two beams and the separation S is the distance beween the thick

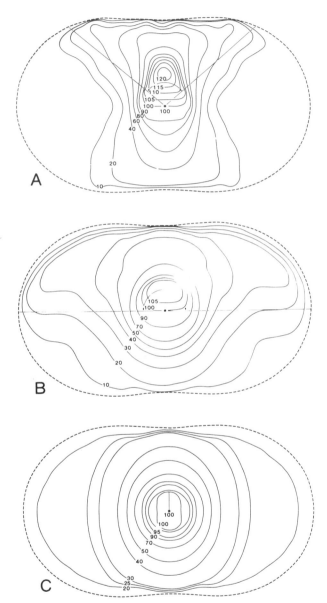

Figure 11.16. Examples of isodose distribution for rotation therapy. A, Arc angle = 100°; B, arc angle = 180°, C, full 360° rotation. 4 MV, field size = 7 × 12 cm at isocenter, SAD = 100 cm.

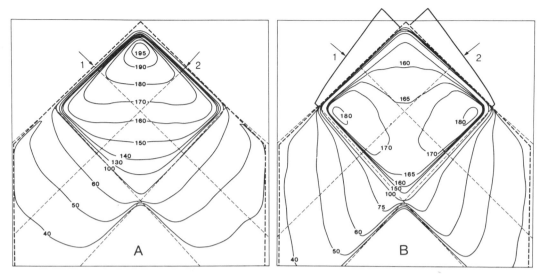

Figure 11.17. Isodose distribution for two angle beams. A, Without wedges; B, With wedges. 4 MV, field size = 10 × 10 cm, SSD = 100 cm, wedge angle = 45°.

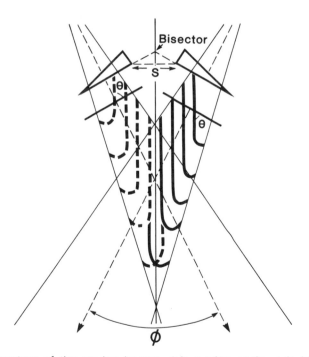

Figure 11.18. Parameters of the wedge beams. θ is wedge angle, ϕ is hinge angle, and S is separation. Isodose curves for each wedge field are parallel to the bisector.

ends of the wedge filters as projected on the surface. Cohen and Martin (3) have discussed in detail how θ, ϕ, and S can be adjusted to achieve a desired plateau.

There is an optimum relationship between the wedge angle θ and the hinge angle ϕ which provides the most uniform distribution of radiation dose in the plateau:

$$\theta = 90° - \phi/2 \qquad (11.5)$$

This equation is based on the principle that for a given hinge angle, the wedge angle should be such that the isodose curves from each field are parallel to the bisector of the hinge angle (see Fig. 11.18). Under these conditions, when the isodoses are combined, the resultant distribution is uniform.

The above equation, although helpful in treatment planning, may not yield an optimum plan for a given patient contour. The relationship assumes that the wedge isodose curves are not modified by the surface contour. In practice, however, contours are usually curved or irregular in shape and thus modify the isodose distribution for the wedged beams. As a result, the isodose curves for the individual fields are no longer parallel to the bisector of the hinge angle, thus giving rise to a nonuniform distribution in the overlap region. This problem can be solved by using *compensators* (to be discussed in Section 12.4) which make the skin surface effectively flat and perpendicular to each beam. An alternative approach is to modify the wedge angle (using a different wedge angle filter than that given by Equation 11.5) so that a part of the wedge angle acts as a compensator and the rest as a true wedge filter. The main objective is to make the isodose curves parallel to the hinge angle bisector. Although the latter approach obviates the need for a compensator, the determination of an optimum wedge angle may not be easy if planning is done manually. The former method, on the other hand, is well suited for manual calculations since all you need is a compensator and an atlas of precalculated isodose distributions for a variety of θ, ϕ, and S values. This method, however, becomes technically difficult to implement if complicated secondary blocking is required in addition to the compensator and the wedge filter.

Equation 11.5 suggests that, for each hinge angle, one should use a different wedge angle. However, in practice, selected wedge angles, *i.e.* 15°, 30°, 45°, and 60°, are adequate over a fairly wide range of hinge angles.

In modern radiotherapy, complex treatment techniques are frequently used, which may involve wedge filters, compensators, field blocking, and field reductions, all for the same patient. Manual treatment planning is difficult for such cases. For this reason, in many institutions, all complex treatments including wedged fields are planned by computer as a matter of standard practice.

A. Uniformity of Dose Distribution

Since wedge pair techniques are normally used for treating small superficial tumor volumes, a high dose region ("hot spot") of up to +10% within the treatment volume is usually acceptable. These hot spots occur under the thin ends of the wedges and their magnitude increases with field size and wedge angle. This effect is related to the differential attenuation of the beam under the thick end relative to the thin end.

Generally, the wedge filter technique is suitable where the tumor is approximately from 0 to 7 cm deep and when it is necessary to irradiate from one side of the skin surface. The most desirable feature of this technique is the rapid dose fall-off beyond the region of overlap. This falloff can be exploited to protect a critical organ such as the spinal cord. Although wedge filters are invaluable in radiotherapy, some of these techniques are being replaced by electron beam techniques (Chapter 14).

B. Open and Wedged Field Combinations

Although wedge filters were originally designed for use in conjunction with the wedge-pair arrangement, it is possible to combine open and wedged beams

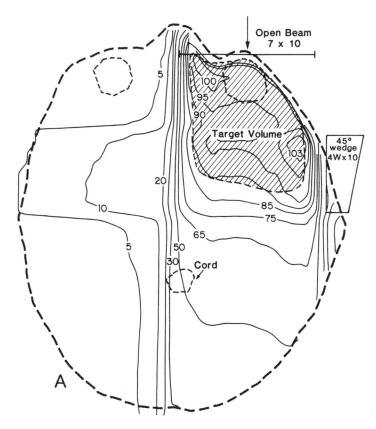

Figure 11.19. Treatment plans using open and wedged field combinations. A, Isocentric plan with anterior open field weighted 100 and lateral wedged field weighted 15 at the isocenter. B, A combination of anterior open beam and two lateral wedged beams. 4 MV x-ray beam from ATC-400 linac.

to obtain a particular dose distribution. One such arrangement which uses an open field anteriorly and wedged field laterally in the treatment of some tumors is shown in Fig. 11.19A. The anterior field is weighted to deliver 100 units to the lateral 15 units to the isocenter (these beams could be weighted in terms of D_{max} in the SSD technique). The weights and wedge angle are usually adjusted for an individual case to obtain an acceptable distribution. The principle of this technique is that as the dose contribution from the anterior field decreases with depth, the lateral beam provides a boost to offset this decrease. As seen in Fig. 11.19A, a wedged beam with the thick end positioned superiorly provides the desired compensation for the dose drop-off. Thus, such a combination of open and wedged beams give rise to a distribution which remains constant with depth within certain limits.

Figure 11.19B shows another technique in which the anterior open beam is combined with the two lateral wedged beams. Again the beam weights and wedge angles are chosen so as to make the open beam distribution remain constant throughout the tumor volume.

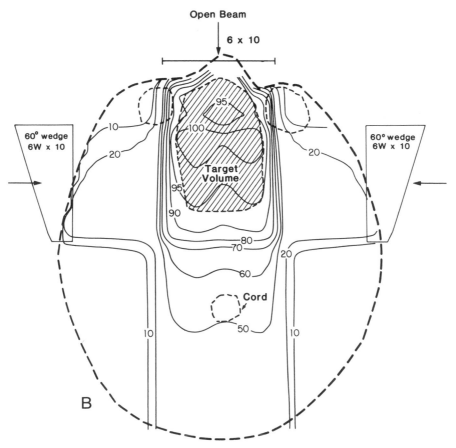

Figure 11.19 continued

11.8 TUMOR DOSE SPECIFICATION FOR EXTERNAL PHOTON BEAMS

The results of treatments can be meaningfully interpreted only if sufficient information is provided regarding the irradiation technique and the distribution of dose in space and time. In the absence of this information, recording of only the so-called "tumor dose" serves little purpose. Unfortunately, this important problem is often ignored. More often than not, treatment summaries and records are ambiguous, and even incomprehensible, to other people. Therefore, one cannot overemphasize the need for a dose-recording system which is sufficiently explicit and detailed to enable other centers to reproduce the treatment.

The ICRU (23) recognized the need for a general dose specification system which could be adopted universally. Although the system proposed by the ICRU has not received a complete consensus, there is a substantial advantage in adopting a common method of dose specification. In this section, we present the highlights of the ICRU proposal. For details the reader is referred to the original document (23).

A. Terminology

A.1. TARGET VOLUME

The *target volume* consists of the demonstrated tumor(s), if present, and any other tissue with presumed tumor. This is the volume which needs to be irradiated to a specified absorbed dose.

In delineating the target volume, consideration must be given to the local invasive capacity of the tumor and its potential spread to the regional lymph nodes. Thus, the target volume should include sufficient margins to allow for the uncertainty in anatomic localization of this volume.

A.2. TREATMENT VOLUME

Additional margins must be provided around the target volume to allow for limitations of the treatment technique. Thus, the minimum target dose should be represented by an isodose surface which adequately covers the target volume in order to provide that margin. The volume enclosed by this isodose surface is called the *treatment volume*. The treatment volume is, in general, larger than the target volume and depends on a particular treatment technique.

A.3. IRRADIATED VOLUME

The volume of tissue receiving a significant dose (*e.g.* ≥50% of the specified target dose) is called the irradiated volume. The irradiated volume is larger than the treatment volume and depends on the treatment technique used.

A.4. MAXIMUM TARGET DOSE

The highest dose in the target area is called the *maximum target dose* provided this dose covers a minimum area of 2 cm^2. Higher dose areas of less than 2 cm^2 may be ignored in designating the value of maximum target dose.

A.5. MINIMUM TARGET DOSE

The minimum target dose is the lowest absorbed dose in the target area.

A.6. MEAN TARGET DOSE

If dose is calculated at a large number of discrete points uniformly distributed in the target area, the *mean target dose* is the mean of the absorbed dose values at these points.

Mathematically:

$$\text{Mean target dose} = \frac{1}{N} \sum_{A_T} D_{i,j}$$

where N is the number of points in the matrix and $D_{i,j}$ is the dose at lattice point i, j located inside the target area A_T.

A.7 MEDIAN TARGET DOSE

This is simply the midvalue between the maximum and the minimum absorbed dose values within the target.

A.8. MODAL TARGET DOSE

This is the absorbed dose that occurs most frequently within the target area. If the dose distribution over a grid of points covering the target area is plotted as a frequency histogram, the dose value showing the highest frequency is called the modal dose. In Fig. 11.20 the modal dose corresponds to the peak of the frequency curve.

A.9. HOT SPOTS

A *hot spot* is an area, outside the target area, which receives a higher dose than the specified target dose. Like the maximum target dose, a hot spot is considered clinically meaningful only if it covers an area of at least 2 cm^2.

B. Specification of Target Dose

The absorbed dose distribution in the target volume is usually not uniform. Although a complete dosimetric specification is not possible without the entire dose distribution, there is value in having one figure as the main statement of *target dose*. The use of the term "tumor dose" is not recommended (23).

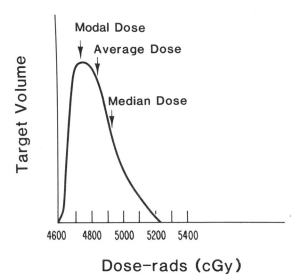

Figure 11.20.   Target volume-dose frequency curve. (Reprinted with permission from: Ellis F, Oliver R: The specification of tumor dose. *Br J Radiol* 34:258, 1961.

The quantity maximum target dose alone cannot be used for reporting since it can conceal serious underdosages in some part of the target volume. Although local tumor control depends on the minimum target dose, this quantity alone is not recommended by the ICRU (23) since it is difficult to determine the extent of the tumor, and, therefore, the selection of the minimum target dose becomes difficult if not arbitrary. Moreover, if most of the target volume receives a dose that is appreciably different from the minimum, this may also reduce its clinical significance. A statement of both the maximum and minimum values is useful but it is not always representative of the dose distribution. Moreover, this would do away with the simplicity of having one quantity for reporting target dose.

The mean, median, and modal doses are not to be generally recommended since they usually require elaborate calculations for their accurate determination and may not be feasible by institutions having limited computational facilities.

The ICRU (23) recommends the following system of dose specification.

B.1. STATIONARY PHOTON BEAMS

(a) For a single beam, the target absorbed dose should be specified on the central axis of the beam at the center of the target area.

(b) For parallel opposed equally weighted beams, the point of target dose specification should be on the central axis midway between the beam entrances.

(c) For parallel opposed unequally weighted beams, the target dose should be specified on the central axis at the center of the target area.

(d) For any other arrangement of two or more intersecting beams, the point of target dose specification should be at the intersection of the central axes of the beams.

B.2. ROTATION THERAPY

For full rotation or arcs of at least 270°, the target dose should be specified at the center of rotation in the principal plane. For smaller arcs, the target dose should be stated in the principal plane, first, at the center of rotation and second, at the center of the target area. This dual point specification is required because in a small arc therapy, *past-pointing* techniques are used which give maximum absorbed dose close to the center of the target area. The dose at the isocenter in these cases, although important to specify, is somewhat less.

B.3. ADDITIONAL INFORMATION

The specification of target dose is meaningful only if sufficient information is provided regarding the irradiation technique. The description of technique should include radiation quality, SSD or SAD, field sizes, beam modification devices (wedges, shielding blocks, etc.), beam weighting, correction for tissue heterogeneities, dose fractionation, and patient positioning. Many of the above treatment parameters are listed with the treatment plan (isodose pattern) and can be attached to the patient chart. "*In vivo*" absorbed dose measurements can also provide useful information and should be recorded in the chart.

Finally, the main objectives of a dose specification and reporting system are to achieve uniformity of dose reporting among institutions, to provide meaningful data for assessing the results of treatments, and to enable the treatment to be repeated elsewhere without having recourse to the original institution for further information.

References

1. International Commission on Radiation Units and Measurements (ICRU): *Report No. 23. Measurement of Absorbed Dose in a Phantom Irradiated by a Single Beam of X or Gamma Rays.* Washington, DC, National Bureau of Standards, 1973.
2. Webster EW, Tsien KC (eds): *Atlas of Radiation Dose Distributions*, vol I, *Single-Field Isodose Charts.* Vienna, International Atomic Energy Agency, 1965.
3. Cohen, M, Martin SM (eds): *Atlas of Radiation Dose Distributions*, vol II, *Multiple-Field Isodose Charts.* Vienna, International Atomic Energy Agency, 1966.
4. Tsien KC, Cunningham JR, Wright DJ, Jones DEA, Pfalzner PM (eds): *Atlas of Radiation Dose Distributions*, vol III, *Moving Field Isodose Charts.* Vienna, International Atomic Energy Agency, 1967.
5. Sterling TD, Perry H, Katz L: Automation of radiation treatment planning. IV. Derivation of a mathematical expression for the percent depth dose surface of cobalt 60 beams and visualization of multiple field dose distributions. *Br J Radiol* 37:544, 1964.
6. Khan FM (Ph.D. thesis, University of Minnesota, 1969): Computer dosimetry of partially blocked fields in cobalt teletherapy. *Radiology* 97:405, 1970.
7. Van de Geijn J: A computer program for 3-D planning in external beam radiation therapy, EXTDϕS. *Comput Prog Biomed* 1:47, 1970.
8. Cunningham JR, Shrivastava PN, Wilkinson JM: Program IRREG—calculation of dose from irregularly shaped radiation beams. *Comput Prog Biomed* 2:192, 1972.
9. Weinkam JJ, Kolde RA, Sterling TD: Extending the general field equation to fit the dose distributions of a variety of therapy units. *Br J Radiol* 46:983, 1973.

10. Nordic Association of Clinical Physics (NACP): Procedures in external beam radiation therapy dosimetry with electron and photon beams with maximum energies between 1 and 50 MeV. *Acta Radiol Oncol* 19:58, 1980.
11. International Commission on Radiation Units and Measurements (ICRU): *Report No. 24. Determination of Absorbed Dose in a Patient Irradiated by Beams of X or Gamma Rays in Radiotherapy Procedures.* Washington, DC, National Bureau of Standards, 1976.
12. Sewchand W, Khan FM, Williamson J: Variation in depth dose data between open and wedge fields for 4 MV X-rays. *Radiology* 127:789, 1978.
13. Cohen M, Burns JE, Sears R: Physical aspects of cobalt 60 teletherapy using wedge filters. I. Physical Investigation. *Acta Radiol* 53:401, 1960. *II. Dosimetric considerations. Acta Radiol* 53:486, 1960.
14. Tranter FW: Design of wedge filters for use with 4 MeV linear accelerator. *Br J Radiol* 30:329, 1957.
15. Van de Geijn J: A simple wedge filter technique for cobalt 60 teletherapy. *Br J Radiol* 35:710, 1962.
16. Aron BS, Scapicchio M: Design of universal wedge filter system for a cobalt 60 unit. *Am J Roentgenol* 96:70, 1966.
17. Wilson CS, Hall EJ: On the advisability of treating all fields at each radiotherapy session. *Radiology* 98:419, 1971.
18. Ellis F: Nominal standard dose and the ret. *Br J Radiol* 44:101, 1971.
19. Orton CG, Ellis F: A simplification in the use of the NSD concept in practical radiotherapy. *Br J Radiol* 46:529, 1973.
20. Tapley N: Parallel opposing portals technique. In Fletcher GH, (ed): *Text Book of Radiotherapy*, 3rd ed. Philadelphia, Lea and Febiger, 1980, p 60.
21. Mayneord WV: The measurement of radiation for medical purposes. *Proc Phys Soc* 54:405, 1942.
22. Podgorsak EB, Rawlinson JA, Johns HE: X-Ray depth doses for linear accelerators in the energy range from 10 to 32 MeV. *Am J Roentgenol* 123:182, 1975.
23. International Commission on Radiation Units and Measurements (ICRU): *Report No. 29. Dose Specification for Reporting External Beam Therapy with Photons and Electrons.* Washington, DC, National Bureau of Standards, 1978.

CHAPTER 12

Treatment Planning II: Patient Data, Corrections, and Setup

Basic depth dose data and isodose curves are usually measured in a cubic water phantom having dimensions much larger than the field sizes used clinically. Phantom irradiations for this purpose are carried out under standard conditions, *e.g.* beams incident normally on the flat surface at specified distances. The patient's body, however, is neither homogeneous nor flat in surface contour. Thus, the dose distribution in a patient may differ significantly from the standard distribution. This chapter discusses several aspects of treatment planning including acquisition of patient data, correction for contour curvature, and tissue inhomogeneities and patient positioning.

12.1 ACQUISITION OF PATIENT DATA

Accurate patient dosimetry is only possible when sufficiently accurate patient data are available. Such data include body contour, outline and density of relevant internal structures, and location as well as extent of the target volume. Acquisition of these data is necessary whether the dosimetric calculations are performed manually or with a computer. However, this important aspect of treatment planning is often executed poorly. For example, in a busy department there may be an inordinate amount of pressure to begin the patient's treatment without adequate dosimetric planning. In other cases, lack of sufficient physics support and/or equipment is the cause of this problem. In such a case, it must be realized that the final accuracy of the treatment plan is strongly dependent on the availability of the patient data and that great effort is needed to improve its quality.

A. Body Contours

A number of devices have been made to obtain patient contours. Some of these are commercially available while others can be fabricated in the department machine shop. The most common and the simplest of the devices is a solder wire or a lead wire imbedded in plastic. Since the wire may not faithfully retain the contour dimensions when transferring it from the patient to the paper, one must independently measure anteroposterior and/or lateral diameters of the contour with a caliper.

Another kind of simple device (1) consists of an array of rods, the tips of which are made to touch the patient's skin and then placed on a sheet of paper for contour drawing. Perhaps the most accurate of the mechanical devices is a pantograph type apparatus (Fig. 12.1) in which a rod can be moved laterally as well as up and down. When the rod is moved over the patient contour, its motion is followed by a pen which records the outline on paper.

Clarke (2) has described an electromechanical device in which motion of the rod over the patient contour is read by a sensing device and transferred to an X-Y recorder. Such a device can also be used for digitizing the patient contour for direct input to the treatment planning computer.

More recently optical (3) and ultrasonic (4) methods have been devised to obtain the contour information. Computer tomography (CT) can also be used to obtain transverse contours in addition to the internal structure information for which it is primarily intended.

Although any of the above methods can be used with sufficient accuracy if carefully used, some important points must be considered with regard to contour making.

(a) The patient contour must be obtained with the patient in the same position as used in the actual treatment. For this reason, probably the best place for obtaining the contour information is with the patient properly positioned on the treatment simulatour couch.

(b) A line representing the table top must be indicated in the contour so that this horizontal line can be used as a reference for beam angles.

(c) Important bony landmarks as well as beam entry points, if available, must be indicated on the contour.

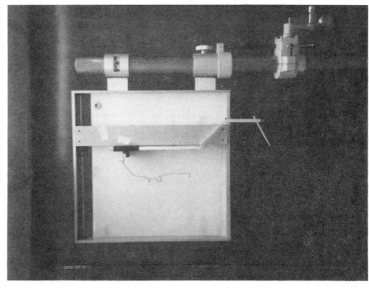

Figure 12.1. Photograph of a contour plotter. (Courtesy of Radiation Products Design, Buffalo, MN.)

(d) Checks of body contour are recommended during the treatment course if the contour is expected to change due to a reduction of tumor volume or a change in patient weight.

(e) If body thickness varies significantly within the treatment field, contours should be determined in more than one plane.

B. Internal Structures

Localization of internal structures for treatment planning should provide quantitative information with regard to the size and location of critical organs or inhomogeneities. Although qualitative information can be obtained from diagnostic radiographs or atlases of cross-sectional anatomy, they cannot be used directly for precise localization of organs relative to the external contour. In order for the contour and the internal structure data to be realistic for a given patient, the localization must be obtained under conditions similar to those of the actual treatment position and on a couch similar to the treatment couch.

The following devices are used for the localization of internal structures and the target volume. A brief discussion regarding their operation and function will be presented.

B.1. TRANSVERSE TOMOGRAPHY

A transverse tomography unit (Fig. 12.2) consists of a diagnostic x-ray tube and a film cassette which rotates simultaneously with the x-ray tube. The tube is set in such a position that the central axis of the beam makes an angle of about 20° with the film surface. The patient is positioned on the table so that the x-ray beam can pass through a desired body cross section. As the gantry rotates, structures in only one transverse plane are "in focus." The structures in regions other than that plane are blurred because of the motion of the x-ray tube and the film cassette.

The difference between conventional tomography and transverse tomography is the orientation of the plane in focus. Whereas a conventional tomographic image is parallel to the long axis of the patient, the transverse tomogram provides a cross-sectional image perpendicular to the body axis.

Transverse tomograms have been used in radiotherapy to provide cross-sectional information of internal structures in relation to the external contour (5, 6). Although the method can be used for localizing bone, lung, air cavities, and organs with contrast media, the tomograms have poor contrast and spatial resolution. In addition, the images are marred by artifacts and require interpretation.

B.2. COMPUTED TOMOGRAPHY

The main disadvantage of conventional transverse tomography is the presence of blurred images resulting from structures outside the plane of interest. In CT, the x-rays used for reconstructing the image enter only the layer under

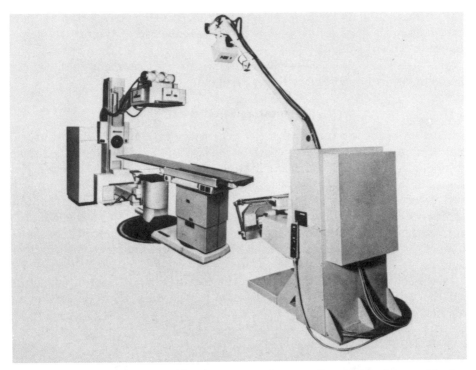

Figure 12.2.   Photograph of a conventional transverse tomography unit (right) in combination with a treatment simulator. (Courtesy of Toshiba Medical Systems, Chicago, IL.)

examination, so that unwanted planes are completely omitted. Basically a narrow beam of x-rays scans across a patient in synchrony with a radiation detector on the opposite side of the patient. If a sufficient number of transmission measurements are taken at different orientations of the x-ray source and detector (Fig. 12.3A), the distribution of attenuation coefficients within the layer may be determined. By assigning different levels to different attenuation coefficients, an image can be reconstructed that represents various structures with different attenuation properties. Such a representaion of attenuation coefficients constitutes a CT image.

Since CT scanning was introduced about 10 years ago, there has been a rapid development in both the software and hardware. Most of the improvements in hardware had to do with the scanner motion and the multiplicity of detectors to decrease the scan time. Fig. 12.3B shows a third generation scanner in which the x-ray tube rotates within a circular array of 600 or more detectors. With such a scanner, scan times as fast as 2 sec are achievable. Fig. 12.4 shows a typical CT image.

The reconstruction of an image by CT is a mathematical process of considerable complexity, generally performed by a computer. For a review of various mathematical approaches for image reconstruction, the reader is referred to a

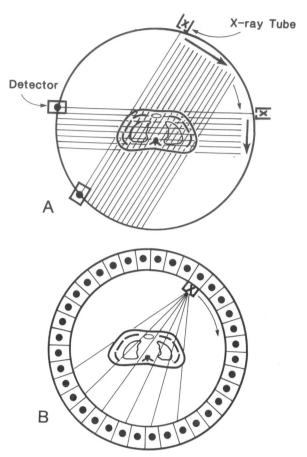

Figure 12.3. Illustration of scan motions in CT. (A) An early design in which the x-ray source and the detector performed a combination of translational and rotational motion. (B) A modern scanner in which the x-ray tube rotates within a stationary circular array of detectors.

paper by Brooks and Di Chiro (7). The reconstruction algorithm generates what is known as *CT numbers* which are related to attenuation coefficients. The CT numbers range from −1000 for air to +1000 for bone, with that for water set at 0. The CT numbers normalized in this manner are called Hounsfield numbers (H).

$$H = \frac{\mu_{\text{tissue}} - \mu_{\text{water}}}{\mu_{\text{water}}} \times 1000 \qquad (12.1)$$

where μ is the linear attenuation coefficient. Thus, a Hounsfield unit represents a change of 0.1% in the attenuation coefficient of water.

Since the CT numbers bear a linear relationship with the attenuation coefficients, it is possible to infer electron density (electrons cm^{-3}) and atomic

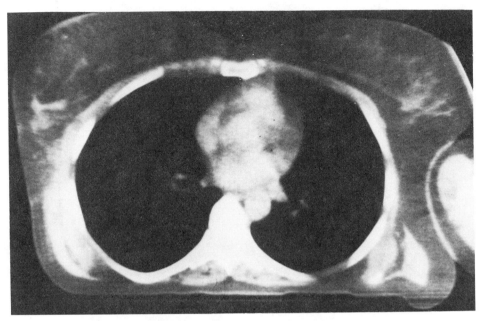

Figure 12.4 Typical CT image.

number information if attenuation coefficients are measured at two different x-ray energies (8). Also it is possible to transform the attenuation coefficients measured by CT at diagnostic energies to therapeutic energies (9). However, for low atomic number materials such as fat, air, lung, and muscle, this transformation is not necessary for the purpose of calculating dose distributions and inhomogeneity corrections (9).

Application of CT in radiotherapy treatment planning has been the subject of many papers (9–21). The CT information is useful in two aspects of treatment planning: (a) delineation of target volume and the surrounding structures in relation to the external contour; and (b) providing quantitative data (in the form of CT numbers) for tissue heterogeneity corrections. From a practical point of view, the first aspect is more important than the second. Accurate delineation of surface contour, internal structures, and target volume is not only crucial for optimizing a treatment technique, but also necessary for accurate calculation of dose distribution. Even the tissue heterogeneity corrections for megavoltage photon beams can be made with acceptable accuracy by using the CT cross-sectional image to determine the extent of the inhomogeneity and employing published values of electron density. To quote Sontag *et al.* (12), "The most severe errors in computing the dose distribution are caused by inaccurate delineation of the geometric outlines of tissue inhomogeneities. Less severe errors in the dose calculation are caused by using an inaccurate relative electron density for the inhomogeneity, provided the outline is accurate." Similar observations were also made by Geise and McCullough (11).

From these investigations, it seems that more sophisticated inhomogeneity correction algorithms such as those using "pixel-by-pixel" CT data produce only small improvements in dose accuracy compared to the traditional methods using equivalent depth, provided the extent of the inhomogeneity is accurately known. However, greater precision in the inhomogeneity outline and electron density may be required in regions where severe dose gradients exist in the direction of the beam. For example, the electron density information may be critical for some cases of electron beam therapy and, for high energy photons, in regions where electronic equilibrium is not established. In such instances, methods using pixel-by-pixel correction methods may be required (16, 22, 23).

There are several commerically available computer treatment planning systems which allow display and use of CT images for treatment planning. Once the CT image has been produced, the data can be transferred to the treatment planning computer either directly or the outlines of the contour and internal structures can be traced by hand and then entered into the computer. In direct systems, the CT scan is displayed in gray-scale mode on the TV monitor of the treatment planning system and relevant structures can be outlined on the basis of CT number distribution. After the treatment plan is finalized, it can be superimposed on the CT image for visual display.

B.3. ULTRASOUND

Ultrasonic imaging for delineating patient contours and internal structure is becoming widely recognized as an important tool in radiotherapy. Tomographic views provide cross-sectional information which is always helpful for treatment planning. Although in most cases the image quality or clinical reliability is not as good as that of the CT, ultrasonic procedure does not involve ionizing radiation, is less expensive, and, in some cases, yields data of comparable usefulness.

Ultrasound can provide useful information in localizing many malignancy-prone structures in the lower pelvis, retroperitoneum, upper abdomen, breast, and chest wall (24). A detailed review of these techniques in the context of radiotherapy planning has been presented by Carson *et al.* (24, 25).

An ultrasound (or ultrasonic) wave is a sound wave having a frequency greater than 20,000 cycles per sec or hertz (Hz). At this frequency, the sound is inaudible to the human ear. Ultrasound waves of frequencies 1–20 MHz are used in diagnostic radiology.

Ultrasound may be used to produce images either by means of transmission or reflection. However, in most clinical applications, use is made of ultrasonic waves reflected from different tissue interfaces. These reflections or echoes are caused by variations in *acoustic impedance* of materials on opposite sides of the interfaces. The acoustic impedance (Z) of a medium is defined as the product of the density of the medium and the velocity of ultrasound in the medium. The larger the difference in Z between the two media, the greater is the fraction of ultrasound energy reflected at the interface. For example, strong reflections of ultrasound occur at the air-tissue, tissue-bone, and chest wall-lung interfaces due to high impedance mismatch. However, since lung contains millions of air-tissue interfaces, strong reflections at the numerous interfaces prevents its use in lung imaging.

Attenuation of the ultrasound by the medium also plays an important role in ultrasound imaging. This attenuation takes place as the energy is removed from the beam by absorption, scattering, and reflection. The energy remaining in the beam decreases approximately exponentially with the depth of penetration into the medium, allowing attenuation in different media to be characterized by attenuation coefficients. Since the attenuation coefficient of ultrasound is very high for bone compared to soft tissue, together with the large reflection coefficient of a tissue-bone interface, it is difficult to visualize structures lying beyond bone. On the other hand, water, blood, fat, and muscle are very good transmitters of ultrasound energy.

Ultrasonic waves are generated as well as detected by an *ultrasonic probe* or *transducer*. A transducer is a device that converts one form of energy into another. An ultrasonic transducer converts electrical energy into ultrasound energy, and vice versa. This is accomplished by a process known as the *piezoelectric effect*. This effect is exhibited by certain crystals in which a variation of an electric field across the crystal causes it to oscillate mechanically, thus generating acoustic waves. Conversely, pressure variations across a piezoelectric material (in response to an incident ultrasound wave) result in a varying electrical potential across opposite surfaces of the crystal.

Although the piezoelectric effect is exhibited by a number of naturally occurring crystals, most common crystals used clinically are made artificially such as barium titanate, lead zirconium titanate, and lead metaniobate. The piezoelectric effect produced by these materials is mediated by their electric dipole moment, the magnitude of which can be varied by addition of suitable impurities.

As the ultrasound wave reflected from tissue interfaces is received by the transducer, voltage pulses are produced which are processed and displayed on the cathode ray tube (CRT), usually in one of three display modes: A (amplitude) mode, B (brightness) mode, and M (motion) mode. A mode consists of displaying the signal amplitude on the ordinate and time on the abscissa. The time, in this case, is related to distance or tissue depth, given the speed of sound in the medium. In the B mode, a signal from a point in the medium is displayed by an echo dot on the CRT. The (x, y) position of the dot on the CRT indicates the location of the reflecting point at the interface and its proportional brightness reveals the amplitude of the echo. By scanning across the patient, the B-mode viewer sees an apparent cross section through the patient. Such cross-sectional images are called *ultrasonic tomograms*.

In the M mode of presentation, the ultrasound images display the motion of internal structures of the patient's antomy. The most frequent application of M mode scanning is echocardiography. In radiotherapy, the cross-sectional information used for treatment planning is exclusively derived from the B scan images (Fig. 12.5).

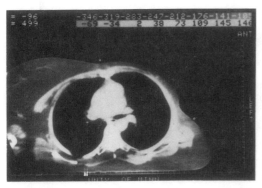 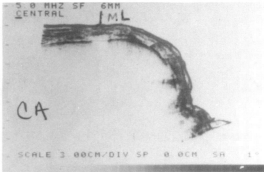

Figure 12.5.   Ultrasonic tomogram showing chest wall thickness (right) compared with the CT image (left).

B.4. TREATMENT SIMULATORS

A treatment simulator (Fig. 12.6) is an apparatus which uses a diagnostic x-ray tube but duplicates a radiation treatment unit in terms of its geometrical, mechanical, and optical properties. The main function of a simulator is to display the treatment fields so that the target volume may be accurately encompassed without delivering excessive irradiation to surrounding normal tissues. By radiographic visualization of internal organs, correct positioning of fields and shielding blocks can be obtained in relation to external landmarks. Most commercially available simulators have fluoroscopic capability for dynamic visualization before a hard copy is obtained in terms of the simulator radiography.

Specifications of a treatment simulator must closely match those of the treatment unit. Several authors (26–30) have discussed these aspects. For a comprehensive discussion, the reader is referred to the paper by McCullough and Earl (30).

The need for simulators arises from four facts. 1) Geometrical relationship between the radiation beam and the external and internal anatomy of the patient cannot be duplicated by an ordinary diagnostic x-ray unit. 2) Although field localization can be achieved directly with a therapy machine by taking a port film, the radiographic quality is poor because of very high beam energy, and, additionally for cobalt-60, a large source size. 3) Field localization is a time consuming process which, if carried out in the treatment room, could engage a therapy machine for a prohibitive length of time. 4) Unforeseen problems with a patient setup or treatment technique can be solved during simulation, thus conserving time within the treatment room.

Although the practical use of simulators varies widely from institution to institution, the simulator room is increasingly assuming the role of a treatment planning room. Besides localizing treatment volume and setting up fields, other necessary data can also be obtained at the time of simulation. Since the simulator table is supposed to be similar to the treatment table, various patient

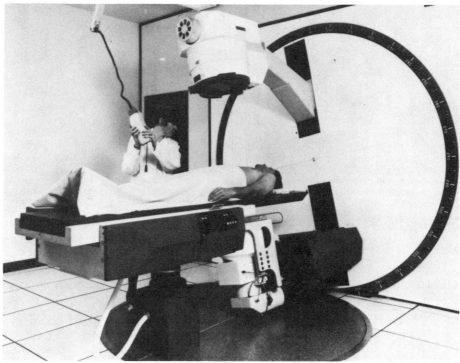

Figure 12.6.   Varian (TEM) Ximatron 5 treatment simulator. (Courtesy of Varian Associates, Minneapolis, MN.)

measurements such as contours and thicknesses including those related to compensator or bolus design, can be obtained under appropriate setup conditions. Fabrication and testing of individualized shielding blocks can also be accomplished with a simulator. In order to facilitate such measurements, modern simulators are equipped with accessories such as laser lights, contour maker, and shadow tray.

Some simulators have a tomography attachment in which the image from the image intensifier is analyzed and reconstructed using either analog[1] or digital[2] processing. Although image quality at present is rather poor, this is an area of active development.

An exciting development in the area of simulation is that of converting a CT scanner into a simulator. A commerical device, known as PZ-SIM,[3] uses a Pfizer 0200 FS CT scanner to localize the treatment fields on the basis of the patient's CT scans. A computer program, specifically written for simulation, automatically positions the patient couch and the laser cross hairs to define the scans and the treatment fields. The software provides automatic outlining

---

[1] Oldelft Corporation of America, 2735 Dorr Ave., Fairfax, Virginia.
[2] TEM Instruments Ltd., Gatwick Road, Crawley, Sussex, England.
[3] Columbia Scientific Incorporated, 8940 Old Annapolis Road, Columbia, Maryland 21045.

of external contours and critical structures, interactive portal displays and placement, display of isodose distribution, and review of multiple treatment plans. Such an integrated approach to treatment planning, although still in its infancy, has the potential of becoming the simulator cum treatment planning system of the future.

B.5. PORT FILMS

The primary purpose of port filming is to verify the treatment volume under actual conditions of treatment. Although the image quality with the megavoltage x-ray beam is poorer than with the diagnostic or the simulator film, a port film is considered mandatory not only as a good clinical practice but also as a legal record.

As a treatment record a port film must be of sufficiently good quality so that the field boundaries can be described anatomically. However, this may not always be possible due to either very high beam energy (10 MV or higher), large source size (cobalt-60), large patient thickness (>20 cm), or poor radiographic technique. In such a case, the availability of a simulator film and/or a treatment diagram with adequate anatomic description of the field is helpful. Anatomic interpretation of a port film is sometimes helped by obtaining a full field exposure on top of the treatment port exposure.

Radiographic technique significantly influences image quality of a port film. The choice of film and screeen as well as the exposure technique is important in this regard. Droege and Bjärngard (31) have analyzed the film screen combinations commonly used for port filming at megavoltage x-ray energies. Their investigation shows that the use of a single emulsion film with the emulsion adjacent to a single lead screen[4] between the film and the patient is preferable to a double emulsion film or a film with more than one screen. Thus, for optimum resolution, one needs a single emulsion film with a front lead screen and no rear screen. Conventional nonmetallic screens are not recommended at megavoltage energies. Although thicker metallic screens produce a better response, an increase in thickness beyond the maximum electron range produces no further changes in resolution (31).

Certain slow speed films, ready packed but without a screen, can be exposed during the entire treatment duration. A therapy verification film such as Kodak XV-2 is sufficiently slow to allow an exposure of up to 200 rad without reaching saturation. In addition, such films can be used to construct compensators for both the contours and tissue heterogeneity (32).

12.2 CORRECTIONS FOR CONTOUR IRREGULARITIES

As mentioned in the beginning of this chapter, basic dose distribution data are obtained under standard conditions which include homogeneous unit

---

[4] Such a sheet of lead acts as an intensifying screen by means of electrons ejected from the screen by photon interactions. These electrons provide an image on the film which reflects the variation of beam intensity transmitted through the patient.

density phantom, perpendicular beam incidence, and flat surface. During treatment, however, the beam may be obliquely incident with respect to the surface and, in addition, the surface may be curved or irregular in shape. Under such conditions, the standard dose distributions cannot be applied without proper modifications or corrections.

Contour corrections may be avoided by using a bolus or a compensator (to be discussed in Section 12.4) but under some circumstances it is permissible, or even desirable, to determine the actual dose distribution by calculation. The following three methods are recommended for angles of incidence of up to 45° for megavoltage beams and of up to 30° from the surface normal for orthovoltage x-rays (33).

A. Effective SSD Method

Consider Fig. 12.7 in which SS is an irregularly shaped patient contour. It is desired to calculate the percent depth dose at point A (*i.e.* dose at A as a percentage of D_{max} dose at point Q). The diagram shows that the tissue deficit above point A is h cm and the depth of D_{max} is d_m. If we note that the percent depth dose does not change rapidly with SSD (provided that the SSD is large), the relative depth dose distribution along the line joining the source with point A is unchanged when the isodose chart is moved down by the distance h and positioned with its surface line at S'-S'. Suppose D_A is the dose at point A. Assuming beam to be incident on a flat surface located at S'-S',

$$D_A = D'_{max} \cdot P' \tag{12.2}$$

where P' is percent depth dose at A relative to D'_{max} at point Q'. Suppose P_{corr} is the correct percent depth dose at A relative to D_{max} at point Q. Then

$$D_A = D_{max} \cdot P_{corr} \tag{12.3}$$

From Equations 12.2 and 12.3,

$$P_{corr} = P' \cdot \left(\frac{D'_{max}}{D_{max}}\right) \tag{12.4}$$

Since, when the distribution is moved, the SSD is increased by a distance h, we have:

$$\frac{D'_{max}}{D_{max}} = \left(\frac{SSD + d_m}{SSD + h + d_m}\right)^2 \tag{12.5}$$

Therefore,

$$P_{corr} = P' \cdot \left(\frac{SSD + d_m}{SSD + h + d_m}\right)^2 \tag{12.6}$$

Thus, the effective SSD method consists of sliding the isodose chart down so

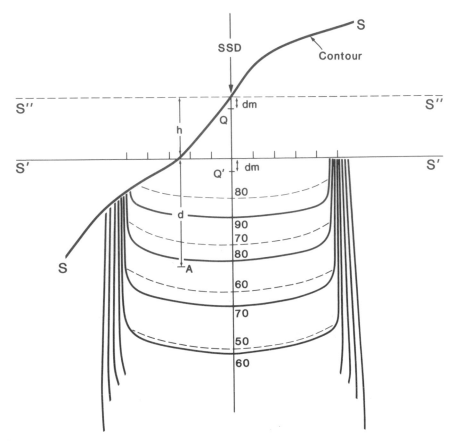

Figure 12.7.   Diagram illustrating methods of correcting dose distribution under an irregular surface such as $S - S$. The solid isodose curves are from an isodose chart which assumes a flat surface located at $S' - S'$. The dashed isodose curves assume a flat surface at $S'' - S''$ without any air gap.

that its surface line is at S'–S', reading off the percent dose value at A and multiplying it by the inverse square law factor to give the corrected percent depth dose value.

The above method applies the same way when there is excess tissue above A instead of tissue deficit. In such a case, the isodose chart is moved up so that its surface line passes through the point of intersection of the contour line and the ray line through A. The value of h is assigned a negative value in this case.

B. Tissue-Air (or Tissue-Maximum) Ratio Method

This method depends on the principle that the tissue-air or tissue-maximum ratio does not depend upon the SSD and is a function only of the depth and the field size at that depth. Suppose, in Fig. 12.7, the surface is located at S''–S'' and the air space between S–S and S''–S'' is filled with tissue-like material. Now, if a standard isodose chart for the given beam and SSD is placed with its surface at S''–S'', the percent depth dose value at A will correspond to the depth $d + h$. But the actual value at A is greater than this since there is a tissue deficit. The correction factor can be obtained by the ratio of tissue-air or tissue-maximum ratios for depths d and $d + h$.

$$\text{Correction factor } (CF) = \frac{T(d,\, r_A)}{T(d + h,\, r_A)} \qquad (12.7)$$

where T stands for tissue-air ratio or tissue-maximum ratio and r_A is the field size projected at point A (*i.e.* at a distance of SSD $+ d + h$ from the source).

Thus, if the uncorrected value of percent depth dose at A with the surface line of the isodose chart at S''–S'', is P'', then the corrected value P_{corr} is given by

$$P_{\text{corr}} = P'' \cdot CF$$

C. Isodose Shift Method

The preceding methods are useful for making individual point dose calculations. However, for manual treatment planning, it is convenient to correct the entire isodose chart for contour irregularities. This can be done by an empirical method, known as the isodose shift method. The procedure is illustrated in Fig. 12.8. Suppose S–S is the patient contour drawn on a transparent paper and S'–S' is a flat surface line passing through the point of intersection of the central axis with the contour. From the line S'–S', draw vertical grid lines, parallel to the central axis and spaced about 1 cm apart to cover the full field width. Place the standard isodose chart underneath this paper and align the central line of the chart with that of the grid. Mark the percent depth dose values on the central axis. For each grid line, slide the isodose chart up or down, depending on whether there is tissue excess or deficit along that line, by an amount $k \times h$ were k is a factor less than 1 (given in Table 12.1). Then mark the isodose values at points of intersection of the given grid line and the shifted isodose curves. After all the isodose positions along all the gridlines have been marked, new isodose curves are drawn by joining the marked points having the same isodose values.

The factor k depends on the radiation quality, field size, depth of interest, and SSD. Table 12.1 gives approximate values recommended for clinical use when manual corrections are needed.

Of the three methods discussed above, the tissue-air or tissue-maximum ratio method gives the most accurate results. The first two methods are especially useful in computer treatment planning.

Example 1. For point A in Fig. 12.7, $h = 3$ cm and $d = 5$ cm. Calculate the percent depth dose at point A using (a) the effective SSD method and (b) the tissue-air ratio method.

Given ^{60}Co beam, TAR(5, 11 × 11) = 0.910 and TAR(8, 11 × 11) = 0.795

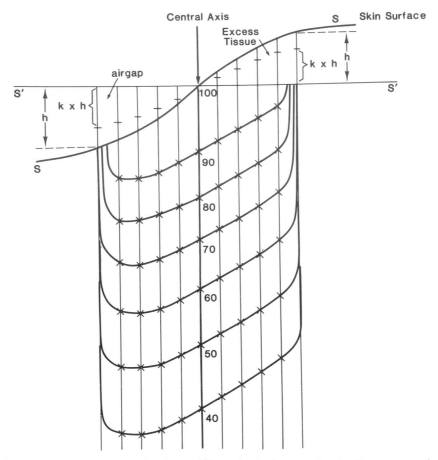

Figure 12.8. Diagram illustrating isodose shift method of correcting isodose curves for surface contour irregularity.

Table 12.1.
Isodose shift factors for different beam energies

Photon Energy (MV)	Approximate Factor k
Up to 1	0.8
^{60}Co-5	0.7
5–15	0.6
15–30	0.5
Above 30	0.4

Data are from Giessen PH: *Br J Radiol* 46:978, 1973.

and SSD = 80 cm

(a) using solid isodose curve lines in Fig. 12.7,

Percent depth dose at A = 78.1

$$\text{Inverse square law factor} = \left(\frac{80 + 0.5}{80 + 3 + 0.5}\right)^2$$

$$= 0.929$$

Corrected percent depth dose at A = 78.1 × 0.929

$$= 72.6$$

(b) Field dimension projected at $A = 10 \times \dfrac{88}{80}$ = 11 cm. Thus field size at A = 11 × 11 cm:

$$CF = \frac{\text{TAR}(5, \ 11 \times 11)}{\text{TAR}(8, \ 11 \times 11)} = \frac{0.910}{0.795} = 1.145$$

Using dashed isodose lines in Fig. 12.7, uncorrected percent depth dose = 65.2.

Corrected percent depth dose = 65.2 × 1.145

$$= 74.6$$

Comparing the results for (a) and (b), the agreement beween the two methods is within 3%.

12.3 CORRECTIONS FOR TISSUE INHOMOGENEITIES

Applications of standard isodose charts and depth dose tables assume homogeneous unit density medium. In a patient however, the beam may traverse layers of fat, bone, muscle, lung, and air. The presence of these inhomogeneities will produce changes in the dose distribution depending on the amount and type of material present and on the quality of radiation.

The effects of tissue inhomogeneities may be classified into two general categories: (a) changes in the absorption of the primary beam and the associated pattern of scattered photons; and (b) changes in the secondary electron fluence. The relative importance of these effects depends on the region of interest where alterations in absorbed dose are considered. For points which lie beyond the inhomogeneity, the predominant effect is the attenuation of the primary beam. Changes in the associated photon scatter distribution alters the dose distribution more strongly near the inhomogeneity than farther beyond it. The changes in the secondary electron fluence, on the other hand, affects the tissues within the inhomogeneity and at the boundaries.

For x-ray beams in the megavoltage range, where Compton effect is a predominant mode of interaction, the attenuation of the beam in any medium is governed by electron density (number of electrons per cm^3). Thus, an effective depth can be used for calculating transmission through nonwaterequivalent materials. However, close to the boundary or interface, the distribution is more complex. For example, for megavoltage beams, there may be loss of electronic equilibrium close to the boundaries of low density materials or air cavities. For orthovoltage and superficial x-rays, the major problem is the bone. Absorbed dose within the bone or in the immediate vicinity of it may be several times higher than the dose in the soft tissue in the absence of bone. This increased energy absorption is caused by the increase in the electron fluence arising from the photoelectric absorption in the mineral contents of the bone.

A. Corrections for Beam Attenuation and Scattering

Figure 12.9 is a schematic diagram showing an inhomogeneity of electron density ρ_e relative to that of water. The material preceding and following the inhomogeneity is water equivalent (relative $\rho_e = 1$). Lateral dimensions of this composite phantom are assumed infinite or much larger than the field size. Calculation is to be made at point P which is located at a distance d_3 from the lower boundary, distance $(d_2 + d_3)$ from the front boundary of the inhomogeneity and distance $d = d_1 + d_2 + d_3$ from the surface.

Three methods of correcting for inhomogeneities are illustrated with reference to Fig. 12.9.

A.1. TISSUE-AIR RATIO METHOD

The following CF applies to the dose at P if the entire phantom was water equivalent:

$$CF = \frac{T(d', r_d)}{T(d, r_d)} \tag{12.8}$$

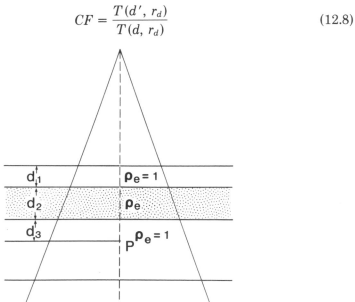

Figure 12.9. Schematic diagram showing a water equivalent phantom containing an inhomogeneity of electron density ρ_e relative to that of water. P is the point of dose calculation.

where d' is the equivalent water depth, *i.e.* $d' = d_1 + \rho_e\, d_2 + d_3$ and d is the actual depth of P from the surface. r_d is the field size projected at point P.

The above correction method does not take into account the position of the inhomogeneity relative to point P. In other words, the correction factor will not change with d_3 as long as d and d' remain constant.

For more details and three-dimensional aspects of the problem, the reader is referred to the paper by Sontag and Cunningham (21). The above method remains valid if tissue-maximum ratios are substituted for tissue-air ratios.

A.2. POWER LAW TISSUE-AIR RATIO METHOD

Batho (34) and Young and Gaylord (35) have proposed a method in which the ratio of the tissue-air ratios is raised to a power. Referring again to Fig. 12.9, the correction factor at point P is

$$CF = \left[\frac{T(d_2 + d_3,\, r_d)}{T(d_3,\, r_d)} \right]^{\rho_e - 1} \tag{12.9}$$

Here ρ_e is the electron density (number of electrons/cm^3) of the heterogeneity relative to that of water.

As seen in Equation 12.9, the correction factor does depend on the location of the inhomogeneity relative to point P but not relative to the surface. This formulation is based on theoretical considerations assuming Compton interactions only. It does not apply to points inside the inhomogeneity or in the buildup region. Experimental verification of the model has been provided for ^{60}Co γ ray beams (34, 35).

A.3. ISODOSE SHIFT METHOD

This method, proposed by Greene and Stewart (36) and Sundblom (37), is convenient for correcting isodose charts for the presence of inhomogeneities. The isodose curves beyond the inhomogeneity are moved by an amount equal to n times the thickness of the inhomogeneity as measured along a line parallel to the central axis and passing through the point of interest. The shift is toward the skin for bone and away from the skin for lung or air cavities. Table 12.2 gives experimentally determined values of n which apply to ^{60}Co radiation and 4-MV x-rays. The factors are believed to be independent of field size.

Table 12.2.
Isodose shift factors* for inhomogeneities

Inhomogeneity	Shift Factor n
Air cavity	−0.6
Lung	−0.4
Hard bone	0.5
Spongy bone	0.25

* Approximate factors, determined empirically for ^{60}Co and 4-MV x-rays (36, 37).

A.4. EXAMPLES: TYPICAL CORRECTION FACTORS

Table 12.3 gives some examples of increase in dose beyond healty lung for various beam energies. These correction factors have been calculated by using Equation 12.8, assuming $d_1 = 6$ cm, $d_2 = 8$ cm, and $d_3 = 3$ cm, relative ρ_e for lung $= 0.25$, and field size $= 10 \times 10$ cm. The values were rounded off to represent approximate factors for typical lung corrections. More detailed tables of the beyond-lung and in-lung correction factors have been calculated by McDonald *et al.* (67) for several representative beam energies and field sizes.

Table 12.4 gives the decrease in dose beyond bone that might be expected with beams of different energies. These are approximate values since the shielding effect of bone depends on the size of the bone, field size, and other parameters that affect scattering. It should be noted that the shielding effect of bone diminishes quite rapidly as the beam energy increases. The shielding effect of bone for x-rays generated between 500 kV and 4 MV is entirely due to its greater electron density (electrons per cm^3) since all the attenuation is due to the Compton process. In the megavoltage range, the corrections for bone attenuation in most clinical situations are small and are usually neglected. However, as the x-ray energy increases beyond 10 MV, the shielding effect begins to increase because pair production becomes significant. Recall that the absorption of radiation due to pair production depends on the atomic number.

Table 12.3.
Increase in dose to tissues beyond healthy lung*

Beam Quality	Correction Factor
Orthovoltage	+10%/cm of lung
^{60}Co γ rays	+5%/cm of lung
4-MV x-rays	+4%/cm of lung
10-MV x-rays	+3%/cm of lung
20-MV x-rays	+2%/cm of lung

* Approximate values calculated by Equation 12.8 for typical clinical situations.

Table 12.4.
Reduction in dose beyond 1 cm of hard bone*

Beam Quality	Correction Factor (%)
1 mm Cu HVL	−15†
3 mm Cu HVL	−7
^{60}Co	−3.5
4 MV	−3
10 MV	−2

* Approximate values calculated by Equation 12.8 for typical clinical situations. Assumed electron density of bone relative to water = 1.65.
† Estimated from measured data by Haas LL, Sandberg GH: *Br J Radiol* 30:19, 1957.

B. Absorbed Dose within an Inhomogeneity

As mentioned earlier, the absorbed dose within an inhomogeneity or in the soft tissues adjacent to it is strongly influenced by alterations in the secondary electron fluence. For example, for x-rays generated at potentials less than 250 kVp, there is a substantial increase in absorbed dose inside bone because of increased electron fluence arising from photoelectric absorption. Spiers (38, 39) has made a comprehensive study of absorbed dose within mineral bone as well as within soft tissue components of bone. The interested reader is referred to the original work or Chapter XIII of Johns and Cunningham (40) for details. Some practical aspects of the problem will be discussed in this section.

B.1. BONE

Under the conditions of electronic equilibrium, the ratio of absorbed doses in different media, for a given photon energy fluence, is given by the ratio of their energy absorption coefficients (see Chapter 8). Since the rad/R or the f factor is proportional to the energy absorption coefficient relative to air, the ratio of f factors also reflects the relative absorbed dose. Thus, for a given quality radiation and the energy fluence, the absorbed dose in bone relative to absorbed dose in muscle is the ratio

$$\frac{f_{\text{bone}}}{f_{\text{muscle}}} \text{ or } \left(\frac{\mu_{\text{en}}}{\rho}\right)^{\text{bone}}_{\text{muscle}}$$

under electronic equilibrium conditions.

Figure 12.10A shows a plot of absorbed dose as a function of depth for an orthovoltage beam incident on a composite phantom containing 2-cm thick bone. Since for this quality radiation $f_{\text{bone}}/f_{\text{muscle}} = 1.9/0.94 = 2.0$, the dose in the first layer of bone will be about twice as much as in soft tissue. In the subsequent layers, the dose will drop from this value due to increased attenuation by bone. The dose within the bone or just beyond it is difficult to calculate since it requires the knowledge of both the energy fluence and the energy absorption coefficient. However, approximate calculations can be made by using empirically derived transmission factors (Table 12.4).

Calculations are simplified in the case of megavoltage beams where photon interactions are entirely Compton. Figure 12.10B compares the above situation with ^{60}Co beam. Since $f_{\text{bone}}/f_{\text{muscle}} = 0.955/0.957 = 0.96$ for this energy, the dose inside the bone for a ^{60}Co beam is slightly less than that expected in the soft tissue. Beyond the bone, the dose is reduced due to the shielding effect of bone since the electron density of bone is higher than that of the muscle tissue (Section 12.3A). Thus the presence of bone in ^{60}Co or higher energy beams produces only small alterations in the depth dose distribution. The dosimetric effects of bone in megavoltage therapy are usually ignored.

Table 12.5 gives the change in dose expected in the bone for different energy beams. These estimates are made on the basis of the f factor ratios of bone to muscle or the ratio of energy absorption coefficients. For orthovoltage beams,

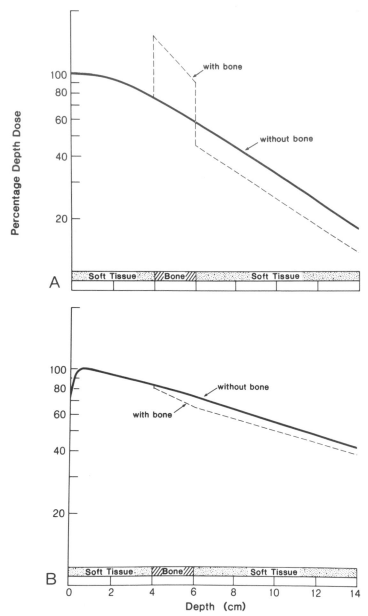

Figure 12.10. Percentage depth dose as a function of depth in a phantom containing 2 cm of bone. (A) HVL = 1 mm Cu; SSD = 50 cm and field size 10 × 10 cm. (B) ^{60}Co γ ray beam; SSD = 80 cm and field size 10 × 10 cm.

Table 12.5.
Absorbed dose to compact bone relative to soft tissue for different energy beams*

Radiation Quality		f Factor†		Rads in Bone/Rad in Soft Tissue†:
HVL	Approximate Effective Energy	Muscle Rad/R	Bone Rad/R	$\left(\dfrac{f_{bone}}{f_{muscle}}\right)$ or $\left(\dfrac{\mu_{en}}{\rho}\right)^{bone}_{muscle}$
1 mm Al	20 keV	0.90	4.2	4.7
3 mm Al	30 keV	0.90	4.2	4.7
1 mm Cu	80 keV	0.94	1.9	2.0
2 mm Cu	110 keV	0.95	1.4	1.45
3 mm Cu	135 keV	0.95	1.1	1.15
10.4 mm Pb(^{60}Co γ rays)	1.25 MeV	0.96	0.92	0.96
11.8 mm Pb (4-MV x-rays)	1.5 MeV	0.96	0.92	0.96
14.7 mm Pb (10-MV x-rays)	4 MeV	—‡	—	0.98
13.7 mm Pb (20-MV x-rays)	8 MeV	—	—	1.02
12.3 mm Pb (40-MV x-rays)	10 MeV	—	—	1.03

* HVL and approximate effective energies calculated using attenuation coefficients (Chapter 7).
† Derived from data given in Johns HE, Cunningham JR: *The Physics of Radiology*, 3rd ed., Springfield, IL, Charles C Thomas, 1969.
‡ —, roentgen not defined for this quality radiation.

these values represent the maximal enhancement in dose occurring just inside bone on the entrance side of the beam.

B.2. LUNG TISSUE

Dose within the lung tissue is primarily governed by its density. As discussed in Section 12.3A, lower lung density gives rise to higher dose within and beyond the lung. Figure 12.11 gives the increase in lung dose as a function of depth in the lung for selected energies using a 10 × 10 cm field. But in the first layers of soft tissue beyond a large thickness of lung, there is some loss of secondary electrons (41). This gives rise to a slight decrease in dose relative to that calculated on the basis of lung transmission.

B.3. AIR CAVITY

The most important effect of air cavities in megavoltage beam dosimetry is the partial loss of electronic equilibrium at the cavity surface. The actual dose to tissue beyond and in front of the cavity may be appreciably lower than expected. This phenomenon of dose buildup at the air cavities has been extensively studied by Epp *et al.* (42, 43). The most significant decrease in dose occurs at the surface beyond the cavity, for large cavities (4 cm deep) and the smallest field (4 × 4 cm). Epp *et al.* (42) have estimated that in the case of ^{60}Co the reduction in dose in practical cases, such as the lesions located in the upper respiratory air passages, will not be greater than 10% unless field sizes smaller than 4 × 4 cm are used. The underdosage is expected to be greater for higher energy radiation (43).

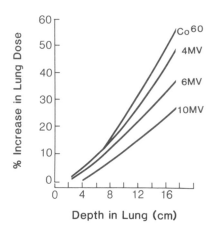

Figure 12.11.   Percentage increase in lung dose as a function of depth in the lung for selected energies. Field size 10 × 10 cm. [Reprinted with permission from: McDonald *et al.* (65).]

12.4 TISSUE COMPENSATION

A radiation beam incident on an irregular or sloping surface produces skewing of the isodose curves. Corrections for this effect have been discussed in Section 12.2. In certain treatment situations, however, the surface irregularity gives rise to unacceptable nonuniformity of dose within the target volume or causes excessive irradiation of sensitive structures such as the spinal cord. Many techniques have been devised to overcome this problem, including the use of wedged fields or multiple fields and the addition of bolus material or compensators. Areas having a smaller thickness of tissue can also be blocked for the last few treatments to reduce the dose in these areas.

Bolus is a tissue-equivalent material placed directly on the skin surface to even out the irregular contours of a patient in order to present a flat surface normal to the beam. This use of bolus should be distinguished from that of a bolus layer which is thick enough to provide adequate dose buildup over the skin surface. The latter should be termed as the *buildup bolus.*

Placing bolus directly on the skin surface is satisfactory for orthovoltage radiation, but for higher energy beams results in the loss of the *skin sparing* advantage. For such radiations, a *compensating filter* should be used, which approximates the effect of the bolus as well as preserves the skin sparing effect. In order to preserve the skin sparing properties of the megavoltage photon beams, the compensator is placed a suitable distance (15–20 cm) away from the patient's skin. Yet, the compensator is so designed that its introduction in the beam gives rise to isodose curves within the patient that duplicate, as closely as possible, those for the bolus.

A. Design of Compensators

Figure 12.12 illustrates schematically the use of a compensator to provide the required beam attenuation which would otherwise occur in the "missing"

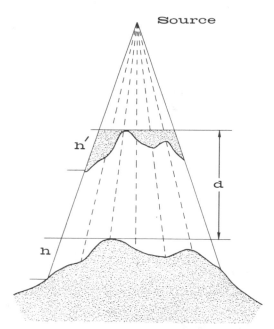

Figure 12.12. Schematic representation of a compensator designed for an irregular surface. [Reprinted with permission from: Khan *et al.* (49).]

tissue when the body surface is irregular or curved. Since the compensator is designed to be positioned at a distance from the surface, the dimensions and shape of the compensator must be adjusted because of (a) the beam divergence, (b) the relative linear attenuation coefficients of the filter material and soft tissues, and (c) the reduction in scatter at various depths when the compensator is placed at a distance from the skin rather than in contact with it. In order to compensate for this scatter, the compensator is designed such that the attenuation of the filter is less than that required for primary radiation only. These considerations and others have been discussed in the literature (44–50).

Minification of the compensating material for geometric divergence of the beam has been achieved in many ways. One method (44, 46–48) constructs the compensator out of aluminum or brass blocks, using a matrix of square columns corresponding to the irregular surface. The dimension of each column is minified according to the geometric divergence correction which is calculated from the SSD and the filter-surface distance. Khan *et al.* (51) described an apparatus which uses thin rods duplicating the diverging rays of the therapy beam (Fig. 12.13). The rods move freely in rigid shafts along the diverging paths and can be locked or released by a locking device. The apparatus is positioned over the patient so that the lower ends of the rods touch the skin surface. When the rods are locked, the upper ends of the rods generate a surface that is similar to the skin surface but corrected for divergence. A

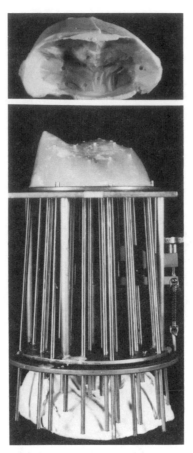

Figure 12.13. An apparatus for the construction of three-dimensional compensator in one piece. [Reprinted with permission from: Khan *et al.* (51).]

plastic compensator can then be built over this surface (49). Beck *et al.* (52) and Boge *et al.* (53) have described styrofoam cutters (Fig. 12.14) which use a heating element or a routing tool mechanism for the hollowing of the styrofoam. The cavity thus produced is a minified version of the patient surface which can be filled with the compensator material.

A tissue equivalent compensator designed with the same thickness as that of the missing tissue will overcompensate, *i.e.* the dose to the underlying tissues will be less than that indicated by the standard isodose chart. This decrease in depth dose, which is due to the reduction in scatter reaching a point at depth, depends on the distance of the compensator from the patient, field size, depth, and beam quality. In order to compensate for this decrease in scatter, one may reduce the thickness of the compensator to increase the primary beam transmission. The compensator thickness should be such that the dose at a given depth is the same whether the missing tissue is replaced

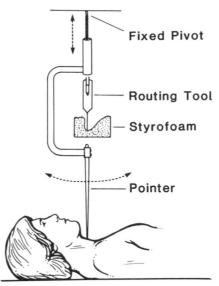

Figure 12.14. Schematic diagram of a styrofoam cutter fitted with a routing tool for constructing compensators. Redrawn from Boge *et al.* (53).

with the bolus in contact or with the compensator at the given distance from the skin surface. The required thickness of a tissue-equivalent compensator along a ray divided by the missing tissue thickness along the same ray may be called the *density ratio* or *thickness ratio* (49) (h'/h in Fig. 12.12). Figure 12.15 gives a plot of thickness ratio, τ, as a function of compensator-surface distance, d. τ is unity at the surface and decreases as d increases.

Thickness ratio depends, in a complex way, on compensator-surface distance, thickness of missing tissue, field size, depth, and beam quality. However, a detailed study of this parameter has shown that τ is primarily a function of d (for $d \leq 20$ cm) and that its dependence on other parameters is relatively less critical (49, 54). Thus, a fixed value of τ, based on a given d (usually 20 cm), 10 × 10 cm field, 7-cm depth, and a tissue deficit of 5 cm can be used for most compensator work.

The concept of thickness ratios also reveals that a compensator cannot be designed to provide absorbed dose compensation exactly at all depths. If, for given irradiation conditions, τ is chosen for a certain compensation depth, the compensator overcompensates at shallower depths and undercompensates at greater depths. Considering the limitations of the theory and too many variables affecting τ, we have found that an average value of 0.7 for τ may be used for all irradiation conditions provided $d \geq 20$ cm. The same value has been tested to yield satisfactory results (errors in depth dose within ±5%) for ^{60}Co, 4-MV and 10-MV x-rays (54).

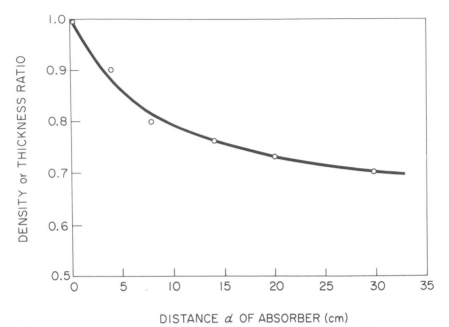

Figure 12.15. A plot of density ratio or thickness ratio as a function of compensator distance for a uniformly thick compensator. ^{60}Co γ rays, field size 10 × 10 cm, SSD = 80 cm, compensation depth = 7 cm, and tissue deficit = 5.0 cm. [Reprinted with permission from: Khan *et al.* (49).]

B. Two-Dimensional Compensators

Designing a three-dimensional compensator is a time consuming procedure. In a well equipped mold or machine shop, a trained technician can probably construct such compensators routinely with a reasonable expenditure of time. In the absence of such facilities and personnel, however, most situations requiring compensation can be handled satisfactorily with simple two-dimensional compensators. In many treatment situations, the contour varies significantly in only one direction: along the field width or length. In such cases, a compensator can be constructed in which the thickness varies only along this dimension. For example, if anterior and posterior fields are incident upon a sloping mediastinum, compensation is usually not required in the lateral direction but only in the craniocaudal direction.

One simple way of constructing a two-dimensional compensator is to use thin sheets of lead (with known thickness ratio or effective attenuation coefficient) and gluing them together in a stepwise fashion to form a laminated filter. The total thickness of the filter at any point is calculated to compensate for the air gap at the point below it. Another method, used routinely at the University of Minnesota, is to construct the compensator in one piece from a block of Lucite. The patient contour is taken showing body thickness at at least three reference points: central axis, inferior margin, and superior margins of the field. Tissue deficits, Δt, are calculated by subtracting thicknesses at the reference points from the maximum thickness. A thickness minification factor is calculated by dividing the thickness ratio τ by the electron density (e^- per cm^3) of Lucite relative to that of tissue. The geometric minification factor is calculated by $(f - d)/f$ where f is the SSD at the point of maximum thickness and d is the filter-surface distance. The compensator dimensions can now be drawn by multiplying the Δt values with the thickness minification factor and the spacing between the reference points with the geometric minification factor. A Lucite block is then machined and glued on a thin Lucite plate for placement in the beam.

C. Compensating Wedges

For oblique beam incidence or curved surfaces where the contour can be approximated with a straight line, standard compensating wedges are very convenient (49, 50). Compensating wedges, or C-wedges for short, are fabricated from a metal such as copper, brass, or lead. They are designed to compensate for a "missing" wedge of tissue, using the same design principles as discussed in Section 12.4B.

Distinction needs to be made between a wedge filter and a compensating wedge. Although a wedge filter can be used effectively as a compensator, it is primarily designed to tilt the standard isodose curves through a certain wedge angle in conjunction with the wedge-pair technique (Section 11.7). The wedge filter isodose curves must be available and used to obtain the composite isodose curves before the filter is used in a treatment setup. The C-wedge, on the other hand, is used just as a compensator, so that the standard isodose charts can be used without modification. In addition, no wedge transmission factors are required for the C-wedges.

An important advantage of C-wedges over wedge filters used as compensators is that the C-wedges can be used for partial field compensation, *i.e.* the C-wedge is used to compensate only a part of the contour which is irregular in shape. A wedge filter, in this case, could not be used as a compensator since it is designed to be placed in the field in a fixed position.

D. Other Applications

Compensating filters can be designed to compensate for tissue heterogeneity. Most of this work was done by Ellis and his coworkers (32) in which compensators were designed from the knowledge of cross-sectional anatomy using transaxial tomography or a photographic film. More recently, Khan *et al.* (55) have described compensators for total body irradiation including compensation for lungs.

Compensators have also been used to improve dose uniformity in the fields where nonuniformity of the dose distribution arises from sources other than contour irregularity: reduced scatter near the field edges and unacceptable high dose regions or "horns" in the beam profile. Leung *et al.* (56) have discussed the design of filters for the mantle technique in which the compensator is designed on the basis of calculated dose distribution in the absence of a compensator. Boge *et al.* (57) have described a special compensator filter to reduce the "horns" present in large fields of a 4-MV linear accelerator.

E. Compensator Setup

As mentioned earlier, the compensator should be placed at a distance of 15 cm or more away from the skin surface in order to preserve the skin sparing properties of the megavoltage beams. Since the dimensions of the compensator are reduced (compared to the bolus) in the plane perpendicular to the beam axis to allow for beam divergence, the filter must be placed at the filter-surface distance for which it is designed. In addition, the nominal SSD should be measured from the plane perpendicular to the beam axis, containing the most elevated point on the contour included in the field (see Fig. 12.12). For isocentric treatments, it is most convenient to use field dimensions projected at the isocenter in compensator design. Accordingly, the depth of the isocenter is measured from the level of the most elevated point on the contour to be compensated.

12.5 PATIENT POSITIONING

Availability of isocentric treatment machines, simulators, CT scanners, and computers has made it possible to achieve a high degree of precision in radiotherapy. However, one of the weakest links in the treatment planning process is the problem of patient positioning and immobilization. It is frequently observed that some of the treatment techniques in current practice are outdated or do not take advantage of the accuracy available with the modern equipment. For example, the patients are treated in less than a stable position, are moved between different fields, and set up primarily by marks inked or tattooed on the skin surface. But, as any experienced observer knows, such practices are prone to serious errors. Skin marks are vulnerable to variation in skin sag and body position on the treatment table.

The problem of precise patient positioning and immobilization has been addressed by a number of investigators (58–63). But this problem still remains the area of greatest variance in actual treatment. The following ideas are presented to focus attention on this important area and offer some guidelines for precise patient positioning.

A. General Guidelines

1) If technically feasible, treatments should be set up isocentrically. The principal advantage of isocentric technique over SSD technique is that the patient is not moved between fields. Once the isocenter is positioned accurately within the patient, the remaining fields are arranged simply by gantry rotation or couch movement, not by displacing the patient relative to the couch.

2) Isocenter position within the patient can be established using the treat-

ment simulator. This is usually accomplished by anterior and lateral radiographs, using the radiographically visible structures to define the target volume.

3) In order to accurately define the patient's position, pads or mattresses should not be used on the simulator table or the treatment table. This is essential for accurate measurement of setup parameters as well as reproducibility.

4) For head and neck treatments, flexible head rests, such as pillows or sponges, should be avoided. The head should rest on a rigid surface such as a block of hard styrofoam or a plastic "head-neck" support (Fig. 12.16).

5) Many methods of head immobilization are available such as partial body casts (62), bite block system (64),[5] nose bridges, [5] head clamps,[5] or simple masking tape. Choice of any of the above will depend upon the location of the treatment fields.

6) As far as possible, the patient should be treated in the supine position. An overhead sagittal laser line is useful in aligning the sagittal axis of the patient with the axis of gantry rotation.

7) For head and neck treatments, the chin extension should be defined anatomically, *e.g.* distance between the sternal notch and the chin bone. This measurement should be accurately made after the head position has been established on the basis of stability and field localization.

8) During simulation as well as treatment, the depth of isocenter should be defined by either the setup SSD (usually measured anteriorly or posteriorly) or by setting the distance between the tabletop distance and lateral beam axis. Side laser lights may also be used for this purpose. In the latter case, the laser lights should be checked frequently for alignment accuracy since these lights are known to drift presumably by expansion and contraction of the walls on which they are mounted.

9) Skin marks should not be relied on for daily localization of the treatment field. The field boundaries should be defined relative to the bony landmarks established during simulation. Do not force the field to fit the skin marks!

10) For lateral portals, the Mylar section of the couch or tennis racket should be removed and the patient placed on a solid surface to avoid sag. These should be used only for anterioposterior (AP) treatments where skin sparing is to be achieved. For example, if the four-field pelvis technique is used, one can use two fields a day in which case AP treatments are given isocentrically on a Mylar window using anterior or posterior setup SSD, and lateral fields are treated on a flat tabletop section using the tabletop distance to lateral beam axis. Or, if four fields are treated the same day, the posterior field can be treated through the rigid Plexiglas section of the couch instead of the Mylar window. Or, AP treatments can be given on the Mylar window and then the window can be replaced by the Plexiglas section for the lateral treatments. The last alternative involves two separate setups, one for the AP

---

[5] Such devices are commercially available, for example, from Radiation Products Design, Inc., Buffalo, Minnesota.

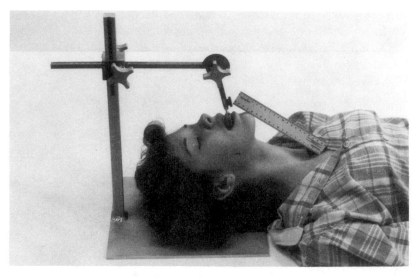

Figure 12.16.   Bite block system for head and neck immobilization. (Courtesy of Radiation Products Design, Buffalo, MN.)

and the other for the lateral fields. It should be used only when skin dose from the posterior fields is to be reduced to a minimum.

11) For isocentric techniques, field sizes must be defined at the isocenter which will, in most cases, be at the center of the treatment volume and not on the skin surface. Physicians who are accustomed to using standard field sizes (*e.g.* pelvic fields) defined at the skin surface should make adjustments in field sizes so that the fields encompass the same irradiated volume.

Some institutions have developed elaborate casting techniques to immobolize patients during treatments. This requires a well equipped mold room as well as personnel trained in mold technology. Some of these techniques have been shown to be quite effective in minimizing patient motion (62). However, patients are known, to move within a cast especially if the fit is not good or if there is a change in the surfaces contour due to regression of the tumor or weight loss.

Detection of patient motion is possible by using small dots of reflective tape on the patient with a pencil light ray and photocell device. Laser localization lights can also be used for this purpose. The signal received from the photocell can be further processed to activate an interlock to interrupt treatment or sound an alarm if pertinent motion exceeds a preset limit. Thus, a good motion detection system can complement patient positioning and immobilization techniques by monitoring the stability of patient position as well as the effectiveness of immobilization.

B. The "XYZ" Method of Isocenter Setup

In the isocentric technique, the isocenter is placed inside the patient, usually at the center of the target volume. Once this point has been localized by simulation, a good treatment setup should reproduce it quickly and accurately. The following steps outline a procedure, hereby called the XYZ method, for the localization of this important point.

B.1. SIMULATION PROCEDURE

1) The patient is positioned on the simulator couch following the general guidelines discussed in Section 12.5A.

2) The patient is leveled using the side lasers (or a bubble level) and the sagittal laser beam to define the sagittal axis of the patient. The patient is then constrained from movement by a suitable immobilization device. For head and neck positioning, chin extension (distance between chin bone and the sternal notch) should be accurately measured.

3) The treatment fields are simulated using anterior and lateral radiographs and the isocenter is established according to the treatment plan.

4) A *reference anatomical point* is chosen on the sagittal axis, somewhere in the neighborhood of the treatment area, to represent a stable anatomical landmark. For example, nasion for head and neck, sternal notch for neck and thorax, tip of xyphoid for thorax and abdomen, and bottom of pubic ramus or tip of coccyx for pelvis, can be chosen as reasonably stable reference points.

5) The coordinates of the treatment isocenter are represented by (X,Y,Z) where X is the lateral distance and Y is the longitudinal distance (along patient axis) of the isocenter from the reference point and Z is the tabletop to isocenter distance (see Fig. 12.17). Beam angle θ is recorded.

B.2. TREATMENT SETUP

1) Position and level the patient on the treatment couch as in simulation.

2) With the gantry vertical, place the central axis at the reference anatomical point and mark it with ink.

3) Move the couch: up or down to obtain Z using the side laser; laterally through X and longitudinally through distance Y. Rotate the gantry through angle θ. This gives the required central axis of the field and the isocenter location.

4) Make secondary checks according to the field diagram such as SSD, location of field borders, etc.

5) For isocentric setup, other fields are positioned by simply rotating the gantry and positioning it at predetermined angles.

One potential advantage of this method is that the setup parameters X, Y, Z, and θ could be computer controlled, thereby decreasing the setup time and minimizing human errors. The technician, in this case, will position the patient as usual and place the central axis vertically at the reference point. Then, with a switch on the hand pendant, the computer control could be initiated to move the couch and the gantry to the X, Y, Z, and θ coordinates. Such a method could be adopted by some of the existing treatment monitoring systems which are capable of moving the couch and the gantry.

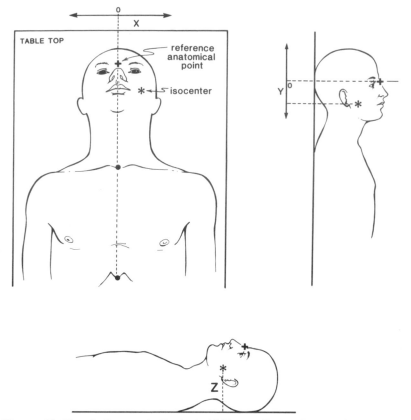

Figure 12.17. A diagram to illustrate XYZ coordinates for a patient setup.

Even manually, the XYZ method can greatly economize setup time as well as enhance setup precision. Most modern couches are motor driven and equipped with motion sensing devices. Videographic display of the couch motions could be conveniently used to position the couch. A reset switch for the X, Y, and Z coordinates would make it easier to move the couch through the X, Y, and Z distances.

References

1. Kuisk H: "Contour maker" eliminating body casting in radiotherapy planning. *Radiology* 101:203, 1971.
2. Clarke HC: A contouring device for use in radiation treatment planning. *Br J Radiol* 42:858, 1969.
3. Clayton C, Thompson D: An optical apparatus for reproducing surface outlines of body-cross sections. *Br J Radiol* 43:489, 1970.
4. Carson PL, Wenzel WW, Avery P, Hendee WR: Ultrasound imaging as an aid to cancer therapy—Part I. *Int J Radiat Oncol Biol Phys* 1:119, 1975; Part II. *Int J Radiat Oncol Biol Phys* 2:335, 1976.
5. Takahashi S, Matsuda T: Axial transverse laminography applied to rotation therapy. *Radiology* 74:61, 1960.

6. Pierquin B: La tomographie transversale: technique de routine en radiotherapie. *J Radiol Electrol* 42:131, 1961.
7. Brooks RA, Di Chiro G: Principles of computer assisted tomography (CAT) in radiographic and radioisotopic imaging. *Phys Med Biol* 21:689, 1976.
8. Rutherford RA, Pullan BR, Isherwood I: Measurement of effective atomic number and electron density using an EMI scanner. *Neuroradiology* 11:15, 1976.
9. Kijewski PK, Bjärngard BE: The use of computed tomography data for radiotherapy dose calculations. *Int J Radiat Oncol Biol Phys* 4:429, 1978.
10. Munzenrider JE, Pilepich M, Ferrero JBR, Tchakarova IT, Carter BL: Use of body scanners in radiotherapy treatment planning. *Cancer* 40:170, 1977.
11. Geise RA, McCullough EC: The use of CT scanners in megavoltage photon-beam therapy planning. *Radiology* 124:133, 1977.
12. Sontag MR, Battista JJ, Bronskill MJ, Cunningham JR: Implications of computed tomography for inhomogeneity corrections in photon beam dose calculations. *Radiology* 124:143, 1977.
13. Chernak, ES, Antunez RA, Jelden GL, Dhaliwal RS, Lavik PS: The use of computed tomography for radiation therapy treatment planning. *Radiology* 117:613, 1975.
14. Sternick ES, Lane FW, Curran B: Comparison of computed tomography and conventional transverse axial tomography in radiotherapy treatment planning. *Radiology* 124:835, 1977.
15. Fullerton GD, Sewchand W, Payne JT, Levitt SH: CT determination of parameters for inhomogeneity corrections in radiation therapy of the esophagus. *Radiology* 124:167, 1978.
16. Parker RP, Hobday PA, Cassell KJ: The direct use of CT numbers in radiotherapy dosage calculations for inhomogeneous media. *Phys Med Biol* 24:802, 1979.
17. Hobday P, Hodson NJ, Husband J, Parker RP, Macdonald JS: Computed tomography applied to radiotherapy treatment planning: techniques and results. *Radiology* 133:477, 1979.
18. Ragan DP, Perez CA: Efficacy of CT-assisted two-dimensional treatment planning: analysis of 45 patients. *Am J Roentgenol* 131:75, 1978.
19. Goitein M: The utility of computed tomography in radiation therapy: an estimate of outcome. *Int J Radiat Oncol Biol Phys* 5:1799, 1979.
20. Goitein M: Computed tomography in planning radiation therapy. *Int J Radiat Oncol Biol Phys* 5:445, 1979.
21. Sontag MR, Cunningham JR: The equivalent tissue-air ratio method for making absorbed dose calculations in a heterogeneous medium. *Radiology* 129:787, 1978.
22. Hogstrom KR, Mills MD, Almond PR: Electron beam dose calculations. *Phys Med Biol* 26:445, 1981.
23. Cassell KJ, Hobday PA, Parker RP: The implementation of a generalized batho inhomogeneity correction for radiotherapy planning with direct use of CT numbers. *Phys Med Biol* 26:825, 1981.
24. Carson PL, Wenzel WW, Hendee WR: Ultrasound imaging as an aid to cancer therapy—I. *Int J Radiat Oncol Biol Phys* 1:119, 1975.
25. Carson PL, Wenzel WW, Avery P, Hendee WR: Ultrasound imaging as an aid to cancer therapy—II. *Int J Radiat Oncol Biol Phys* 1:335, 1976.
26. Green, D, Nelson KA, Gibb R: The use of a linear accelerator "simulator" in radiotherapy. *Br J Radiol* 37:394, 1964.
27. Ovadia J, Karzmark CJ, Hendrickson FR: *Radiation Therapy Simulation and Transverse Tomography: Apparatus Bibliography and Tumor Localization.* Houston, American Association of Physicists in Medicine Radiological Physics Center, 1971.
28. Karzmark CJ, Rust DC: Radiotherapy simulators and automation. *Radiology* 105:157, 1972.
29. Bomford CK, Craig LM, Hanna, FA, et al: *Treatment Simulators. Report No. 10.* London, British Institute of Radiology, 1976.
30. McCullough EC, Earl JD: The selection, acceptance testing, and quality control of radiotherapy treatment simulators. *Radiology* 131:221, 1979.
31. Droege RT, Bjärngard BE: Metal screen-film detector MTF at megavoltage x-ray energies *Med Phys* 6:515, 1979.
32. Ellis F, Lescrenier C: Combined compensation for contours and heterogeneity. *Radiology* 106:191, 1973.
33. International Commission on Radiation Units and Measurements (ICRU): *Report 24. Determination of Absorbed Dose in a Patient Irradiated by Beams of X or Gamma Rays in Radiotherapy Procedures.* Washington, DC, United States National Bureau of Standards, 1976.
34. Batho HF: Lung corrections in cobalt 60 beam therapy. *J Can Assn Radiol* 15:79, 1964.
35. Young MEJ, Gaylord JD: Experimental tests of corrections for tissue inhomogeneities in

radiotherapy. *Br J Radiol* 43:349, 1970.

36. Greene D, Stewart JR: Isodose curves in non-uniform phantoms. *Br J Radiol* 38:378, 1965.
37. Sundblom L: Dose planning for irradiation of thorax with cobalt in fixed beam therapy. *Acta Radiol* 3:342, 1965.
38. Spires SW: Dosage in irradiated soft tissue and bone. *Br J Radiol* 24:365, 1951.
39. International Commission on Radiological Units and Measurements (ICRU): *Report 10d. Clinical Dosimetry.* Washington, DC, United States Bureau of Standards, 1963.
40. Johns HE, Cunningham JR: *The Physics of Radiology,* 2nd ed Springfield, IL, Charles C Thomas, 1969, p 455.
41. Leung PMK, Seaman, B, Robinson P: Low-density inhomogeneity corrections for 22-MeV x-ray therapy. *Radiology* 94:449 1970.
42. Epp ER, Lougheed MN, McKay JW: Ionization buildup in upper respiratory air passages during teletherapy units with cobalt 60 radiation. *Br J Radiol* 31:361, 1958.
43. Epp ER, Boyer AL, Doppke KP: Underdosing of lesions resulting from lack of electronic equilibrium in upper respiratory air cavities irradiated by 10 MV x-ray beam. *Int J Radiat Oncol Biol Phys* 2:613, 1977.
44. Ellis F, Hall EJ, Oliver R: A compensator for variations in tissue thickness for high energy beam. *Br J Radiol* 32:421, 1959.
45. Cohen, M, Burns JE, Sear R: Physical aspects of cobalt 60 teletherapy using wedge filters. II. Dosimetric considerations. *Acta Radiol* 53:486, 1960.
46. Hall EJ, Oliver R: The use of standard isodose distributions with high energy radiation beams—the accuracy of a compensator technique in correcting for body contours. *Br J Radiol* 34:43, 1961.
47. Sundblom L: Individually designed filters in cobalt-60 teletherapy. *Acta Radiol Ther Phys Biol* 2:189, 1964.
48. Van De Geijn J: The construction of individualized intensity modifying filters in cobalt 60 teletherapy. *Br J Radiol* 38:865 1965.
49. Khan FM, Moore VC Burns DJ: The construction of compensators for cobalt teletherapy. *Radiology* 96:187, 1970.
50. Sewchand W, Bautro N, Scott RM: Basic data of tissue-equivalent compensators for 4 MV x-rays. *Int J Radiat Oncol Biol Phys* 6:327, 1980.
51. Khan FM, Moore VC, Burns DJ: An apparatus for the construction of irregular surface compensators for use in radiotherapy. *Radiology* 90:593, 1968.
52. Beck GG, McGonnagle WJ, Sullivan CA: Use of styrofoam block cutter to make tissue-equivalent compensators. *Radiology* 100:694, 1971.
53. Boge RJ, Edland RW, Matthes, DC: Tissue compensators for megavoltage radiotherapy fabricated from hollowed styrofoam filled with wax. *Radiology* 111:193, 1974.
54. Khan FM, Sewchand W, Williamson JF: unpublished data.
55. Khan FM, Williamson JF, Sewchand W, Kim TH: Basic data for dosage calculation and compensation. *Int J Radiat Oncol Biol Phys* 6:745, 1980.
56. Leung PMK, Van Dyke J, Robins, J: A method for large irregular field compensation. *Br J Radiol* 47:805, 1974.
57. Boge RJ, Tolbert DD, Edland RW: Accessory beam flattening filter for the Varian Clinac-4 linear accelerator. *Radiology* 115:475, 1975.
58. Chung-Bin A, Kartha P, Wachtor T, Hendrickson FR: Development and experience in computer monitoring and the verification of daily patient treatment parameters. In Sternick ES (ed): *Proceedings of the 5th International Conference on Use of Computers in Radiation Therapy.* Hanover, New Hampshire: University Press of New England, 1976, p. 551.
59. Haus A, Marks J: Detection and evaluation of localization errors in patient radiation therapy. *Invest Radiol* 8:384, 1973.
60. Kartha PKI, Chung-Bin A, Wachtor T, Hendrickson FR: Accuracy in patient setup and its consequence in dosimetry. *Med Phys* 2:331, 1975.
61. Williamson TJ: Improving the reproducibility of lateral therapy portal placement. *Int J Radiat Oncol Biol Phys* 5:407, 1979.
62. Verhey LJ, Goitein M, McNulty P, Muzenrider JE, Suit HD: Precise positioning of patients for radiation therapy. *Int J Radiat Oncol Biol Phys* 8:289, 1982.
63. Hendrickson FR: Precision in radiation oncology. *Int J Radiat Oncol Biol Phys* 8:311, 1981.
64. Huaskins LA, Thomson RW: Patient positioning device for external-beam radiation therapy of the head and neck. *Radiology* 106:706, 1973.
65. McDonald SC, Keller BE, Rubin P: Method for calculating dose when lung tissue lies in the treatment field. *Med Phys* 3:210, 1976.

CHAPTER 13

Treatment Planning III: Field Shaping, Skin Dose, and Field Separation

Shielding of vital organs within a radiation field is one of the major concerns of radiotherapy. Considerable time and effort are spent in shaping fields not only to protect critical organs but also to avoid unnecessary irradiation of the surrounding normal tissue. Attendant to this problem is its effect on skin dose and the buildup of dose in the subcutaneous tissue. Skin sparing is an important property of megavoltage photon beams and every effort should be directed to maintaining this effect when irradiating normal skin.

Another problem frequently encountered in radiotherapy is the matching of adjacent fields. This situation arises when radiation fields available with the equipment are not large enough to encompass the entire target volume. In some cases, the target volume is divided into two parts such that the treatment to the second part does not commence until the treatment course to the first part has been completed. Such a scheme is designed to avoid toxicity due to irradiating an excessive volume of tissue. Multiple adjacent fields are also used when tumor distribution or patient anatomy does not allow coplanar fields (fields with central axes in the same plane). The main problem with these techniques is the possibility of extreme dose inhomogeneity in the junctional region. Since radiation beams are divergent, adjacent fields can overlap at depth and give rise to regions of excessive dose or hot spots. Overlaps can be avoided by separating the fields but this in turn can give rise to areas of reduced dose or "cold spots."

This chapter on treatment planning focuses on the above problems and discusses their possible solutions.

13.1 FIELD BLOCKS

The shaping of treatment fields is primarily dictated by tumor distribution— local extensions as well as regional metastases. Not only should the dose to vital organs not exceed their tolerance, but the dose to normal tissue, in general, should be minimized. As long as the target volume includes, with adequate margins, the demonstrated tumor as well as its presumed occult spread, significant irradiation of the normal tissue outside this volume must be avoided as much as possible. These restrictions can give rise to complex field shapes which require intricate blocking.

The frequency and complexity of field shaping vary from institution to institution. However, if complex techniques involving elaborate blocking are frequently used, it is necessary to establish a rational system of field shaping.

A. Block Thickness

Shielding blocks are most commonly made of lead. The thickness of lead required to provide adequate protection of the shielded areas depends on the beam quality and the allowed transmission through the block. A primary beam transmission of 5% through the block is considered acceptable for most clinical situations. If n is the number of half-value layers to achieve this transmission,

$$\frac{1}{2^n} = 0.05$$

or

$$2^n = \frac{1}{0.05} = 20$$

or

$$n \log 2 = \log 20$$

or

$$n = \frac{\log 20}{\log 2} = 4.32$$

Thus, a thickness of lead between 4.5 and 5 half-value layers would give less than 5% primary beam transmission and is, therefore, recommended for most clinical shielding.

Shielding against primary radiation for superficial and orthovoltage beams is readily accomplished by thin sheets of lead that can be placed or molded on to the skin surface. However, as the beam energy increases to the megavoltage range, the thickness of lead required for shielding increases substantially. The lead blocks are then placed above the patient supported in the beam on a transparent plastic tray, called the *shadow tray*. Table 13.1 gives the recommended lead shield thicknesses for various quality beams.

Although the primary beam transmission can be reduced further by using extra thick blocks, the reduction in dose in the shielded region may not be that significant due to the predominance of scattered radiation from the adjoining open areas of the field.

Table 13.1
Recommended minimum thickness of lead for shielding*

Beam Quality	Required Lead Thickness
1.0 mm Al HVL	0.2 mm
2.0 mm Al HVL	0.3 mm
3.0 mm Al HVL	0.4 mm
1.0 mm Cu HVL	1.0 mm
3.0 mm Cu HVL	2.0 mm
4.0 mm Cu HVL	2.5 mm
^{137}Cs	3.0 cm
^{60}CO	5.0 cm
4 MV	6.0 cm
6 MV	6.5 cm
10 MV	7.0 cm
25 MV	7.0 cm

* Approximate values to give ≤5% primary transmission.

B. Block Divergence

Ideally, the blocks should be shaped or tapered so that their sides follow the geometric divergence of the beam. This minimizes the block transmission penumbra (partial transmission of the beam at the edges of the block). However, divergent blocks offer little advantage for beams with large geometric penumbra. For example, in the case of ^{60}Co, the sharpness of the beam cutoff at the block edge is not significantly improved by using divergent blocks. Also, for some clinical situations this sharpness is not critical or worth the time required for making divergent blocks which have to be invariably custom designed for a given treatment setup. Therefore, most institutions keep a stock of straight-cut blocks of various shapes and dimensions.

Divergent blocks are most suited for beams having small focal spots. Since the sides of these blocks follow beam divergence, one can reduce the lateral dimensions by designing the shields for smaller source to block distances without increasing the block transmission penumbra.

13.2 A SYSTEM OF FIELD SHAPING

Although a number of systems have been used for field shaping (1–8), the one introduced by Powers *et al.* (1), is most commonly used in radiotherapy. This system uses a low melting point alloy, Lipowitz metal (brand name, Cerrobend) which has a density of 9.4 g/cm^3 at 20°C (~83% of lead density). This material consists of 50.0% bismuth, 26.7% lead, 13.3% tin, and 10.0% cadmium (1). The main advantage of Cerrobend over lead is that it melts at about 70°C (compared to 327°C for lead) and therefore can be easily cast into any shape. At room temperature, it is harder than lead.

The minimum thickness of Cerrobend blocks required for blocking may be calculated from Table 13.1 using its density ratio relative to lead (*e.g.* multiply lead thickness by 1.21). In the megavoltage range of photon beams, the most commonly used thickness is 7.5 cm which is equivalent to about 6 cm of pure lead.

The procedure for constructing Cerrobend blocks starts with a simulator radiograph or a port film on which the radiotherapist draws the outline of the treatment field indicating areas to be shielded. The film is then used to construct divergent cavities in a styrofoam block which are used to cast Cerrobend blocks. Figure 13.1 shows a styrofoam-cutting device which consists of an electrically heated wire which pivots about a point simulating the source or the x-ray target. The film, the styrofoam block, and the wire apparatus are so adjusted that the actual treatment geometry (same source to film and source to block distances) is obtained. The lower end of the wire traces the outline on the film.

If "positive" blocks such as lung blocks are to be made, cavities are cut in the styrofoam with the heated segment of the wire and subsequently filled with melted Cerrobend. If a "negative" block with central area open and peripheral areas blocked is desired, an inner cut is first made to outline the

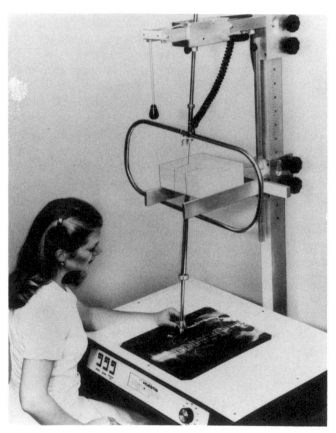

Figure 13.1. Photograph of block cutter. (Courtesy of Huestis Machine Corp., Bristol, Rhode Island.)

field opening. An outer rectangular cut is then made to define the collimator field with 1–2-cm margin. The three styrofoam pieces thus made are placed on a Lucite plate and carefully aligned relative to central axis. The intermediate piece, corresponding to the areas to be shielded, is then removed and Cerrobend is poured into the cavity.

It is important tht the Cerrobend is poured slowly to prevent formation of air bubbles. Also the styrofoam block should be pressed tightly against a rubber pad at the bottom to avoid leakage of the liquid metal. The inside walls of the cavity may be sprayed with silicone for easy release of the styrofoam pieces from the block.

The blocks can be mounted on a Lucite plate which is premarked with the central axis cross hairs. Blocks can also be placed on a template made on a clear film by tracing the outline of the field at the shadow tray position while the port film outline is placed at the distance at which the radiograph was taken.

Figure 13.2, A and B, shows examples of Cerrobend blocks, one constructed for shielding lungs and the other for a head and neck field.

13.3 SKIN DOSE

When a patient is treated with a megavoltage beam, the surface dose or skin dose can be substantially lower than the maximum dose which occurs in the subcutaneous tissues. In contrast to lower energy beams (*e.g.* superficial and orthovoltage x-rays) which give rise to maximum ionization at or close to the skin surface, the megavoltage beams produce an initial electronic buildup with depth, resulting in a reduced dose at the surface and maximum dose at the equilibrium depth. This phenomenon of dose buildup has been discussed in Section 9.3.

Skin sparing is one of the most desirable features of high energy photon beams. However, this effect may be reduced or even lost if the beam is excessively contaminated with secondary electrons or low energy photons. In the following sections, we will discuss the sources of this contamination and the methods used to reduce it.

A. Electron Contamination of Photon Beams

Surface dose is due to electron contamination of the incident beam as well as the backscattered radiation (both electrons and photons) from the medium. It is well known that all x-ray and γ ray beams used in radiotherapy are contaminated with secondary electrons. These electrons arise from photon interactions in the air, in the collimator, and in any other scattering material in the path of the beam. If a shadow tray is used to support beam shaping blocks, secondary electrons produced by photon interactions in the tray and the air column between the tray and the skin surface significantly increases skin dose. The shadow tray is usually thick enough to absorb most of the electrons incident on the tray.

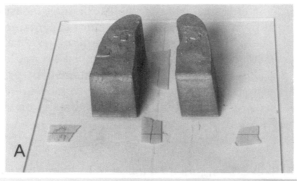

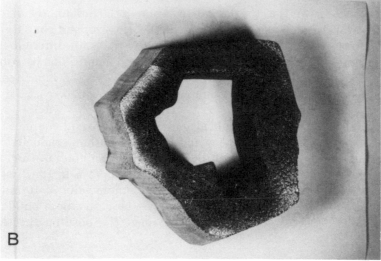

Figure 13.2.   (A) Cerrobend blocks for lung shielding. (B) Custom blocks for head and neck.

There appears to be a controversy as to the relative contribution of secondary electrons *vs.* low energy scattered photons to the dose in the buildup region. It is well known that as the field size increases, the depth dose in the buildup region increases resulting in a shift in the depth of maximum dose, d_{max}, to increasingly shallower depths (9–11). Specifically, the cause of the d_{max} shift with field size has been studied by several investigators (12–14) but the results are not conclusive. Probably the effect is due to both secondary electrons and low energy photons.

B. Measurement of Dose Distribution in the Buildup Region

Because of the steep dose gradient in the buildup region, the size of the dosimeter along the beam direction should be as small as possible. Parallel plate ion chambers with a thin ion collection volume or extrapolation chambers (see Chapter 6) are the instruments of choice for such measurements. Thin layers (<0.5 mm) of thermoluminescent dosimeter (TLD) material can also be used for measuring dose distribution in the buildup region. The TLD phosphor (*e.g.* LiF) can be in the form of chips, crystals imbedded in plastic, or powder layers (15, 17, 20). The surface dose may be obtained by extrapolating the depth dose distribution curve to zero depth. *In vivo* measurements of surface dose can also be made by placing thin TLD chips directly on the skin surface. Such measurements are useful in checking dosimetry if a patient develops an unacceptable degree of skin reaction.

C. Skin Sparing as a Function of Photon Energy

Studies have shown that the dose distribution in the buildup region depends on many variables such as beam energy, SSD, field size, and configuration of secondary blocking tray (15–20). Table 13.2 gives values for different energies. These data are presented here as an example and should not be considered universal for all machines, especially for depths less than 2 mm. Reasonable agreement between different machines has been shown to exist for greater depths.

Examination of Table 13.2 would also indicate that for all energies the dose increases rapidly within the first few millimeters and then gradually achieves its maximum value at the depth of peak dose. For example, in the case of 4 MV, the percent depth dose increases from 14% to 74% in the first 2 mm, reaches 94% at 5-mm depth and achieves its maximum value at 10-mm depth. A practical application of this phenomenon is the case where buildup bolus (Section 12.4) is used intentionally to maximize the dose on the skin (*e.g.*

Table 13.2
Buildup dose distribution in polystyrene for 10 × 10 cm field

Depth (mm)	^{60}Co 80 cm	4 MV 80 cm	10 MV 100 cm	25 MV 100 cm
0	18.0	14.0	12.0	17.0
1	70.5	57.0	30.0	28.0
2	90.0	74.0	46.0	39.5
3	98.0	84.0	55.0	47.0
4	100.0	90.0	63.0	54.5
5	100.0	94.0	72.0	60.5
6		96.5	76.0	66.0
8		99.5	84.0	73.0
10		100.0	91.0	79.0
15			97.0	88.5
20			98.0	95.0
25			100.0	99.0
30				100.0

[60] Co, 4-MV, and 25-MV data are from Velkley *et al.* (20) and 10-MV data are from Khan *et al.* (17).

covering a scar with a strip of bolus). A tissue equivalent bolus of 5–6-mm thickness is usually adequate for 4 MV. Thus, the thickness of bolus required to achieve 90–95% buildup of dose is substantially less than the depth of maximum dose.

Although the skin sparing depends on many conditions, as mentioned earlier, the effect, in general, becomes more and more pronounded as photon energy increases. For higher energy beams, significant sparing can be achieved not only for the skin surface but also for the subcutaneous tissues.

D. Effect of Absorber—Skin Distance

The electron contamination with no absorber placed in the beam is mainly due to the secondary electron emission from the collimator (including source, flattening filter, and air). When an absorber of thickness greater than the range of secondary electrons (equilibrium thickness) is introduced in the beam, the collimator electrons are almost completely absorbed but the absorber itself becomes the principal source of electron contamination of the beam. By increasing the distance between the tray and the surface, the electron fluence incident on the skin is reduced because of divergence as well as absorption and scattering of electrons in the air. Thus, skin sparing is enhanced by placing the shadow tray farther away from the skin. In the case of a ^{60}Co γ ray beam, it has been shown (21, 22) that for small fields an air gap of 15–20 cm between the scatterer and the skin is adequate to keep the skin dose to an acceptable level (<50% of the D_{max}). This has been found to be true for higher energy beams as well (17).

Figure 13.3 shows the effect on dose distribution in the buildup region as a Lucite shadow tray is placed in the beam at various distances from the phantom surface. Not only does the relative surface dose increase with decreasing tray-to-surface distance but the point of maximum dose buildup moves closer to the surface.

Figure 13.3 also illustrates the principle of what is known as the "beam spoiler." A low atomic number absorber, such as a Lucite shadow tray, placed at an appropriate distance from the surface, can be used to modify the buildup curve. Doppke *et al.* (23) have discussed the treatment of certain head and neck cancers with 10-MV x-rays using a beam spoiler to increase the dose to the superficial neck nodes.

E. Effect of Field Size

The relative skin dose depends strongly on field size. As the field dimensions are increased, the dose in the buildup region increases. This increase in dose is due to increased electron emission from the collimator and air. Figure 13.4 is a plot of relative surface dose as a function of field size for ^{60}Co, 4-MV, and 10-MV beams. These data show that skin sparing is significantly reduced for the larger field sizes.

Saylor and Quillin (16) have discussed the relative importance of field size

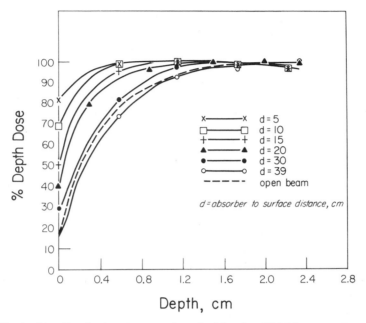

Figure 13.3. Effect of Lucite shadow tray on dose buildup for 10-MV x-rays. Percent depth dose distribution is plotted for various tray-to-surface distances (d). 10-MX x-rays, tray thickness = 1.5 g/cm^2, field size = 15 × 15 cm, SSD = 100 cm, and SDD = 50 cm. [Reprinted with permission from: Khan *et al.* (17).]

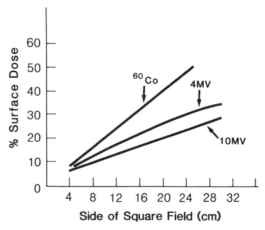

Figure 13.4. Percent surface dose as a function of field size. ^{60}Co, Theratron 80, SSD = 80 cm, SDD = 59 cm. 4 MV, Clinac 4, SSD = 80 cm. 10 MV, LMR 13, SSD = 100 cm, SDD = 50 cm. [^{60}Co and 4-MV data are from Velkley *et al.* (20) and 10-MV data are from Khan *et al.* (17).]

and tray-skin distance for ^{60}Co γ rays. They have shown that the optimum skin sparing occurs for an h/r value of about 4, where h is the tray-surface distance and r is the radius of an equivalent circular field. This ratio can be easily achieved for the 5×5 cm field, since it requires a distance of 12 cm; however, for the 30×30 cm field, the corresponding absorber-surface distance is 67 cm which is hardly possible for isocentric treatments.

When using large fields with the tray-skin distance of 15–20 cm, it becomes necessary to use *electron filters* to maintain the skin sparing effect. These are discussed in the next section.

F. Electron Filters

The skin dose can be reduced by using γ ray absorbers of medium atomic number (Z in the range of 30–80). Such absorbers are commonly known as electron filters since their introduction in the photon beam reduces the secondary electron scatter in the forward direction. Hine (24, 25) studied the scattering of electrons produced by γ rays in materials of various atomic numbers. He showed that the medium atomic number absorbers give less electron scatter in the forward direction than either the low or the very high Z materials. Khan (15) and Saylor Quillin (16) applied the results of Hine's study to the design of electron filters for the purpose of improving skin dose for ^{60}Co teletherapy. Later it was shown that such filters not only reduce the surface dose but also improve the buildup characteristics of large fields (26).

Figure 13.5 is a plot of relative surface dose as a function of log ($Z + 1$). These data are plotted in this manner to show agreement with the theoretical relationship discussed by Hine (24, 25). As Z increases, the surface dose falls to a shallow minimum due to increased electron scattering in the absorbers. Further increases in Z result in increased surface dose due to increased production of photoelectrons and electron pairs in addition to the Compton electrons. The minimum occurs at about $Z = 50$ which is the atomic number of tin. These results qualitatively agree with those obtained for ^{60}Co γ rays (16, 24, 25).

Effectiveness of tin in reducing skin dose is demonstrated in Fig. 13.6. Greater reduction is possible by increasing filter-skin distance as discussed earlier.

In order to preserve the light field, Saylor and Quillin (16) have suggested the use of leaded glass as an electron filter. However, breakability of leaded glass may pose a serious problem. We have used a tin sheet mounted on a pressed wood sheet which could be slipped under the Plexiglas tray at the end of the treatment setup. In this arrangement, the tin filter must face the patient surface.

The thickness of an electron filter, in theory, should be at least equal to the maximum range of secondary electrons. For ^{60}Co, this thickness is about 0.5 g/cm^2 or 0.9 mm of tin (assuming $\rho_{\text{tin}} = 5.75$ g/cm^3). For higher energies,

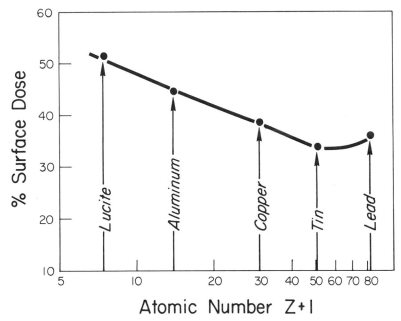

Figure 13.5. Variation of percent surface dose with atomic number of absorber. Each absorber had a thickness of 1.5 g/cm² and was mounted underneath a Lucite shadow tray. 10-MV x-rays, field size = 15 × 15 cm and absorber-to-surface distance = 15 cm. [Reprinted with permission from: Khan *et al.* (17).]

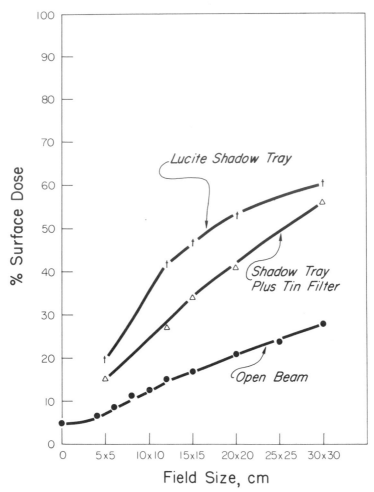

Figure 13.6. Percent surface dose plotted as a function of field size for open beam, Lucite tray and tin filter mounted underneath the tray. 10-MV x-rays, tray-to-surface distance = 15 cm. [Reprinted with permission from: Khan *et al.* (17).]

thicknesses less than the maximum range of electrons may be used for practical reasons.

G. Skin Sparing at Oblique Incidence

Skin dose has been shown to increase with increasing angle of incidence (27–33). Clinically, brisk reactions have been observed in patients when the beam is incident at near glancing angles. Jackson (29) has explained the increase in skin dose with increasing angle of incidence through the concept of electron range surface (e.r.s.) The e.r.s. is a three-dimensional representation of secondary electron range and distribution produced by a pencil beam of photons interacting with the medium (Fig. 13.7). Electrons generated inside the e.r.s. volume will reach P and contribute to the dose there, while those generated outside, because of their inadequate range, make no contribution. The e.r.s. for ^{60}Co γ rays is in the shape of an ellipsoid with axial dimensions of 5 × 2.4 mm (29). As illustrated in the figure, the increase in the angle of incidence of the photon beam results in additional surface dose at P because of electron contribution from the portion of the e.r.s. which appears below the phantom surface (hatched curve). For tangential beam incidence, since half of the e.r.s. is below the phantom surface, an upper estimate of the dose to the skin may be obtained by the following relationship (29, 33):

$$\text{Percent skin dose} = \tfrac{1}{2}(100\% + \text{entrance dose}) \qquad (13.1)$$

where the entrance dose represents the surface dose for normal incidence

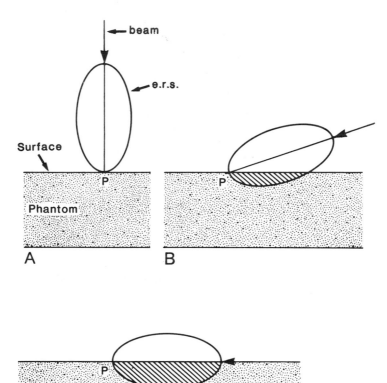

Figure 13.7. The use of e.r.s. to determine surface dose buildup at point P. (A) Perpendicular beam incidence; (B) oblique beam incidence; (C) tangential beam incidence.

expressed as a percentage of D_{max}. The skin dose for other angles of incidence will lie between the values for the normal and the tangential incidence. It should be mentioned that the skin dose at oblique angles also depends on photon attenuation, photon scatter, and the curvature of the surface.

Another important effect associated with oblique angles is that as the surface dose increases with the angle of incidence, the depth of maximum buildup decreases. The dose reaches its maximum value faster at glancing angles than at normal incidence. As a result, the dose buildup region is compressed into a more superficial region. Under these conditions, a high skin reaction becomes much more likely. Jackson (29) has discussed the possibility that if the sensitivity of the skin extends to the first or second millimeter below the surface, at glancing angles skin sparing is practically lost for the cobalt unit and greatly reduced for higher energy beams.

13.4 SEPARATION OF ADJACENT FIELDS

Adjacent treatment fields are commonly employed in external beam radiotherapy, such as the "mantle" and "inverted-Y" fields for the treatment of Hodgkin's disease. In some cases, the adjacent fields are orthogonal such as the craniospinal fields used in the treatment of medulloblastoma. Another example is the irradiation of head and neck tumors when the lateral neck fields are placed adjacent to the anterior supraclavicular field. In each of these situations, there is a possibility of introducing very large dosage errors across the junction. Consequently, this region is at risk for tumor recurrence if it is underdosed or severe complications if it is overdosed.

The problem of adjacent fields has been extensively studied (34–46). A number of techniques have been devised to achieve dose uniformity in the field junction region. Some of the more commonly used techniques are illustrated in Fig. 13.8. Figure 13.8A has been described by Lance and Morgan (34) in which fields are angled away from a common line of abutment to avoid overlap of the fields due to their geometric divergence. Figure 13.8B illustrates the methods in which the fields are separated at the skin surface to provide dose uniformity at a desired depth. The separation or gap between the fields is calculated on the basis of geometric divergence (46) or isodose curve matching (35, 36). A technique using split beams (42, 46) is illustrated in Fig. 13.8C. In this method, the beam is split along the plane containing the central axis by using a "half-beam" block or a "beam-splitter," thus removing the geometric divergence of the beams at the split line. Figure 13.8D uses "penumbra generators" or "spoilers" (39, 40). These lead wedges are custom designed to provide satisfactory dose distribution across the field junction.

In clinical practice, the fields are usually abutted at the surface if the tumor is superficial at the junction point. Care is however taken that the "hot spot" created due to the overlap of the beams at depth is clinically acceptable, considering the magnitude of the overdosage and the volume of the hot spot. In addition, the dosage received by a sensitive structure such as spinal cord must not exceed its tolerance dose.

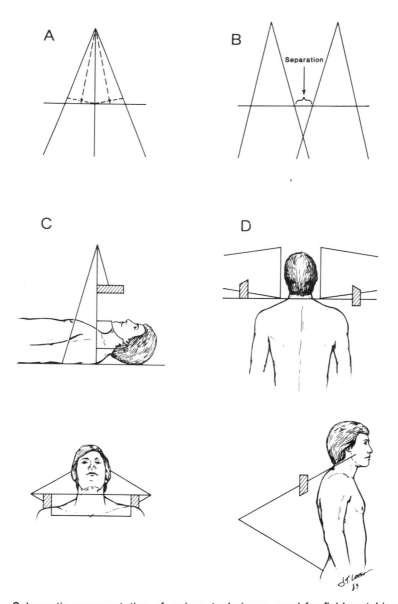

Figure 13.8. Schematic representation of various techniques used for field matching. (A) Angling the beams away from each other so that the two beams abut and are aligned vertically. (B) Fields separated at the skin surface. The junction point is at depth where dose is uniform across the junction. (C) Isocentric split beam technique for head and neck tumors. [Redrawn from: Williamson (42).] (D) Craniospinal irradiation using penumbra generators. [Redrawn from: Griffin *et al.* (41).]

For the treatment of deep-seated lesions such as in the thorax, abdomen, and pelvis, the fields can be separated on the surface. It is assumed in this case that the "cold spots" created by the field separation are located superficially where there is no tumor.

A. Methods of Field Separation

As stated earlier, the fields separation can be accomplished geometrically or dosimetrically.

A.1. GEOMETRIC

If the geometric boundary of the field is defined by the 50% decrement line (line joining the points at depth where the dose is 50% of the central axis value at the same depth), the dose at the point of junction between the beams will add up to be 100%. The dose distribution laterally across the junction is more or less uniform, depending upon the interfield scatter contribution and the penumbra characteristics of the beam.

If the two fields are incident from one side only and made to junction at a given depth (see Fig. 13.9), the dose above the junction will be lower and below the junction higher than the junction dose. In the case of four fields where two fields are incident from one side and two from the parallel opposed direction (Fig. 13.10), the fields are usually made to junction at the midline depth (*e.g.* mantle and inverted Y fields). Such an arrangement can be used to obtain almost a uniform distribution at the midline, but cold spots are created above and below the junction point.

Figure 13.9 shows the geometry of two adjacent beams which are allowed to join at a given depth d. Let L_1 and L_2 be the field lengths and SSD_1 and SSD_2 be the source-surface distances. Since triangles ABC and CDE are similar:

$$\frac{CD}{DE} = \frac{BC}{AB}$$

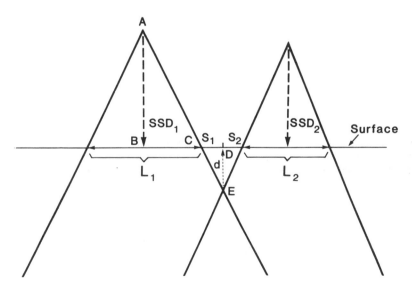

Figure 13.9. Geometry of two adjacent beams, separated by a distance $S_1 + S_2$ on the surface and junctioning of depth d.

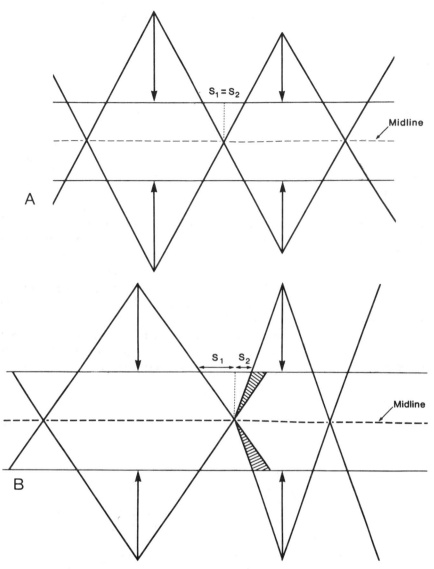

Figure 13.10. Two pairs of parallel opposed fields. Adjacent fields are separated on the surface so that they all join at a point on the midline. (A) Ideal geometry in which there is no three-field overlap. (B) Arrangement in which there are two regions (shaded) of three-field overlap.

or

$$\frac{S_1}{d} = \frac{L_1}{2} \cdot \frac{1}{\text{SSD}_1} \tag{13.2}$$

giving

$$S_1 = \tfrac{1}{2} \cdot L_1 \cdot \frac{d}{\mathrm{SSD}_1} \tag{13.3}$$

Similarly,

$$S_2 = \tfrac{1}{2} \cdot L_2 \cdot \frac{d}{\mathrm{SSD}_2} \tag{13.4}$$

Thus, the total separation S on the surface is given by:

$$S = S_1 + S_2 = \tfrac{1}{2} \cdot L_1 \cdot \frac{d}{\mathrm{SSD}_1} + \tfrac{1}{2} \cdot L_2 \cdot \frac{d}{\mathrm{SSD}_2} \tag{13.5}$$

Figure 13.10A shows an ideal geometry in which there is no overlap between a field and its adjacent opposing neighbor. The arrangement shown in Fig. 13.10B, on the other hand, creates regions of "three-field overlap" (shaded areas) where the bigger fields diverge into the opposing smaller fields. Consequently, the total dose there may exceed the central axis dose at the same depth. This will be of concern if a significant portion of the spinal cord is in the three-field overlap region.

The maximum length of three-field overlap (ΔS) occurs on the surface and is given by

$$\Delta S = S_1 - S_2 \tag{13.6}$$

ΔS can be made equal to zero if

$$\frac{L_1}{L_2} = \frac{\mathrm{SSD}_1}{\mathrm{SSD}_2} \tag{13.7}$$

Thus, if the field lengths are different, the SSDs can be adjusted to eliminate the three-field overlap. Also, if the geometrically calculated gap ($S_1 + S_2$) is increased by ΔS, the three-field overlap is eliminated at the expense of a cold spot at the midline. As a compromise, one could increase the gap ($S_1 + S_2$) by an amount $\Delta S'$ just enough to eliminate the three-field overlap in a specific region such as the spinal cord. $\Delta S'$ can be calculated geometrically:

$$\Delta S' = \Delta S \cdot \frac{d' - d}{d} \tag{13.8}$$

where d' is the depth of the cord from the anterior surface and d is the midline depth.

Example 1. A patient is treated with parallel-opposed mantle and paraortic fields of lengths 30 and 15 cm, respectively. Calculate (a) the gap required on the surface for the beams to intersect at a midline depth of 10 cm and (b) the gap required to just eliminate the three-field overlap on the cord assumed to be at a depth of 15 cm from the anterior surface, given SSD = 100 cm for all the fields.

(a) $S_1 = \frac{1}{2} \cdot L_1 \cdot \dfrac{d}{\text{SSD}} = \frac{1}{2} \times 30 \times \dfrac{10}{100} = 1.5 \text{ cm}$

  $S_2 = \frac{1}{2} \cdot L_2 \cdot \dfrac{d}{\text{SSD}} = \frac{1}{2} \times 15 \times \dfrac{10}{100} = 0.75 \text{ cm}$

  Total gap required = 1.5 + 0.75 = 2.3 cm

(b) $\Delta S = S_1 - S_2 = 1.5 - 0.75 = 0.75 \text{ cm}$

  Length of three-field overlap on the cord

  $\Delta S' = \Delta S \cdot \dfrac{d' - d}{d} = 0.75 \, \dfrac{15 - 10}{10} = 0.4 \text{ cm}$

  New gap required = $S_1 + S_2 + \Delta S' = 2.7$ cm

Although the above geometric considerations provide useful criteria for field separation, one must be aware of their limitations. For example, the actual dose distribution may present a different picture than the predictions based on pure geometry of beam divergence. Patient positioning, beam alignment, field penumbra, and radiation scatter are all relevant factors which make this problem one of the most complex in radiotherapy.

Figure 13.11 shows the dose distribution for the cases discussed in Example 1. The expected three-field hot spot is seen in Fig. 13.11A when the beams intersect in the midline. This hot spot is eliminated when the gap is increased from 2.3 to 3.0 cm (= $S_1 + S_2 + \Delta S$) (Fig. 13.11B). However, the dose in the junction region has dropped considerably. Such a procedure will be justified only if the junctional region is tumor free. Figure 13.11C shows the distribution when the gap is just enough to eliminate the three-field overlap at the cord, i.e. gap = 2.7 cm. This reduces the dose to the cord but also cools down the midjunction area by about 10%.

In practice, the choice between the options shown in Fig. 13.11, A, B, and C, should be based on physical, clinical, and technical considerations. As usual, the guiding principles are that the tumor must receive adequate dosage and sensitive structures must not be treated beyond tolerance. If these conditions are not satisfied, other methods of field matching, discussed earlier in this chapter, may be considered.

A.2. DOSIMETRIC

The separation of fields can be determined by optimizing the placement of fields on the contour so that the composite isodose distribution is uniform at the desired depth and the "hot" and "cold" spots are acceptable. The accuracy

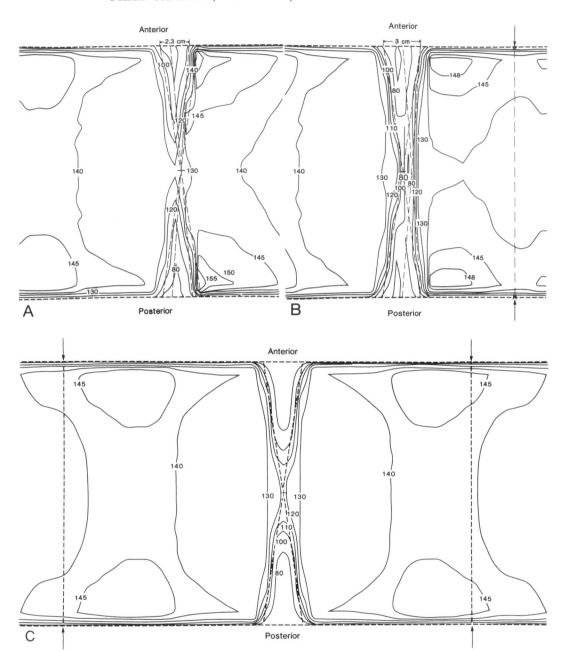

Figure 13.11. Geometric separation of fields with all the four beams intersecting at midpoint. Adjacent field sizes: 30 × 30 cm and 15 × 15 cm; SSD = 100 cm; AP thickness = 20 cm; 4-MV x-ray beams. (A) Field separation at surface = 2.3 cm. A three-field overlap exists in this case because of the fields having different sizes but the same SSD. (B) The adjacent field separation increased to 3 cm to eliminate three-field overlap on the surface. (C) Field separation adjusted 2.7 cm to eliminate three-field overlap at the cord at 15 cm depth from anterior.

of this procedure depends on the accuracy of the individual field isodose curves especially in the penumbra region.

B. Orthogonal Field Junctions

Orthogonal fields denote an arrangement in which the central axes of the adjacent fields are orthogonal (*i.e.* perpendicular to each other). For example, orthogonal fields are used for the treatment of medulloblastoma in which the craniospinal irradiation is accomplished by lateral parallel-opposed brain fields coupled with a posterior spine field. Another common example is treatment of the neck by bilateral fields while an orthogonally adjacent anterior field is used to treat the supraclavicular areas.

The problem of matching orthogonal fields has been discussed by several investigators (41–45). For superficial tumors such as in the head and neck areas, it may be inadvisable to separate the adjacent fields unless the junction area is over a tumor-free region. If separation is not possible, one may use beam splitters and abut the fields along or close to their central axes (43). The matching line should be drawn each time before treatment to avoid overlap of the fields. If a sensitive structure such as the spinal cord exists in the junction region, one may additionally block an appropriate segment of the cord anteriorly or laterally, provided there is no tumor in the shielded region.

As stated earlier, field separation is possible for deep-seated tumors if there is no tumor in the superficial junction region. A geometrical method of orthogonal field separation has been described by Werner *et al.* (45). According to this method, one pair of opposing fields, defined by the collimating light, is allowed to diverge on the skin and the point of intersection of the field borders is marked. From this point, a distance S is calculated to separate the orthogonal fields. The separation S is given by

$$S = \tfrac{1}{2} \cdot L \cdot \frac{d}{\text{SSD}} \tag{13.9}$$

where d is the depth at which the orthogonal fields are allowed to join. A general diagram for orthogonal field separation is illustrated in Fig. 13.12A. Figure 13.12B presents a practical example showing bilateral cranial fields adjacent to a spinal field. The cranial light fields are allowed to diverge on the skin and their inferior borders meet at a point midway on the posterior neck surface. From this point, the spinal field is separated by a distance S which is calculated from Equation 13.9 by substituting depth d of spine (from the posterior surface), length L, and SSD for the spinal field. In this diagram, the solid line represents the light field on the surface. The dashed line shows the field projected at the depth of the spinal cord. Figure 13.12C is the lateral view of B.

Other orthogonal field setups, such as lateral pelvic fields coupled with a spinal field can be treated in a similar way. In the case of orthogonal four-field junctions, the procedure is still the same. Once the third field is placed

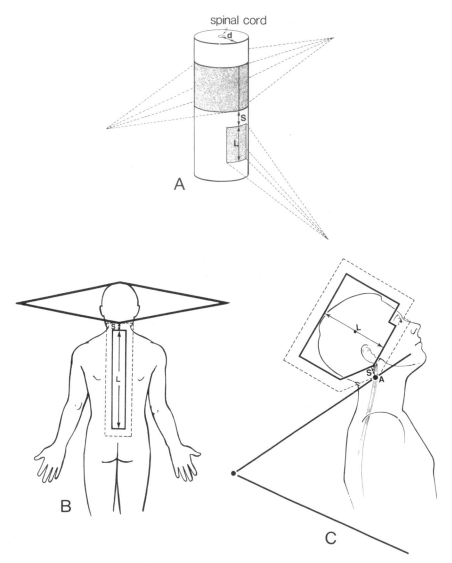

Figure 13.12. (A) A general diagram showing the separation of orthogonal fields. (B) An example of orthogonal fields used for craniospinal irradiation. (C) A lateral view of B, illustrating the geometry of orthogonal fields separation.

at a distance S, then the fourth field is positioned by rotating the gantry through 180°.

C. Guidelines for Field Matching

1) The site of field matching should be chosen, insofar as possible, over an area which does not contain tumor or a critically sensitive organ.

2) If the tumor is superficial at the junction site, the fields should not be separated since a "cold spot" on the tumor will risk recurrence. However, if the diverging fields abut on the skin surface, they will overlap at depth. In some cases, this may be clinically acceptable provided the excessive dosage delivered to the underlying tissues does not exceed their tolerance. In particular, the tolerances of critical structures such as the spinal cord must not be exceeded. In the case of a superficial tumor with a critical organ located at depth, one may abut the fields at the surface but eliminate beam divergence using a beam splitter or by tilting the beams.

3) For deep-seated tumors, the field may be separated on the skin surface so that the junction point lies at the midline. Again, care must be taken with regard to a critical structure near the junction region.

4) The line of field matching must be drawn at each treatment session on the basis of the first field treated. It is not necessary to anatomically reproduce this line every day since variation in its location will only "smear" the junction point, which is desirable. For the same reason some advocate moving the junction site two or three times during a treatment course.

5) A field matching technique must be verified by actual isodose distributions before it is adopted for general clinical use. In addition, beam alignment with the light field and the accuracy of isodose curves in the penumbra region are essential prerequisites.

References

1. Powers WE, Kinzie JJ, Demidecki AJ, Bradfield JS, Feldman A: A new system of field shaping for external-beam radiation therapy. *Radiology* 108:407, 1973.
2. Earl JD, Bagshaw MA: A rapid method for preparation of complex field shapes. *Radiology* 88:1162, 1967.
3. Maruyama Y, Moore VC, Burns D, Hilger MTJ: Individualized lung shields constructed from lead shots embedded in plastic. *Radiology* 92:634, 1969.
4. Edland RW, Hansen H: Irregular field-shaping for ^{60}Co teletherapy. *Radiology* 92:1567, 1969.
5. Jones D: A method for the accurate manufacture of lead shields. *Br J Radiol* 44:398, 1971.
6. Parfitt H: Manufacture of lead shields. *Br J Radiol* 44:895, 1971.
7. Karzmark CJ, Huisman PA: Melting, casting and shaping of lead shielding blocks: method and toxicity aspects. *Am J Roentgenol* 114:636, 1972.
8. Kuisk H: New method to facilitate radiotherapy planning and treatment, including a method for fast production of solid lead blocks with diverging walls for cobalt 60 beam. *Am J Roentgenol* 117:161, 1973.
9. Almond PR, Roosenbeek EV, Browne R, Milcamp J, Williams CB: Variation in the position of the central axis maximum buildup point with field size for high energy photons beams. *Br J Radiol* 43:911, 1970, (correspondence).
10. Marinello G, Dutreix A: Etude dosimétrique d'un faisceau de rayons X de 25 MV (dosimetric study of a 25 MV x-ray beam). *J Radiol Electrol* 54:951, 1973.
11. Johns HE, Rawlinson JA: Desirable characteristics of high-energy photons and electrons. In Kramer S, Suntharalingam N, Zinniger GF (eds): *High Energy Photons and Electrons*. New York, John Wiley and Sons, 1976, p 11.
12. Marbach JR, Almond PR: Scattered photons as the cause of the observed d_{max} shift with field size in high-energy photon beams. *Med Phys* 4:310, 1977.
13. Padikal, TN, Deye JA: Electron contamination of a high energy x-ray beam. *Phys Med Biol* 23:1086, 1978.
14. Biggs PJ, Ling CC: Electrons as the cause of the observed d_{max} shift with field size in high energy photons beams. *Med Phys* 6:291, 1979.

15. Khan FM: Use of electron filter to reduce skin dose in cobalt teletherapy. *Am J Roentgenol* 111:180, 1971.
16. Saylor WL, Quillin RM: Methods for the enhancement of skin sparing in cobalt-60 teletherapy. *Am J Roentgenol* 111:174, 1971.
17. Khan FM, Moore VC, Levitt SH: Effect of various atomic number absorbers on skin dose for 10-MeV x-rays. *Radiology* 109:209, 1973.
18. Gray L: Relative surface doses from supervoltage radiation. *Radiology* 109:437, 1973.
19. Rao PX, Pillai K, Gregg EC: Effect of shadow trays on surface dose and buildup for megavoltage radiation. *Am J Roentgenol* 117:168, 1973.
20. Velkley DE, Manson DJ, Purdy JA, Oliver GD: Buildup region on megavoltage photon radiation sources. *Med Phys* 2:14, 1975.
21. Johns HE, Epp ER, Cormack DV, Fedoruck SO: Depth dose data and diaphragm design for the Saskatchewan 1000 curie cobalt unit. *Br J Radiol* 25:302, 1952.
22. Richardson JE, Kerman HD, Brucer M: Skin dose from cobalt 60 teletherapy unit. *Radiology* 63:25, 1954.
23. Doppke, K, Novack D, Wang CC: Physical considerations in the treatment of advanced carcinomas of the larynx and pyriform sinuses using 10 MV x-rays. *Int J Radiat Oncol Biol Phys* 6:1251, 1980.
24. Hine GD: Scattering of secondary electrons produced by gamma rays in materials of various atomic numbers. *Phys Rev* 82:755, 1951.
25. Hine GJ: Secondary electron emission and effective atomic numbers. *Nucleonics* 10:9, 1952.
26. Leung PMK, Johns HE: Use of electron filters to improve the buildup characteristics of large fields from cobalt-60 beams. *Med Phys* 4:441, 1977.
27. Burkell CC, Watson TA, Johns HE, Horsley RJ: Skin effects of cobalt 60 telecurie therapy. *Br J Radiol* 27:171, 1954.
28. Hughes HA: Measurements of superficial absorbed dose with 2 MV x-rays used at glancing angles. *Br J Radiol* 32:255, 1959.
29. Jackson W: Surface effects of high-energy x-rays at oblique incidence. *Br J Radiol* 44:109, 1971.
30. Orton CG, Seibert JB: Depth dose in skin for obliquely incident ^{60}Co radiation. *Br J Radiol* 45:271, 1972.
31. Hanson WF, Grant W: Use of auxillary collimating devices in the treatment for breast cancer with ^{60}Co teletherapy units. II. Dose to the skin. *Am J Roentgenol* 127:653, 1976.
32. Gagnon WF, Peterson MD: Comparison of skin doses to large fields using tangential beams from cobalt-60 gamma rays and 4 MV x-rays. *Radiology* 127:785, 1978.
33. Gagnon, WF, Horton JL: Physical factors affecting absorbed dose to the skin from cobalt-60 gamma rays and 25-MV x-rays. *Med Phys* 6:285, 1979.
34. Lance JS, Morgan JE: Dose distribution between adjoining therapy fields. *Radiology* 79:24, 1962.
35. Glenn DW, Faw FL, Kagan RA, Johnson RE: Field separation in multiple portal radiation therapy. *Am J Roentgenol* 102:199, 1968.
36. Faw FL, Glenn DW: Further investigations of physical aspects of multiple field radiation therapy. *Am J Roentgenol* 108:184, 1970.
37. Page V, Gardner A, Karzmark, CJ: Physical and dosimetric aspects of the radiotherapy of malignant lymphomas. II. The inverted Y technique. *Radiology* 96:619, 1970.
38. Agarwal SK, Marks RD, Constable WC: Adjacent field separation for homogeneous dosage at a given depth for the 8 MV (Mevatron 8) linear accelerator. *Am J Roentgenol* 114:623, 1972.
39. Armstrong DI, Tait JJ: The matching of adjacent fields in radiotherapy. *Radiology* 108:419, 1973.
40. Hale J, Davis LW, Bloch P: Portal separation for pairs of parallel opposed portals at 2 MV and 6 MV. *Am J Roentgenol* 114:172, 1972.
41. Griffin TW, Schumacher D, Berry HC: A technique for cranial-spinal irradiation. *Br J Radiol* 49:887, 1976.
42. Williamson TJ: A technique for matching orthogonal megavoltage fields. Int J Radiat Oncol Biol Phys 5:111, 1979.
43. Bukovitz A, Deutsch M, Slayton R: Orthogonal fields: variations in dose *vs.* gap size for treatment of the central nervous system. *Radiology* 126:795, 1978.
44. Gillin MT, Kline RW: Field separation between lateral and anterior fields on a 6 MV linear accelerator. *Int J Radiat Oncol Biol Phys* 6:233, 1980.

45. Werner BL, Khan FM, Sharma SC, Lee CKK, Kim TH: A method for calculating field border separation when treating with adjacent orthogonal fields. Abstract presented at the *Annual Meeting of the American Society of Therapeutic Radiologists, Dallas, Texas, Oct. 21–25, 1980.*
46. Hopfan S, Reid A, Simpson L, Ager PJ: Clinical complications arising from overlapping of adjacent radiation fields—phyiscal and technical considerations. *Int J Radiat Oncol Biol Phys* 2:801, 1977.

CHAPTER 14

Electron Beam Therapy

High energy electrons have been used in radiotherapy since the early 1950s. Originally, the beams were extracted mostly from betatrons although a few linear accelerators and Van de Graaf generators with relatively low electron energies were also available. In the 1970s, high energy linear accelerators, having photon and multi-energy electron beam capabilities, became increasingly available for clinical use. The surge in the commercial development of these machines was prompted largely by the clinical experience gained at a few major centers which showed that in some commonly encountered situations "there is no alternative treatment to electron beam therapy" (1).

The most clinically useful energy range for electrons is 4–15 MeV. At these energies, the electron beams can be used for treating superficial tumors (less than 5 cm deep) with a characteristically sharp drop-off in dose beyond the tumor. The principal applications are: 1) the treatment of skin and lip cancers; 2) chest wall irradiation for breast cancer; 3) administering boost dose to nodes; and 4) the treatment of head and neck cancers. Although many of these sites can be treated with superficial x-rays, brachytherapy, or tangential photon beams, the electron beam irradiation offers distinct advantages in terms of dose uniformity in the target volume and in minimizing dose to deeper tissues.

This chapter is intended to provide basic information on electron beam characteristics, dosimetry, and treatment planning. Most of the discussion will pertain to 4–20-MeV electrons although the data at these energies can be qualitatively extrapolated to the lower or the higher energy range.

14.1 ELECTRON INTERACTIONS

As electrons travel through a medium, they interact with atoms by a variety of processes due to coulomb force interactions. The processes are: 1) inelastic collisions with atomic electrons (ionization and excitation); 2) inelastic collisions with nuclei (bremsstrahlung); 3) elastic collisions with atomic electrons; and 4) elastic collisions with nuclei.

In inelastic collisions, some of the kinetic energy is lost as it is used in producing ionization or converted to other forms of energy such as photon energy and excitation energy. In elastic collisions, kinetic energy is not lost although it may be redistributed among the particles emerging from the collision. In low atomic number media such as water or tissues, electrons lose energy predominantly through ionizing events with atomic electrons. In higher atomic number materials, such as lead, bremsstrahlung production is more important. In the collision process with the atomic electrons, if the kinetic energy acquired by the stripped electron is large enough for it to cause further ionization, the electron is known as a secondary electron or a δ-ray. As a beam of electrons travels through a medium, the energy is continually degraded until the electrons reach thermal energies and are captured by the surrounding atoms.

A. Rate of Energy Loss

An electron travelling in a medium loses energy due to collisional and radiative processes. The magnitudes of the two effects for water and lead are shown in Fig. 14.1. The theoretical treatment of this subject is given elsewhere (2–5). It will suffice here to provide some important generalizations:

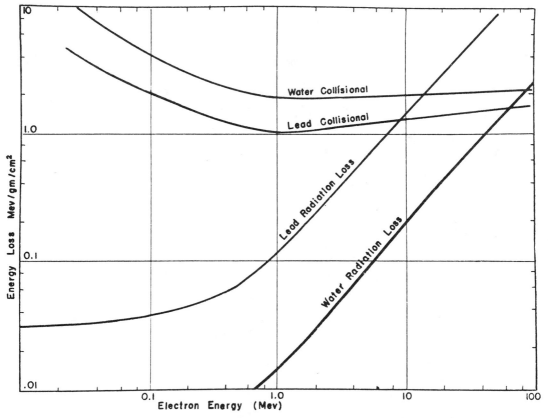

Figure 14.1.   Rate of energy loss in MeV per g/cm² as a function of electron energy for water and lead. (Reprinted with permission from: Johns HE, Cunningham JR: *The Physics of Radiology*, 3rd ed. Springfield, IL, Charles C Thomas, 1969).

A.1. COLLISIONAL LOSSES (IONIZATION AND EXCITATION)

1) The rate of energy loss depends on the electron density of the medium; 2) The rate of energy loss per gram per cm^2, which is called the mass stopping power, is greater for low atomic number (Z) material than for high Z materials (compare the water curve to the lead curve in Fig. 14.1). There are two reasons for this: first, high Z materials have fewer electrons per gram than low Z materials have; second, high Z materials have more tightly bound electrons which are not as available for this type of interaction; 3) as seen in Fig. 14.1, the energy loss rate first decreases and then increases with increase in electron energy with a minimum occurring at about 1 MeV. Above 1 MeV the variation with energy is very gradual; 4) the energy loss rate of an electron in water is roughly 2 MeV/cm.

A.2. RADIATION LOSSES (BREMSSTRAHLUNG)

The rate of energy loss per cm is approximately proportional to the electron energy and to the square of the atomic number (Z^2). Moreover, the probability of radiation loss relative to the collisional loss increases with the electron kinetic energy and with Z. That means that x-ray production is more efficient for higher energy electrons and higher atomic number absorbers.

A.3. POLARIZATION

A high-energy electron loses more energy per gram per square centimeter in a gas than in traversing a more dense medium due to appreciable polarization of the condensed medium. Atoms close to the electron track screen those remote from the track (5). This phenomenon is particularly important in dosimetry with ionization chambers where energy deposition in a solid wall or medium and a gas cavity are compared.

A.4. STOPPING POWER

The total mass stopping power $(S/\rho)_{tot}$ of a material for charged particles is defined in Reference 6 as the quotient of dE by ρdl, where dE is the total energy lost by the particle in traversing a path length dl in the material of density ρ.

$$(S/\rho)_{tot} = (S/\rho)_{col} + (S/\rho)_{rad} \qquad (14.1)$$

where $(S/\rho)_{col}$ and $(S/\rho)_{rad}$ apply respectively to collisional losses and radiation losses, discussed in Sections A.1 and A.2 above.

A.5. ABSORBED DOSE

In calculating the energy absorbed per unit mass (absorbed dose), one needs to know the electron fluence and the "restricted" collision stopping power. Restricted collision stopping power refers to the linear energy transfer (LET) concept, that is, the rate of energy loss per unit path length in collisions in which energy is "locally" absorbed, rather than carried away by energetic secondary electrons. Thus, the restricted collision mass stopping power, $(L/\rho)_{col}$, of a material for charged particles is defined (6) as the quotient of dE by ρdl, where dE is the energy lost by a charged particle in traversing a distance dl due to those collisions with atomic electrons in which the energy loss is less than Δ.

$$\left(\frac{L}{\rho}\right)_{col,\Delta} = \left(\frac{dE}{\rho dl}\right)_{col,\Delta} \tag{14.2}$$

If ϕ_E is the distribution of the fluence in energy, the absorbed dose, D, is closely approximated by

$$D = \int_{\Delta}^{E_0} \phi_E \cdot \left(\frac{L}{\rho}\right)_{col,\Delta} \cdot dE \tag{14.3}$$

The use of stopping powers in photon and electron dosimetry has been discussed in Chapter 8. Quantitative data on stopping powers as a function of electron energy for various elements and materials have been calculated by Berger and Seltzer (7, 8, 100) and tabulated in Table A.8 of the Appendix.

B. Electron Scattering

When a beam of electrons passes through a medium, the electrons suffer multiple scattering due to coulomb force interactions between the incident electrons and, predominantly, the nuclei of the medium. As a result, the electrons acquire velocity components and displacements transverse to their original direction of motion. For most practical applications, the angular and spatial spread of a narrow, collimated beam of electrons can be approximated by a Gaussian distribution (10).

By analogy with mass stopping power, Reference 6 defines the mass angular scattering power of the material as the quotient $\overline{\theta^2}/\rho l$, where $\overline{\theta^2}$ is the mean square scattering angle. Following the calculations of Rossi (10), mass scattering powers for various materials and electron energies have been tabulated in Reference 9.

The scattering power varies approximately as the square of the atomic number and inversely as the square of the kinetic energy. For this reason, high Z materials are used in the construction of scattering foils. Scattering foils spread out the electron beam that emerges from the accelerator tube and are made thin to minimize x-ray contamination of the electron beam.

14.2 ENERGY SPECIFICATION AND MEASUREMENT

Although an electron beam is almost monoenergetic before hitting the accelerator window, the random energy degradation which the electrons suffer as they pass through the exit window, scattering foil, monitor chambers, air, and other materials, results in the beam taking on a spectrum of energies at

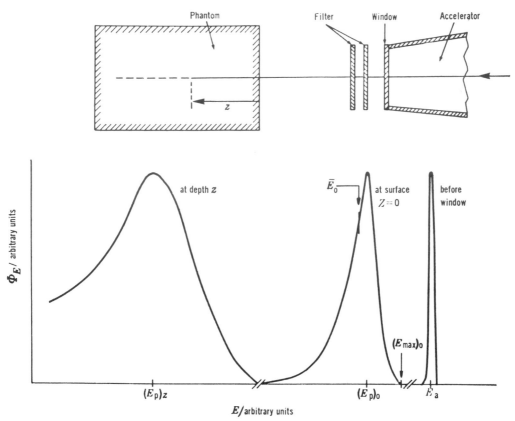

Figure 14.2. Distribution of electron fluence in energy, Φ_E, as the beam passes through the collimation system of the accelerator and the phantom. [Reprinted with permission from: ICRU Report No. 21 (9).]

the phantom surface. Further degradation and spread of beam energy take place with depth in the phantom (Fig. 14.2).

In clinical practice, an electron beam is usually characterized by the energy at the body surface. There are several methods that can be used to determine this energy: measurement of threshold energy for nuclear reactions, range measurements, and the measurement of Cerenkov radiation threshold (9). Of these, the range method is the most practical and convenient for clinical use.

A. Most Probable Energy

The Nordic Association of Clinical Physics (13) recommends the specification of most probable energy, $(E_p)_0$ (defined by the position of the spectral peak in Fig. 14.2) at the phantom surface and the use of the relationship:

$$(E_p)_0 = C_1 + C_2 R_p + C_3 R_p{}^2 \qquad (14.4)$$

where R_p is the practical range in centimeters as defined in Fig. 14.3. For

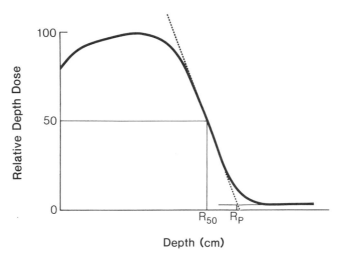

Depth (cm)

Figure 14.3. Depth dose curve illustrating the definition of R_p and R_{50}.

water, $C_1 = 0.22$ MeV, $C_2 = 1.98$ MeV cm^{-1}, and $C_3 = 0.0025$ MeV cm^{-2} (14–16). They further recommend that the field size for range measurements be no less than 12×12 cm for energies up to 10 MeV and no less than 20×20 cm for higher energies.

For the determination of range, ion chambers, diodes, or film may be used. Although the range measurements are usually made using the depth-ionization curve, the result is only slightly different from what would be obtained using depth-dose curves (11). The practical range, R_p, is the depth of the point where the tangent to the descending linear portion of the curve (at the point of inflection) intersects the extrapolated background, as shown in Fig. 14.3.

Each point on the depth-ionization curve should be corrected for beam divergence before the range is determined. The correction factor is $\left(\dfrac{f + z}{f}\right)^2$,

where f is the effective source-to-surface distance (see Section 14.4E for details) and z is the depth.

B. Mean Energy

It has been shown (17) that the mean energy of the electron beam, $\bar{E}_0$, at the phantom surface is related to R_{50} (the depth at which the dose is 50% of the maximum dose) by the following relationship:

$$\bar{E}_0 = C \cdot R_{50} \qquad (14.5)$$

where $C = 2.33$ MeV cm^{-1} for water. Again the divergence correction must be applied to each point on the depth-dose curve before determining R_{50}.

C. Energy at Depth

Harder (18) has shown that the most probable energy and, approximately, the mean energy of the spectrum decreases linearly with depth. This can be expressed by the relationships:

$$(E_p)_z = (E_p)_0 \left(1 - \frac{z}{R_p}\right) \tag{14.6}$$

and approximately

$$\bar{E}_z = \bar{E}_0 \left(1 - \frac{z}{R_p}\right) \tag{14.7}$$

where z is the depth.

Equation 14.7 is important in dosimetry since for absorbed dose measurements it is necessary to know the mean electron energy at the location of the chamber.

14.3 DETERMINATION OF ABSORBED DOSE

Calorimetry is the most basic method for the determination of absorbed dose but because of technical difficulties, the use of calorimeters is not practical in a clinical setting. Ionization chambers and Fricke dosimeters are more commonly used. Film, thermoluminescent dosimeters (TLD), and solid state diodes are used to find the ratio of the dose at one point in a phantom to the dose at another point, but not usually for measuring the absolute absorbed dose at a point.

Ionization chambers should be calibrated by a Regional Calibration Laboratory (RCL) or the National Bureau of Standards. However, an RCL can usually provide calibrations only for high energy photon beams (^{60}Co or 2-MV x-rays) but not for high energy electron beams. The use of ionization chambers calibrated for photon beams for the measurement of absorbed dose in electron beams has been the subject of many national and international protocols (9, 12, 13, 19). The most current recommendations are included in the protocol by the Task Group 21 of the AAPM (20). Elements of this protocol and other related concepts were presented in Chapter 8. Procedures specific to electron dosimetry will be discussed in this section.

A. Output Calibration

The variation of output (absorbed dose at a reference point in phantom) with field size differs considerably from one accelerator to another. Therefore, for every available electron energy, the output of each treatment cone or representative field size should be measured. The output for one cone or field size (often the 10×10 cm field), is often selected as the standard to which the other output measurements are referred. Some of the important considerations in the calibration of electron beams are discussed below.

A.1. ION CHAMBER

The American Association of Physicists in Medicine (AAPM) protocol (20) recommends the use of plane-parallel ionization chambers for the calibration of electron beams with energies less than 10 MeV, and either plane-parallel or cylindrical chambers for higher energy beams. These recommendations are based on the rationale that a plane-parallel chamber with a thin window and a small electrode separation (<2 mm) offers the least perturbation to the electron field and, therefore, should be the instrument of choice for low energy electrons.

Using a chamber of material different than that of the phantom may also cause significant perturbation of the electron fluence due to the electron scatter from the back and side walls of the chamber. Small volume cylindrical chambers with thin walls, such as 0.6-cc Farmer-type chambers, produce negligible wall perturbation but their relatively large cavity size gives rise to significant perturbation at low energies. Correction factors for these perturbations are available (Table 8.4), but the reliability of these factors decreases significantly with decrease in energy.

A.2. PHANTOM

Water is the preferred medium for calibration, although plastic phantoms such as polystyrene and Lucite are commonly used as well. The dose measured in a plastic phantom must be converted into the dose that would have been measured had the phantom been made of water (20). The phantom should have dimensions large enough (*e.g.* 30 × 30 × 30 cm) to provide full scatter for all field sizes and energies.

The chamber should be embedded in the phantom without its buildup cap. A thin (less than 0.5 mm) plastic or rubber sheath may be used to keep the chamber dry in a water phantom.

A.3. REFERENCE DEPTH AND FIELD SIZE

The reference depth for calibration measurements should be the point of maximum dose on the central axis. Since the depth-dose curve for electrons usually has a broad maximum, the chamber should be positioned in the deepest part of the maximum to avoid low energy electron contamination problems close to the phantom surface.

A 10 × 10 cm field size or cone of similar size is usually used as a reference field with the dose per monitor unit (MU) at the depth of maximum dose (d_{max}) for this field set at 1 rad/MU. The rad/MU for another cone or field size is expressed as an output factor defined as the ratio of dose rate at d_{max} for the given field size to that for the reference field size at its own d_{max}.

A.4. CHAMBER VOLTAGE

Because accelerators produce electrons in pulses rather than in a continuous stream, there may be a collection efficiency problem in the ion chamber. It is important to operate the chamber under saturation conditions with a known collection efficiency. The voltage of the chamber should be arranged to give less than 1% loss in charge by ion recombination. It is generally sufficient to set the collection voltage at about 300 V for a 0.6-cc Farmer chamber if the dose per pulse at the center of the chamber volume is 0.1 rad or less.

Methods of calculating collection efficiency for pulsed beams are discussed by Boag (21) and Reference 22. (See Section 6.8 for details.) The collection efficiency can be measured experimentally by plotting current as a function of the reciprocal of the polarizing voltage for collection losses less than 5%. The saturation current is then determined by extrapolation to infinite polarizing voltage. The ratio of current for the given voltage to that for the infinite voltage is the collection efficiency.

A.5. EFFECTS OF CHAMBER POLARITY

It is possible that the charge collected by an ion chamber is different for different polarities of its bias voltage (Section 6.9). It is recommended that the difference between the charges measured at positive and negative polarizing potentials should be less than 0.5%.

A.6 PERTURBATION OR REPLACEMENT CORRECTION

As discussed earlier, the perturbation of the electron fluence caused by the air cavity in the ionization chamber depends on the electron energy as well as on the size of the cavity. Harder (23) has calculated correction factors for thimble chambers of various radii and these are given in Table 8.4. The mean energy of the electrons at the point of measurement can be calculated using Harder's equation (Equation 14.7).

A.7. DISPLACEMENT CORRECTION

It has been shown experimentally and theoretically (24) that for a thimble chamber the effective point of measurement is displaced upstream, *i.e.* toward the source of the electron beam, from the center of the chamber. According to the recent data (25, 26), the displacement of effective point of measurement is about $0.45r$ for 3 to 10 MeV electrons and $0.6r$ for 10–30 MeV electrons, where r is the radius of the chamber. For thin plane-parallel chambers, the effective point of measurement is best taken to be at the front surface of the collecting volume.

For the output calibrations at d_{max}, it is not necessary to make the displacement correction.

A.8. ABSORBED DOSE CALCULATION

The theory of absorbed dose calculation has been discussed in Chapter 8. The dose in water at the point of measurement can be calculated by either the

C_E method or the N_{gas} method. The following notation will be used:

M = chamber reading corrected for temperature and pressure

N_c = exposure calibration factor for ^{60}Co

P_{repl} = perturbation or replacement correction factor

P_{ion} = ion recombination correction (inverse of collection efficiency)

$\dfrac{\overline{L}}{\rho}$ = mean restricted collision stopping power

$\dfrac{\overline{S}}{\rho}$ = mean nonrestricted collision stopping power

D = absorbed dose at the effective point of measurement

W = water

med = any medium or phantom in which the measurement is made

(a) *The C_E Method:*

$$D_{med} = M_{med} \cdot N_c \cdot C_{E,med} \cdot P_{ion} \cdot P_{repl} \tag{14.8}$$

$C_{E,med}$ depends on the electron energy at the point of measurement and the chamber wall composition. The general expression for C_E is given by Equation 8.45.

(b) *The N_{gas} Method:*

$$D_{med} = M_{med} \cdot N_{gas} \cdot \left(\frac{\overline{L}}{\rho}\right)_{air}^{med} \cdot P_{ion} \cdot P_{repl} \tag{14.9}$$

The expression for N_{gas} is given by Equation 8.46.

If measurements are made in a water medium, then the symbol med in the above two equations is replaced by W. However, if the measurements are made in a medium other than water, then D_{med} should be transferred to D_W by the following expression:

$$D_W = D_{med} \cdot \left(\frac{\overline{S}}{\rho}\right)_{med}^{W} \cdot \phi_{med}^{W} \tag{14.10}$$

where ϕ_{med}^{W} is the ratio of electron fluence in water to that in the medium (Chapter 8).

B. Depth-Dose Distribution

The depth-dose and isodose distributions can be determined by ion chambers, diodes, or films. Automatic isodose and isodensity plotters are useful in this regard and are available commercially.

Depth-ionization curves obtained with air-ionization chambers can be converted into depth dose curves by making corrections for change in stopping power ratio of water to air with depth. In addition, perturbation and displacement corrections are required for cylindrical chambers, as discussed in Section A.

Silicon p-n junction diodes offer some advantages in terms of small size and high sensitivity. However, diodes suffer from energy and temperature dependence and can be damaged by radiation. For these reasons absolute dosimetry with diodes is not recommended. Dose distributions obtained with diodes should be checked by ion chamber measurements. Diodes, however, are useful for obtaining quick qualitative scans of a radiation field for checking field flatness and symmetry.

Film dosimetry offers a convenient and rapid method of obtaining a complete set of isodose curves in the plane of the film. Its use for determining electron beam dose distributions is well established (27–29). It has been shown that the depth dose distributions measured by using film agree well with those by ion chambers when the latter measurements are corrected as outlined in Section A (see Fig. 14.4). Good agreement has also been demonstrated between film and $FeSO_4$ dosimeters used for the measurement of depth-dose curve (29). The energy independence of film may be explained by the fact that the ratio of collision stopping power in emulsion and in water varies slowly with electron energy (7). Thus, the optical density of the film can be taken as proportional to the dose with essentially no corrections.

Film is useful for a variety of dosimetry problems such as determining practical range, isodose curves, and beam flatness. However, film cannot be used reliably for absolute dosimetry because the optical density of a film exposed to electrons depends on many variables such as emulsion, processing, conditions, magnitude of absorbed dose, and some measurement conditions which can give rise to serious artifacts. The use of film is therefore restricted to relative dosimetry. Care is required to avoid air gaps adjacent to the film. In addition, the sensitometric curve (optical density as a function of absorbed dose) must be known in order to interpret the optical density in terms of absorbed dose. Wherever possible, a film with a linear response over the range of measured dose should be used. Errors due to changes in the processing conditions can be minimized by developing the films at approximately the same time. Accuracy can also be improved by using films from the same batch.

Film can be positioned either perpendicular or parallel to the beam axis. In the latter case, precautions must be taken to align the top edge of the film with the surface of the phantom or serious artifacts and errors in the depth dose distribution may result (28) (see Fig. 14.5).

To obtain isodose curves, the film is usually placed in a plastic phantom such as polystyrene and oriented parallel to the beam axis. The film can be kept in its original paper jacket and pressed tightly between the phantom slabs. Small holes can be punched in the corners of the jacket for trapped air to escape. The film wrapping that extends beyond the phantom should be folded to one side and taped down. After processing, the film may be analyzed

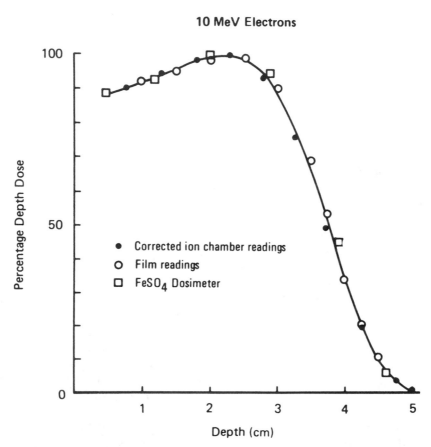

Figure 14.4.   Comparison of central axis depth dose curve measured with an ion chamber, film, and FeSO₄ dosimeter. (Reprinted with permission from: Almond PR: In *Handbook of Medical Physics*, vol 1. Boca Raton, FL, CRC Press, 1982, p 173.)

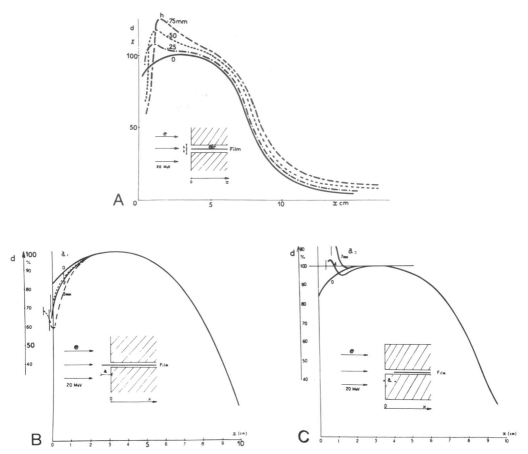

Figure 14.5. Film artifacts created by misalignment of the film in the phantom. The effects of (A) air gaps between the film and the phantom, (B) film edge extending beyond the phantom, and (C) film edge recessed within the phantom. [Reprinted with permission from: Dutreix and Dutreix (28).]

using a densitometer having a light aperture of about 1-mm diameter. Figure 14.6 shows an example of a film exposed to electrons and a set of isodose curves obtained by isodensity scanning. Since the effective density of transparent polystyrene is close to that of water, the resulting isodose curves can be used clinically without further correction.

Because many electron energies are often available with accelerators, an automatic film dosimetry system is a desirable thing to have in a clinical department. Automatic density plotters are commercially available and some of them are interfaced with treatment planning computers. Although hand-processing of films gives the best results, automatic rapid processors can be used in many instances. A strict quality assurance, however, is necessary to maintain consistency in film dosimetry.

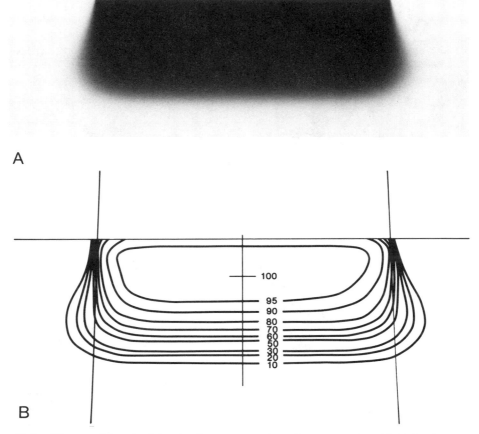

Figure 14.6. Film used for obtaining isodose curves. A, a film exposed to 12-MeV electron beam, 14 × 8 cm cone, in a polystyrene phantom; B, isodensity curves.

14.4 CHARACTERISTICS OF CLINICAL ELECTRON BEAMS

A. Central Axis Depth-Dose Curves

The major attraction of the electron beam irradiation is the shape of the depth-dose curve, especially in the energy range of 4 to 15 MeV. A region of more or less uniform dose followed by a rapid drop-off of dose offers a distinct clinical advantage over the conventional x-ray modalities. This advantage, however, tends to disappear with increasing energy.

It was stated earlier that high energy electrons lose energy at the rate of about 2 MeV/cm of water or soft tissue. Beyond the maximum range of electrons, the dose is contributed only by the x-ray contamination of the beam, indicated by the tail of the depth-dose curve (Fig. 14.7).

The useful depth in centimeters where electrons deliver a dose to the 80–90% isodose level, is equal to about ⅓–¼ of the electron energy in MeV. Thus, a 13-MeV electron beam is useful to a depth of about 3–4 cm, depending upon the isodose level specified. As seen in Fig. 14.7, the depth-dose curve falls off sharply beyond the useful depth and therefore the underlying tissues are spared.

The choice of beam energy is much more critical for electrons than for photons. Since the dose decreases abruptly beyond the 90% dose level, the treatment depth and the required electron energy must be chosen very carefully. The guiding principle is that, when in doubt, use a higher electron energy to make sure that the target volume is well within the specified isodose curve.

The skin sparing effect with the clinical electron beams is only modest or nonexistent. Unlike the photon beams, the percent surface dose for electrons increases with energy. This effect can be explained by the nature of the

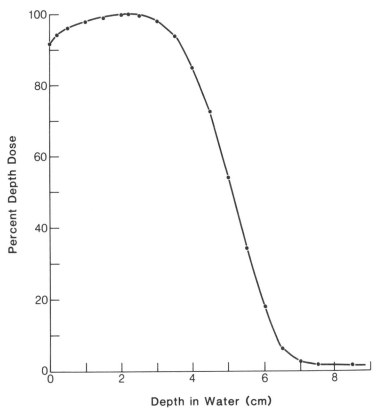

Figure 14.7. Central axis depth dose distribution measured in water with a plane-parallel chamber (beam directed horizontally). Chamber readings were corrected for change in stopping power ratio. 13 MeV, 8 × 10 cm cone, effective source to surface distance = 68 cm.

electron scatter. At the lower energies, the electrons are scattered more easily and through larger angles. This causes the dose to build up more rapidly and over a shorter distance. The ratio of surface dose to maximum dose is, therefore, less for the lower energy electrons than for the higher energy electrons.

Because of differences in beam generation, beam bending, and collimation, the depth-dose distribution as well as the surface dose can be quite different for different machines. Figure 14.8 illustrates this point by comparing central axis depth-dose curves for the Sagittaire linear accelerator and the Siemen's betatron for different beam energies. In clinical practice, therefore, it is not sufficient to specify just beam energy. Isodose distributions for an individual machine, cone, and/or field size are required.

B. Isodose Curves

The scattering of electrons plays an important role in determining the shape of the isodose curves—the central axis distribution, flatness and curvature near the field borders. Significant differences exist between the shapes of the isodose curves for different machines. These differences arise due to different collimation systems that the accelerators employ. The collimation system (*e.g.* scattering foil, monitor chambers, jaws, and cones) and the air column above

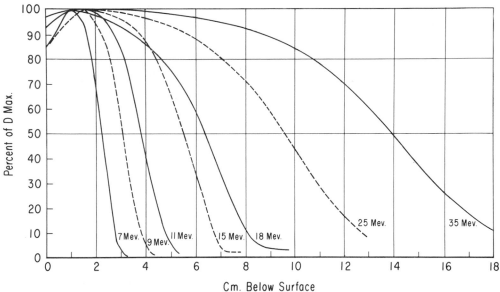

Figure 14.8. Comparison of central axis depth dose distributions of the Sagittaire linear accelerator (continuous curves) and the Siemen's betatron (dashed curve). [Reprinted with permission from: Tapley (35).]

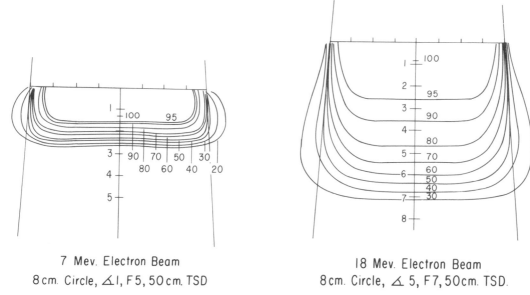

7 Mev. Electron Beam
8 cm. Circle, ∠1, F5, 50 cm. TSD

18 Mev. Electron Beam
8 cm. Circle, ∠ 5, F7, 50 cm. TSD.

Figure 14.9. Comparison of isodose curves for different energy electron beams. [Reprinted with permission from: Tapley, p 86 (35).]

the patient cause an angular dispersion of the beam as well as energy spread. Thus, beams of the same energy, E_0, but passing through different collimation systems give rise to different dose distributions.

As the beam penetrates a medium, the beam expands rapidly below the surface due to scattering. However, individual spread of the isodose curves varies depending upon the isodose level, energy, field size, and collimation. Figure 14.9, A and B, shows isodose patterns for two different energy beams. Whereas for the low energy beams all the isodose curves show some expansion, for the higher energies only the low isodose levels bulge out. The higher isodose levels tend to show lateral constriction which becomes worse with decreasing field size.

C. Field Flatness and Symmetry

Uniformity of the electron beam is usually specified in a plane perpendicular to the beam axis and at a fixed depth. Reference 30 specifies beam flatness in terms of a "uniformity index." This is defined in a reference plane and at a reference depth as the ratio of the area where the dose exceeds 90% of its value at the central axis, to the geometric beam cross section area at the phantom surface. The uniformity index should exceed a given fraction (*e.g.* 0.80 for a 10 × 10 cm field size and at depth of maximum dose). In addition, the dose at any arbitrary point in the reference plane should not exceed 103% of the central axis value.

Figure 14.10 shows isodose curves obtained from a film exposed perpendicular to an electron beam at the depth of maximum dose. The dashed line is the boundary of the geometric beam at the surface. In this example, the homogeneity index is 0.8.

Because of the presence of lower energy electrons in the beam, the flatness changes significantly with depth. Therefore, it has been recommended (83) that the uniformity index be defined at the depth of half the therapeutic range (*e.g.* ½ the depth of 85% depth dose). Furthermore, it is defined as the ratio of the areas inside the 90 and 50% isodose lines at this depth. A uniformity index of 0.70 or higher is acceptable with field sizes larger than 100 cm^2. The peak value in this plane should be less than 103%.

The symmetry specification requires that the integrated dose over any half of the cross-sectional area of the field does not vary more than 2% compared to the integrated dose over the other half.

C.1. BEAM COLLIMATION

Acceptable field flatness and symmetry are obtained with a proper design of beam scatterers and beam defining collimators. Accelerators with magnetically scanned beam do not require scattering foils. Others use one or more

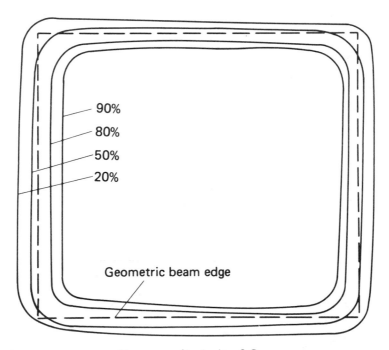

Homogeneity Index 0.8

Figure 14.10.   Isodose curves in a plane perpendicular to central axis, obtained with a film placed in a phantom at the depth of maximum dose. [Reprinted with permission from: Almond, p 50 (40).]

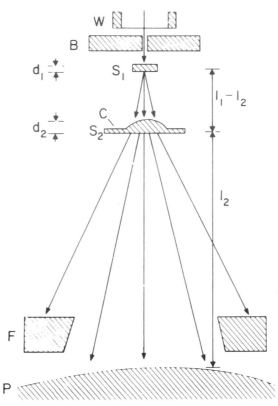

Figure 14.11.   Principle of dual foil system for obtaining uniform electron beam field. (Reprinted with permission from: Almond PR: In *Handbook of Medical Physics*, vol I. Boca Raton, FL, CRC Press, 1982, p 149.

scattering foils, usually made up of lead, to widen the beam as well as give a uniform dose distribution across the treatment field.

The beam collimation has been significantly improved by the recent introduction of dual foil system (31). Figure 14.11 shows a typical arrangement for such a system. Whereas, the first foil widens the beam by multiple scattering, the second foil is designed to make the beam uniform in cross section. The thickness of the second foil is differentially varied across the beam to produce a desired degree of beam widening and flattening. Analysis by Werner *et al.* (32) shows that the dual foil systems compare well with the scanning beam systems in minimizing angular spread and, hence, the effect on dose distribution characteristics.

The beam defining collimators are designed to provide a variety of field sizes and to maintain or improve the flatness of the beam. Basically, all collimators provide a primary collimation close to the source which defines the maximum field size and a secondary collimation close to the patient to define the treatment field. The latter can be in the form of trimmer bars or a series of cones. In the electron therapy mode, the x-ray collimator jaws are usually opened to their maximum extent and the appropriate cone is attached to an adapter fastened to the lower end of the diaphragm. In some collimation systems, the treatment cones augment the flatness of the beam by scattering electrons into the periphery of the field.

D. Field Size Dependence

The output and the central axis depth dose distribution are field size dependent. The dose increases with field size because of the increased scatter from the collimator and the phantom. As stated above, most electron collimators provide a fixed jaw opening and the treatment field size is varied by various size cones, inserts, or movable trimmer bars. Such an arrangement minimizes the variation of collimator scatter and, therefore, the output variation with field size is kept reasonably small. If the collimator aperture (x-ray jaw setting) were allowed to change with the treatment field, the output would vary too widely with field size, especially for lower energy beams. This effect is shown in Fig. 14.12 where the cone size is held fixed while the x-ray jaws

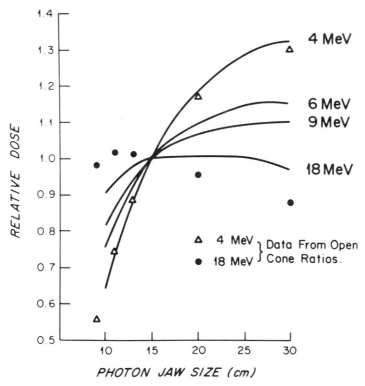

Figure 14.12. Variation of relative dose at d_{max}, through a 10 × 10 cm cone, with change of jaw setting, relative to the recommended jaw setting. [Reprinted with permission from: Biggs *et al.* (33).]

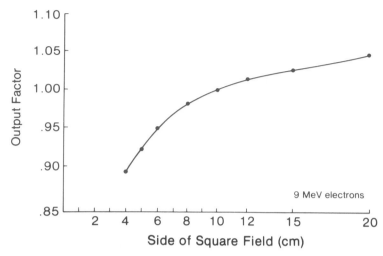

Figure 14.13. Output factors as a function of side of square field. Primary collimator fixed, secondary collimators (trimmers) close to the phantom varied to change the field size. Data are from Therac 20 linear accelerator. [Reprinted with permission from: Mills *et al.* (82).]

are varied (33). Note that the dose rate varies by a factor of greater than 2 between small and large jaw openings at 4 MeV.

The effects of field size on output and the central axis depth-dose curve due to phantom scatter alone is significant as long as the distance between the point of measurement and the edge of the field is shorter than the range of the scattered electrons. When this distance is reached, there is no further increase in depth dose due to phantom scatter. When the field is reduced below what is required for scattering equilibrium, the dose rate decreases rapidly. This is shown in Fig. 14.13. In these measurements, the field size at the phantom was varied without changing the photon collimator opening. For small fields, the output factor as well as depth dose can be significantly reduced compared to the broad beam distribution. In addition, the depth d_{max} shifts toward the surface for the smaller fields. Thus, in clinical practice, depth-dose distribution for small fields should be measured individually in addition to the output calibration.

The concept of equivalent squares, as traditionally applied to photon beams, does not, in general, apply to electron beams. However, it has been shown that, if the change in collimator scatter with field size is not considered, the depth dose for rectangular field sizes can be extracted from square field data by the following relationships (81).

$$D^{X,Y} = [D^{X,X} \cdot D^{Y,Y}]^{1/2}$$

where D is the central axis depth dose and X and Y are the field dimensions. Thus, the dose for a rectangular field size can be determined from the square root of the two square field depth doses where the sides of the two square fields are equal to the two sides of the rectangular field. Referred to as the square root method, this concept has also been applied to the determination of output factors where the primary collimation is fixed and the secondary collimation close to the phantom is varied (82). It may be restated that the collimator scatter is neglected in this model. Thus, the applicability of the square root method is not automatically valid for those machines where collimator scatter varies substantially with field size.

E. Effective SSD

Because of factors such as the fringing magnetic fields of betatrons, scattering foils or scanning magnets, and scattering from the collimator surfaces, the electrons appear to come from a virtual source. One of the methods (40) of determining virtual source position consists of taking readings with an ion chamber at several distances from the assumed source position. A plot of the reciprocal of the square root of the reading as a function of distance should yield a straight line, if the electrons follow the inverse square law. As shown in Fig. 14.14, the virtual source position is the point at which the extrapolated line intersects the abscissa.

The above method of measuring effective SSD requires measurements at large distances from the cone end or trimmers, *e.g.* every 20 cm, up to an SSD of about 200 cm. Consequently, the procedure is relatively insensitive to changes in the beam collimation. Another method (41) is to make measure-

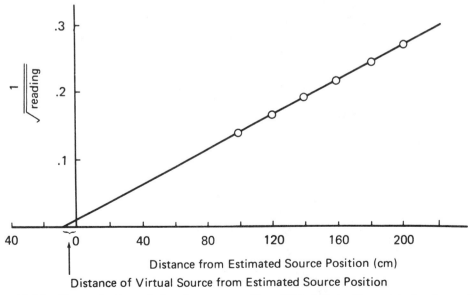

Figure 14.14. Determination of virtual source position. [Reprinted with permission from: Almond (40).]

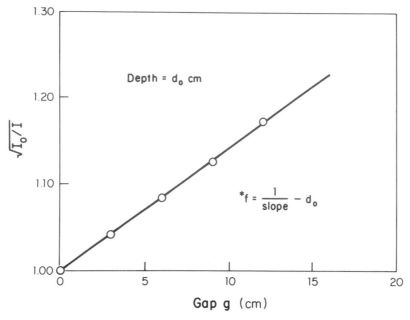

Figure 14.15. Determination of effective SSD. [Reprinted with permission from: Khan *et al.* (41).]

ments at small distances from the cone end, *e.g.* every few centimeters, up to about 10 cm from the cone end. In this method, doses are measured in a phantom at the depth of maximum dose (d_m), with the phantom first in contact with the cone (zero gap) and then at various distances. Suppose $f =$ effective SSD; $I_0 =$ dose with zero gap; $I_g =$ dose with gap g between the end of cone and the phantom surface. Then, if electrons obey inverse square law,

$$\frac{I_0}{I_g} = \left(\frac{f + d_m + g}{f + d_m}\right)^2 \tag{14.11}$$

or

$$\sqrt{\frac{I_0}{I_g}} = \frac{g}{f + d_m} + 1 \tag{14.12}$$

By plotting $\sqrt{\dfrac{I_0}{I_g}}$ as a function of gap g (Fig. 14.15), a straight line is obtained, the slope of which is $\dfrac{1}{f + d_m}$. Thus, $f = \dfrac{1}{\text{slope}} - d_m$.

The above method is recommended since it gives an effective SSD which can be used to correct depth doses when air gaps exist between the treatment applicator and the skin surface (see Section 14.5B).

Although the effective SSD is obtained by making measurements at the depth d_m, its value does not change significantly with the depth of measurement (41). However, the effective SSD does change with energy, collimation, and field size. A table of effective SSDs may be necessary to meet all clinical situations.

F. X-ray Contamination

The x-ray contamination dose at the end of the electron range can be determined from the tail of the depth-dose curve by reading off the dose value at the point where the tail becomes straight (see Fig. 14.3). This dose in a patient is contributed by bremsstrahlung interactions of electrons with the collimation system (scattering foils, chambers, collimator jaws, etc.) and the body tissues.

Table 14.1 gives the x-ray dose for the theoretical beam, with no initial x-ray contamination. These values were extracted from the depth-dose distributions in water calculated by Berger and Seltzer using the Monte Carlo program. The x-ray contamination dose from a medical accelerator depends very much on its collimation system and is usually an order of two greater than the values given in Table 14.1.

For regular treatment field sizes, the dose contributed by the x-ray contamination is not of much concern. However, even small amounts of x-ray contamination become critical for total body electron irradiation such as in the treatment of mycosis fungoides (Section 14.8).

14.5 TREATMENT PLANNING

Most electron beam treatments are planned for a single field technique. For a relatively flat and homogeneous block of tissue the dose distribution can be found by using the appropriate isodose chart. However, this simplicity of treatment planning is the exception rather than the rule. Surface areas are seldom flat and, in many cases, inhomogeneities, such as bone, lung and air cavities, present dosimetric complexities.

Table 14.1.
X-ray contamination dose (D_x) to water, at the end of the electron range as a percentage of D_{max}

Energy (MeV)	D_x (%)
5	0.1
10	0.5
15	0.9
20	1.4
30	2.8
40	4.2
50	6.0

Data are for theoretical beam with no initial x-ray contamination and are extracted from Monte Carlo data of Berger and Selzter.[34]

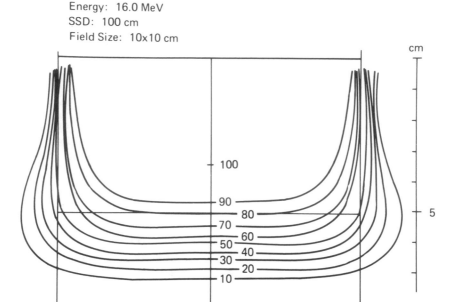

Energy: 16.0 MeV
SSD: 100 cm
Field Size: 10x10 cm

Figure 14.16. Lateral constriction of the 80% isodose curve with depth. [Reprinted with permission from: Almond (40).]

A. Choice of Energy and Field Size

The energy of beam is dictated, in general, by the depth of the target volume, minimum target dose required, and clinically acceptable dose to a critical organ, if present in the path of the beam. In most cases, where there is no danger of overdosing a critical structure beyond the target volume, the beam energy may be set so that the target volume lies entirely within the 90% isodose curve. However, in the treatment of breast, the energy is often chosen so that the depth dose at the chest wall-lung interface is 80% (35). The rationale for this lowering of the energy is to spare the lung, with the belief that the target volume for the chest wall irradiation is quite superficial and that a minimum of 80% (and some even advocate 70%) isodose curve is sufficient for the chest wall. Beyond the 80% depth dose, the dose fall-off is characteristically rapid at these beam energies.

The choice of field size in electron beam therapy should be strictly based on the isodose coverage of the target volume. Examination of the electron isodose curves (Fig. 14.16) reveals that there is a significant tapering of the 80% isodose curve at energies above 7 MeV (35). The constriction of the useful treatment volume also depends on the field size and is worse for the smaller fields. Thus, with electrons, a larger field at the surface may be necessary to adequately cover a target area than one is usually accustomed to in the case of photon beams.

B. Corrections for Air Gaps and Beam Obliquity

In electron beam therapy, there is a frequent problem of treatment cone end[1] not being parallel to the skin surface. These uneven air gaps can sometimes be large due to the extreme curvature of the sloping surface. In these cases, it is a common practice to calculate dose distribution simply by applying inverse square law correction to the dose distribution along fan lines emanating from a virtual or effective electron source (38, 84, 96). As a result of this correction, the relative depth dose distribution for a sloping contour remains almost unchanged but the absolute value of the dose is decreased at all depths because of beam divergence. This method, however, does not take into account changes in side scatter due to beam obliquity. This has been pointed out by Ekstrand and Dixon (97) who showed that the beam obliquity tends to 1) increase side scatter at the depth of maximum dose (d_{max}); 2) shift d_{max} toward the surface; and 3) decrease the depth of penetration (as measured by the depth of the 80% dose).

A broad electron beam can be represented by a summation of a large number of pencil or slit beams placed adjacent to each other. When the beam is incident obliquely on the patient surface, the point at the shallow depth receives greater side scatter from the adjacent pencil beams which have traversed a greater amount of material, while the point at the greater depth receives less scatter. This is schematically illustrated by Fig. 14.17A. As a result of these changes in the relative orientation of the pencils, one would expect an increase in dose at shallow depths and a decrease in dose at greater depths. However, since the beam is divergent, the dose will also decrease at all depths due to the inverse square law effect, as the air gap between the cone end and the surface increases with the increase in the angle of obliquity. Thus, the depth dose at a point in an obliquely incident beam is affected both by the "pencil effect" and the beam divergence.

Figure 14.17B schematically represents an arrangement used frequently for the treatment of chest wall. The beam is incident vertically on a sloping surface, thus increasing the angle of obliquity as well as the air gap between the end of the cone and the surface. Let $D_0(f,d)$ be the dose at a point at depth d for a beam incident normally on a flat surfaced phantom with an effective SSD $= f$. When the cone is placed on the chest wall, the depth dose $D(f + g,d)$ will be given by

$$D(f + g,d) = D_0(f,d)\left(\frac{f + d}{f + g + d}\right)^2 \times OF(\theta,d)$$

---

[1] In a general sense, the cone end means a plane perpendicular to the beam axis at the nominal SSD.

where g is the air gap and $OF(\theta,d)$ is the obliquity factor for the pencil beam effect discussed above. $OF(\theta,d)$ accounts for the change in depth dose at a point if the beam angle θ changes relative to the surface without change in the distance from the point to the effective source.

The obliquity factor becomes significant for angles of incidence approaching 45° or higher. For example, a 60° angle of obliquity for a 9-MeV beam gives rise to $OF = 1.18$ at the d_{max}, a shift of the d_{max} to about 0.5 cm, and a shift of the 80% depth to about 1.5 cm (97). Of course, in a given clinical situation, these effects are compounded by the inverse square law effect when significantly large air gaps are caused by the sloping surface.

Computer algorithms have been developed (81, 98, 99, 103) in which broad beam distribution is calculated by placing a set of narrow or pencil beams

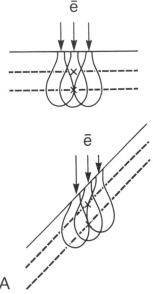

Figure 14.17. A, a schematic illustration of how the relative orientation of pencil beams changes with the angle of obliquity. For a parallel beam, this effect would increase dose at the shallower points and decrease dose at the deeper points as the angle of obliquity is increased. (Redrawn from Reference 97.) B, a diagrammatic representation of irradiation of a chest wall with sloping surface. The gap g and depth d for a point are measured along the fan line (the line joining the point to the effective source location). Θ is the angle between the fan line and the tangent to the sloping surface. The figure on the right represents the reference setup, with beam incident normal, with no air gaps between the cone end and the phantom. C, comparison of measured (solid lines) and calculated (dashed lines) isodose distribution for a beam incident on a polystyrene cylindrical phantom. The measured distribution represents isodensity distribution obtained with a film sandwiched in the phantom according to the procedure outlined in Section 14.3B. The calculated distribution was obtained with a computer using a divergent pencil beam algorithm. Both distributions are normalized to the D_{max} in a reference setup in which the beam is incident normally on a flat phantom with no air gaps between the cone end and the phantom. 12-MeV electrons, field size 18 × 12 cm, effective SSD = 70 cm.

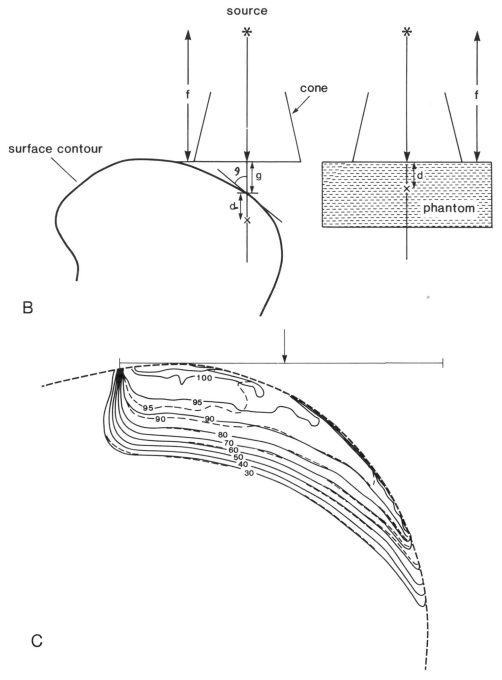

Figure 14.17B–C.

along the contour. The divergence correction can be taken into account by aligning central axes of the pencil beams along the fan lines and normalizing the resulting dose distribution to the dose at d_{max} for the beam incident normally on a flat surfaced phantom. Figure 14.17C compares the calculated distribution using a pencil beam algorithm with the measured distribution obtained in a cylindrical polystyrene phantom.

Sharp surface irregularities produce localized "hot spots" and "cold spots" in the underlying medium due to scattering. Electrons are predominantly scattered outward by steep projections and inwards by steep depressions. This can be seen in Fig. 14.18 (47). In practice, such sharp edges may be smoothed with an appropriately shaped bolus. Also, if a bolus is used to reduce beam penetration in a selected part of the field, its edges should be tapered to minimize the effect shown in Fig. 14.18.

C. Tissue Inhomogeneities

Electron beam dose distribution can be significantly altered in the presence of tissue inhomogeneities such as bone, lung, and air cavities. It is difficult to determine dose distribution within or around small inhomogeneities because of enhanced scattering effects. However, for large and uniform slabs, dose distribution beyond the inhomogeneity can be corrected by using the "coefficient of equivalent thickness" (CET) method (36, 37, 43, 44, 96). It is assumed that the attenuation by a given thickness z of the inhomogeneity is equivalent to the attenuation ($z \times$ CET) of water. The CET for a given material is approximately given by its electron density (electron/cc) relative to that of water. The dose at a point beyond the inhomogeneity is determined by calculating the effective depth, d_{eff}, along the ray joining the point and the virtual source of the electrons.

$$d_{eff} = d - z(1 - \text{CET}) \qquad (14.13)$$

where d is the actual depth of point P from the surface. The depth dose is read from dose distribution data for water at the effective depth. An additional correction may be applied due to the inverse square law, *i.e.* $\left(\dfrac{f + d_{eff}}{f + d}\right)^2$, where f is the effective SSD.

C.1. BONE

The CET method is in good agreement with *in vivo* measurements in patients for the dose behind the mandible (40). The electron density (or CET) of a compact bone (*e.g.* mandible) relative to that of water is taken as 1.65. For spongy bone, such as sternum, which has a density of 1.1 g/cm^3, the electron densities are not much different from water and therefore CET can be assumed to be unity.

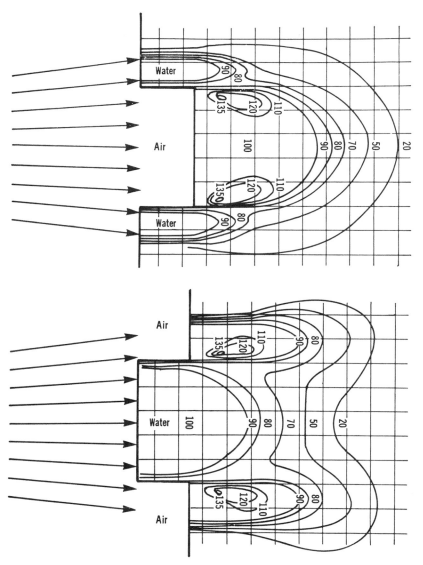

Figure 14.18. Effect of sharp surface irregularities on electron beam isodose distributions. [Reprinted with permission from: Dutreix (47).]

C.2. LUNG

The problem of lung inhomogeneity has been studied by many investigators (36, 37, 43, 44). Results of *in vivo* measurements in the lungs of dogs have shown that there is a considerable variation of CET with depth in the lung (45). This is illustrated by Fig. 14.19 for a water-cork system (simulating chest wall and lung interface). The dose near the interface is decreased due to reduced scatter from the low density cork. Beyond a certain depth, the dose to the cork begins to increase relative to the reference curve (measured in water) as the increased penetration overtakes the reduced scatter.

Thus, in general, the CET values for lung are dependent on depth within the lung. Empirical equations for the CET values derived from *in vivo* measurements have been proposed to take this variation into account (40). An average lung CET value of 0.5 has also been suggested (36). Recent measurements (46) in anthropomorphic phantoms have shown that a CET value based on electron density gives an accuracy of about 10% for typical chest wall irradiations.

The relative electron density of lung may be equated to its mass density. The studies with computed tomography (CT) have shown that the electron density of lung varies between 0.20 and 0.25 relative to that of water. Therefore, if CET is assumed equal to electron density, Equation 14.13 may be used to calculate lung correction by substituting lung density in place of CET. Figure 14.20 shows examples of uncorrected and corrected isodose distributions obtained by using pencil beams. In the case of the corrected distribution, the effective depth was calculated assuming CET equal to the lung density.

In routine treatment planning, any of the above methods may be used as approximations. Obviously, the effective depth calculation based on electron density or some empirically derived CET is only a rough approximation in which scattering effects are not fully taken into account.

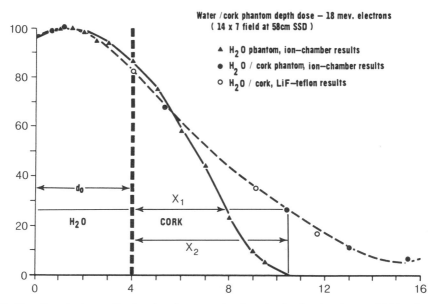

Figure 14.19. Depth dose distribution in water and water/cork phantoms. CET values may be calculated from these data. CET $= X_1/X_2$. (Modified from Reference 43.)

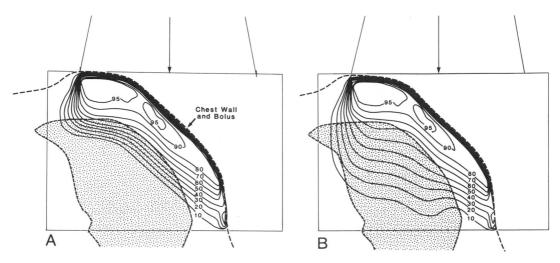

Figure 14.20.   An example of chest wall irradiation with electrons. The surface contour was irregular in shape, so bolus was used to even out chest wall thickness as well as maximize surface dose. A, calculated isodose curves uncorrected for lung density; B, calculated isodose curves corrected for lung density ($\rho = 0.25$ gm^3). 10-MeV electron beam, effective SSD = 68 cm, field size = 13 × 15 cm.

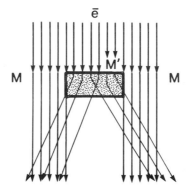

Figure 14.21.   Schematic illustration of electron scatter behind edges between materials M and M'. The scattering power of M is greater than that of M′.

C.3. SMALL INHOMOGENEITIES

Small inhomogeneities present a more complex situation because of electron scattering behind edges. Figure 14.21 schematically illustrates the effect at a single edge. For simplicity, it is assumed that the path of the electrons in medium M is along straight lines. If a material M' of a higher mass scattering power is introduced, electrons are scattered at larger angles. This causes a decrease in the electron fluence behind the slab, thus reducing the dose there.

The scattered electrons, on the other hand, increase the dose in the medium M. Thus, a small inhomogeneity causes cold spots and hot spots behind its edges.

Pohlit and Manegold (48) have made a systematic analysis of dose distributions behind edges of different materials. Their method can be used to get a rough estimate of the maximum values for increase and decrease of dose behind such inhomogeneities. Figure 14.22 defines angles α and β of dose perturbation. The mean angle α gives the position of the maxima of reduction and of increase of dose and β represents the mean angle where the effect of the inhomogeneity is practically negligible. These angles, which are related to the scattering of electrons in the medium, depend mainly on the mean electron energy $\bar{E}$ at the edge. Figure 14.23 gives these angles as a function of $\bar{E}$.

The dose distribution under the inhomogeneity but outside angle β may be calculated according to the regular CET method discussed earlier. The maxima and minima of dose along the boundaries of angle α may be estimated by defining a maximum change, P_{max}, in dose.

$$P_{max} = \frac{D_m - D_0}{D_0}$$

where D_m is the dose at the highest increase or depression and D_0 is the dose

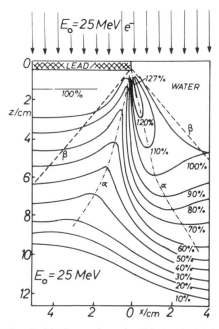

Figure 14.22. Isodose distribution behind an edge of a thin lead slab in water. Angle α denotes the maxima of dose change and angle β of negligible change. [Reprinted with permission from: Pohlit and Manegold (48).]

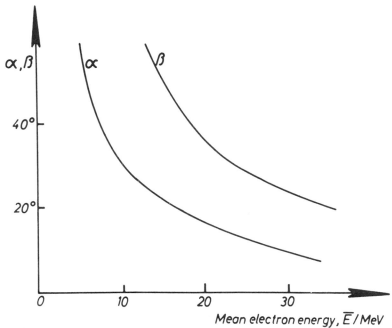

Figure 14.23. Plot of angles α and β as a function of mean energy at the edge for inhomogeneities in water (or tissue). [Reprinted with permission from: Pohlit and Manegold (48).]

in the homogeneous water phantom at that point. Figure 14.24 may be used to estimate P_{max} for different energies and materials. It is important to note that the influence of an edge increases with increasing electron energy.

Scattering effects can be enhanced by adjoining scattering edges and, therefore, small inhomogeneities produce complex effects resulting in large changes in dose due to the overlapping of these regions.

The above method is useful for quick and rough calculations. More accurate calculations will require more sophisticated methods based on multiple scattering theory. Some work along these lines has been reported recently in the literature (23, 32, 51, 52, 81, 103).

D. Use of Bolus and Absorbers

Bolus is often used in electron beam therapy to (a) flatten out an irregular surface, (b) reduce the penetration of the electrons in parts of the field, and (c) increase the surface dose. Ideally, the bolus material should be equivalent to tissue in stopping power and scattering power. A given bolus material should be checked by comparing depth-dose distribution in the bolus with that in the water. If a scaling factor is required, it should be documented and used in treatment planning whenever the bolus is used.

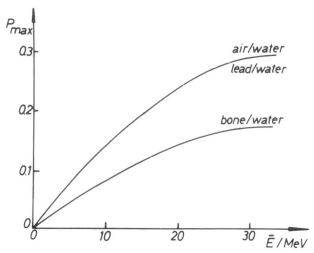

Figure 14.24. Plot of maximum change in dose P_{max} as a function of mean electron energy at the edge of various inhomogeneities in water. [Reprinted with permission from: Pohlit and Manegold (48).]

A number of commercially available materials can be used as bolus, *e.g.* paraffin wax, polystyrene, Lucite, "Superstuff," "Superflab." Usefulness of some of these materials for electron bolusing have been discussed in the literature (49, 50). In my experience, Superflab[2] is excellent for bolusing. This material is transparent, flexible, and almost water equivalent.

A plate of low atomic number material such as Lucite and polystyrene is sometimes used to reduce the energy of an electron beam. Such plates are known as decelerators. The decelerator should be placed in close contact with the patient surface as with a bolus. Large air gaps between the absorber and the surface would result in reduction in dose which may not be easily predictable unless specifically measured for those conditions. For these reasons, a flexible bolus which conforms to the surface contour is more desirable.

E. Problems of Adjacent Fields

When two adjacent electron fields are overlapping or abutting, there is a danger of delivering excessively high doses in the junction region. On the other hand, separating the fields may seriously underdose parts of the tumor. Examples of combined isodose distributions for different field separations are shown in Fig. 14.25. In a clinical situation, the decision as to whether the fields should be abutted or separated should be based on the uniformity of the combined dose distribution across the target volume. Since the tumors treated

---

[2] Developed by G. R. Feaster, University of Kansas, Kansas City, KS and supplied by Mick Radio-Nuclear Instruments, Inc., 1470 Outlook Avenue, Bronx, NY 10465.

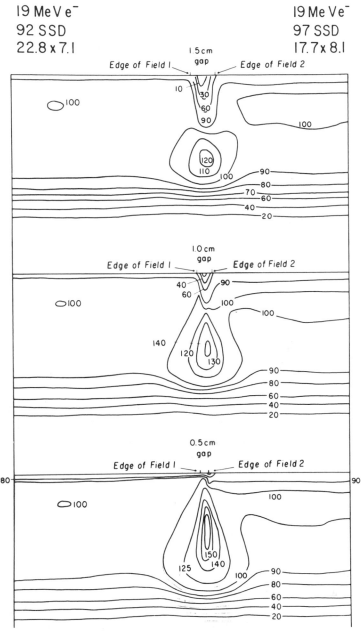

Figure 14.25.   Isodose distributions for adjacent electron fields with different gaps widths. [Reprinted with permission from: Almond (40).]

with electrons are mostly superficial, the electron fields are usually abutted. The hot spots can be accepted depending on their magnitude, extent, and location. Similar considerations apply to electron fields adjacent to x-ray fields.

14.6 FIELD SHAPING

Extensive field shaping is sometimes required in electron beam therapy. Lead cutouts are often used to give shape to the treatment area and to protect the surrounding normal tissue or a critical organ. These cutouts are placed either directly on the skin or at the end of the treatment cone.

For lower energy electrons (<10 MeV), less than 3 mm thickness of lead is required for adequate shielding (*e.g.* ≤5% transmission). Lead sheets of this thickness can be easily molded to conform more or less to the surface contour and therefore can be placed directly on the skin surface. For higher energy electrons, however, thicker lead is required and cannot be so easily contoured. Moreover, a heavy lead mask may cause discomfort to the patient. The alternative method is to support a lead cutout at the end of the treatment cone or the field trimmers. Shields to be used in such a configuration can be designed from pure lead sheets or a low melting alloy such as Lipowitz metal (trade names: Cerrobend, Ostalloy, and Lometoy).

A. External Shielding

Several publications have reported the thickness of lead or low melting point lead alloy required for shielding in electron beam therapy (53–57). Figure 14.26 shows a set of transmission measurements through lead. The thickness for shielding can be chosen on the basis of allowable transmission (*e.g.* 5%). The shield thickness should be neither overly large nor so critical in measurement that a small change in thickness would cause a large change in the transmitted dose.

An important consideration in electron beam shielding is to make certain that the thickness is appropriate to reduce the dose to an acceptable value. As seen in Fig. 14.26, if the lead is too thin, the transmitted dose may even be enhanced directly behind the shield. Normally, if weight or thickness is no problem, one can use a shield of thickness greater than the required minimum. But there are practical limits on the amount of lead that can be used. For example, in the case of eyeshields (58) and internal shields, it is important to use the minimum thickness of lead to obtain the desired reduction in dose.

B. Measurement of Transmission Curves

Transmission curves for a shielding material may be obtained with an ion chamber embedded in a phantom. A suitable arrangement for such measurements consists of a parallel-plate ion chamber in a polystyrene phantom. Since the maximum transmitted dose through lead occurs at a point close to the patient's surface, the measurement depth in the phantom should not exceed 5 mm (59).

The transmission curve is a plot of ionization current as a function of shield thickness. Generally, the shielding measurements made with broad beams gives an upper limit to the shielding requirements for all field sizes (53, 57). However, if minimum thickness shields are needed, as for internal shielding,

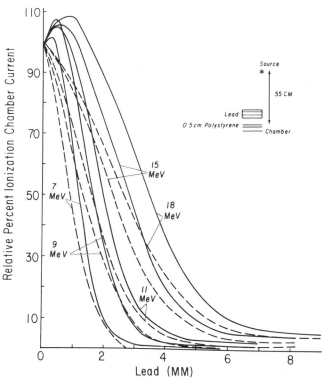

Figure 14.26. Transmission curves through lead for 7-, 9-, 11-, 15-, and 18-MeV electrons. Measurements made with a plane-parallel chamber in a polystyrene phantom, at a depth of 0.5 cm. Solid lines are 10.5 × 10.5 cm effective field size and dashed lines are for 6.3 × 6.3 cm effective field size. (Redrawn from Reference 53.)

a transmission curve may be measured especially for the given field size and the depth of the structure to be shielded.

Although it is desirable to make measurements with the shields in the same configuration relative to the applicator and the phantom as used clinically, this is not a critical consideration. Purdy *et al.* (57) made measurements with the shield placed at the end of the treatment cone and at the phantom surface. They did not find significant differences in the percent transmission for the two arrangements.

C. Effect of Blocking on Dose Rate

Blocking a portion of the electron beam field, in general, produces changes in the dose rate and dose distribution. The magnitude of the change depends on the extent of blocking, the thickness of lead, and the electron energy. Figure 14.27 shows increase in output factor at d_{max} when a field is blocked down to a smaller size (56). However, if a field produced by a lead cutout is smaller than the minimum size required for maximum lateral dose buildup, the dose

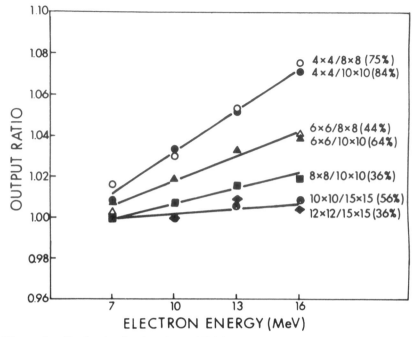

Figure 14.27. ratio of ionization for the shaped field to the ionization for the open cone (output ratio) as a function of beam energy. The field sizes for the reduced fields were defined by a lead cutout placed at the phantom surface. [Reprinted with permission from: Choi *et al.* (56).]

in the open portion may be reduced (54) (Fig. 14.28). The increase or reduction in dose also depends on the depth of measurement. Thus, field shaping affects output factor as well as depth-dose distribution in a complex manner.

If the field is large and the blocking is minimal, the normal calibration for the field size set by the collimator can be used. If the blocking is over more than 25% of the field area, a special calibration should be carried out (40). In severe cases of blocking, it may be necessary to determine the entire isodose distribution in addition to the output factor.

D. Internal Shielding

In some situations such as the treatment of lip, buccal mucosa, and eyelid lesions, internal shielding is useful to protect the normal structures beyond the target volume. Lead shielding may be used to reduce the transmitted dose to an acceptable value. However, the electron backscatter from lead enhances the dose to the tissue near the shield. This effect has been discussed by several investigators (54, 60–65).

The enhancement in dose at the tissue-lead interface can be quite substantial, *e.g.* 30–70% in the range of 1–20 MeV. Figure 14.29 shows the increase in dose (relative to homogeneous phantom) as a function of the mean energy

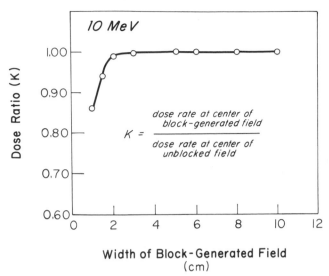

Figure 14.28. Change of dose at D_{max} as the field size is changed using a lead cutout at the phantom surface. Discussed in Reference 54.

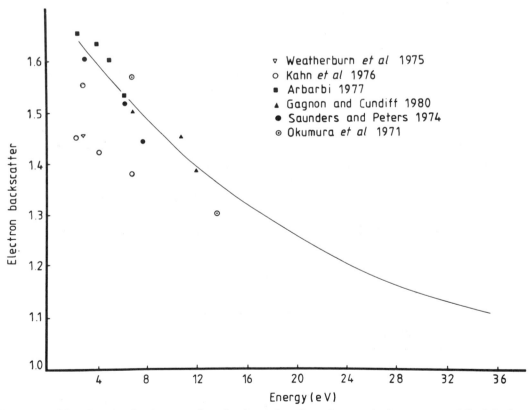

Figure 14.29. Electron backscatter from lead as a function of mean electron energy at the interface. The solid line represents the best fit to experimental data of Klevenhagen *et al.* (65). [Reprinted with permission from: Klevenhagen *et al.* (65).]

incident at the tissue-lead interface. The scatter in the experimental data is probably due to differences in the measurement techniques and the state of angular spread of the electron beam before incidence at the interface. The curve by Klevenhagen *et al.* (65) represents the best fit to his experimental data for polystyrene-lead interface and has been characterized by the following equation (65):

$$\text{EBF} = 1 + 0.735 \exp(-0.052 \, \bar{E}_Z)$$

where EBF is the electron backscatter factor, defined as the quotient of the dose at the interface with the lead present to that with a homogeneous polystyrene phantom at the same point. $\bar{E}_Z$ is the average electron energy incident at the interface.

Variation of electron backscatter with atomic number Z of the scattering material has also been studied (64, 65). Figure 14.30 gives the data by Klevenhagen *et al.* (65).

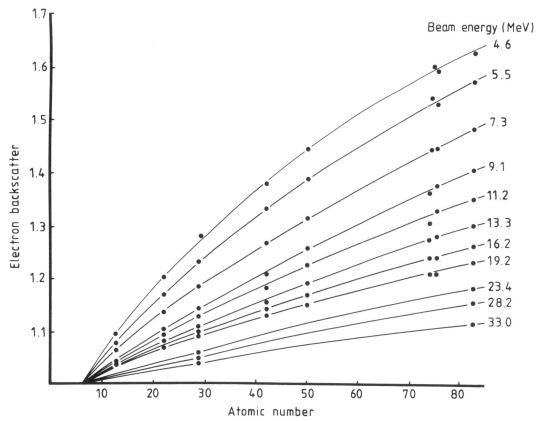

Figure 14.30. Variation of electron backscatter with atomic number Z of scattering material for different electron energies at the interface. [Reprinted with permission from: Klevenhagen *et al.* (65).]

An important aspect of the electron backscatter problem is the range of the backscattered electrons. Measurements of dose in the phantom layers preceding the lead have shown (54, 64) that for electrons in the range of 8–20 MeV the range of the backscattered electrons is about 1–2 g/cm^2 of polystyrene, depending on the energy of the incident electrons. The dose enhancement drops off exponentially with the distance from the interface on the entrance side of the beam. Figure 14.31 illustrates this effect for 10-MeV beam incident on a phantom with a sheet of lead placed at various depths.

In order to dissipate the effect of electron backscatter, a suitable thickness of low atomic number absorber such as bolus may be placed between the lead shield and the preceding tissue surface. Saunders and Peters (62) recommend the use of an aluminum sheath around any lead used for internal shielding. Oral shielding has also been accomplished by special oral stents made of dental acrylic which encompasses the lead (35). Such a shield provides lead protection for the tongue and other structures as well as reduces the electron backscatter from lead reaching the buccal mucosa.

Eyeshields are designed to protect the lens. Minimum thickness of lead is used to provide acceptable transmission value. Since a significant thickness of low Z material is required to absorb the electron backscatter, eyeshields cannot be coated with an adequate thickness of such materials without exceeding the size requirements. In such cases, it is desirable to coat the lead shield with a

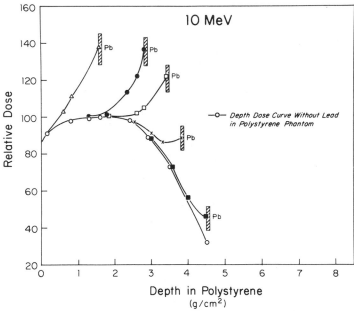

Figure 14.31. Modification of depth dose by lead placed at various depths in a polystyrene phantom. Lead thickness = 1.7 mm. [Reprinted with permission from: Khan *et al.* (54).]

thin film of wax or dental acrylic (to absorb the very low energy electrons) and calibrate the setup for actual dose received by the lid.

14.7 ELECTRON ARC THERAPY

Electron beam arch technique gives excellent dose distribution for treating superficial tumors along curved surfaces. The technique was first described by Becker and Weitzel (85) in 1956. Several papers (86–93) have since appeared in the literature describing the various technical and physical aspects of electron arc therapy. For details, the reader is referred to the Proceedings of the Symposium on Electron Dosimetry and Arc Therapy (94).

On the basis of isodose distribution, electron arc therapy is most suited for treating superficial volumes which follow curved surfaces such as chest wall, ribs, and entire limbs. Although all chest wall irradiations can be done with electron arcing, this technique is mostly useful in cases where the tumor involves a large chest wall span and extends posteriorly beyond the midaxillary line. The conventional technique of using tangential photon beams in this case will irradiate too much of the underlying lung. The alternative approach of using multiple abutting electron fields is fraught with field junction problems especially when angled beams are used. In short, it appears that for a certain class of cases, electron arc therapy has no reasonable alternative.

Not all electron accelerators are equipped with electron arc mode. However, with increasing interest in this technique, more and more linear accelerators are being made with this capability. Besides the arcing capability, certain modifications in electron collimation are necessary to make this technique feasible. For example, one needs a beam-defining aperture with adequate clearance from the patient and collimation close to the patient surface to sharpen the dose fall-off at the arc limits (88).

Machines that cannot rotate in the electron mode may still be used to perform what is called a "pseudoarc" technique (101). In this technique, the field is defined by the x-ray jaws and the electron collimation is provided on the patient's skin surface. The beam is directed isocentrically through equally spaced large number of angles. The fields are overlapped by aligning the center of a given fixed field with the edge of its next neighboring field. Thus, the pseudoarc technique is designed to achieve the results of a continuous arc by using sufficiently large number of overlapping fields directed isocentrically.

A. Calibration of Arc Therapy Beam

Calibration of an electron arc therapy procedure requires special considerations in addition to those required for stationary beam treatments. Dose per arc can be determined in two ways: (a) integration of the stationary beam profiles; and (b) direct measurement. The first method requires an isodose distribution as well as the dose rate calibration of the field (under stationary beam conditions) used for arcing. The integration procedure is illustrated in Fig. 14.32. Radii are drawn from the isocenter at a fixed angular interval $\Delta\theta$

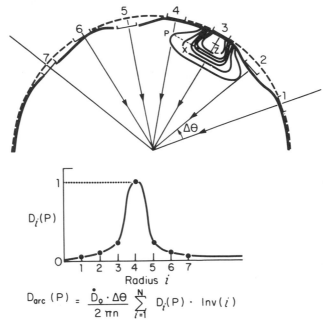

Figure 14.32. Integration of dose per arc at a point P. Solid line represents an irregularly shaped patient contour and the dotted line is a circle approximating the contour. Isodose curves for the scanning field are placed along each radius to integrate the dose at point P. [Reprinted with permission from: Khan (102).]

(*e.g.* 10°). The isodose chart is placed along each radius while the dose at point P as a fraction of the maximum dose on the central axis is recorded. Let $D_i(P)$ be this dose as the isodose chart is placed at the radius. The dose per arc at P is given by (102)

$$D_{\mathrm{arc}}(P) = \frac{\dot{D}_0 \cdot \Delta\theta}{2\pi n} \sum_{i=1}^{N} D_i(P) \cdot \mathrm{Inv}(i)$$

where $\dot{D}_0$ is the dose rate per minute in the stationary field at the depth of $d_{\max}$, n is the speed of rotation (number of revolutions per minute), and $\mathrm{Inv}(i)$ is the inverse square law correction for an air gap between the dotted circle, and the beam entry point. The term $\Delta\theta \cdot \sum_{i=1}^{N} D_i(P)$ can also be evaluated graphically as shown in the figure inset.

The direct measurement of dose per arc requires a cylindrical phantom of a suitable material such as polystyrene or Lucite. A hole is drilled in the phantom to accommodate the chamber at a depth corresponding to the $d_{\max}$. The radius of the phantom need only be approximately equal to the radius of curvature of the patient since only a small part of the arc contributes dose to the chamber reading (102). The integrated reading per arc can be converted to dose per arc by using correction factors normally applicable to a stationary beam.

B. Treatment Planning

The treatment planning for electron arc therapy includes (a) choice of beam energy, (b) choice of isocenter, (c) choice of field size, (d) field shaping, and (e) isodose distribution. These are briefly considered below.

BEAM ENERGY

The central axis dose distribution is somewhat altered due to field motion. For a small scanning field width, the depth dose curve shifts slightly and the beam appears to penetrate somewhat farther than for a stationary beam (Fig. 14.33). The surface dose is reduced and the bremsstrahlung dose at the isocenter is increased. This phenomenon is known as the "velocity effect": a deeper point is exposed to the beam longer than a shallower point, resulting in apparent enhancement of beam penetration.

SCANNING FIELD WIDTH

Although any field width may be used to produce acceptable isodose distribution, smaller scanning fields (*e.g.* width of 5 cm or less) give lower dose rate and greater x-ray contamination (88, 90). However, small field widths allow almost normal incidence of the beam on the surface, thus simplifying dosimetry. Another advantage of the smaller field width is that the dose per arc is less dependent on the total arc angle. For these reasons, a geometric field width of 4–8 cm at the isocenter is recommended for most clinical situations.

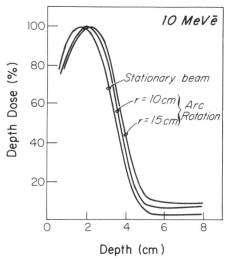

Figure 14.33. Effect of isocenter depth-dose distribution compared with a stationary beam. Cylindrical polystyrene phantoms were used: SAD = 100 cm, SSD = 64 cm, diaphragm opening = 3 × 6 cm, arc angle = 120°. [Reprinted with permission from: Khan *et al.* (88).]

LOCATION OF ISOCENTER

The isocenter should be placed at a point approximately equidistant from the surface contour for all beam angles. In addition, the depth of isocenter must be greater than the maximum range of electrons so that there is no accumulation of electron dose at the isocenter.

FIELD SHAPING

Without electron collimation at the patient surface, the dose fall-off at the treatment field borders is rather gradual. In order to sharpen the distribution, lead strips should be used to define the arc limits as well as the field limits in the length direction (Fig. 14.34). Cast shielding has been found to be useful for routine electron arc therapy (93).

ISODOSE DISTRIBUTION

This crucial information for arc therapy is not as easily available for electrons as it is for photons. Until computer programs of adequate sophistication are routinely available for electron arc therapy, this modality of treatment will probably remain inaccessible to most institutions. Of course, this problem is part of the general problem of electron beam treatment planning. However, the current surge of activity in this area as well as the CT development provides an optimistic future for the development of sophisticated electron beam therapy techniques including the arc.

14.8 TOTAL SKIN IRRADIATION

Electrons in the energy range of 2–6 MeV have been found useful for treating superficial lesions covering large areas of the body, such as mycosis fungoides and other cutaneous lymphomas. At these energies, electron beams are characterized by a rapid fall-off in dose beyond a shallow depth and a minimal x-ray background (1% or less). Thus, superficial skin lesions extending to about 1 cm depth can be effectively treated without exceeding bone marrow tolerance.

The treatment of mycosis fungoides with total skin irradiation was suggested at least 30 years ago (66). Since that time, various techniques have been developed and applied with success to the treatment of this disease (67–70). Basically, the methods fall into two general categories: 1) translational technique in which a horizontal patient is translated relative to a beam of electrons of sufficient width to cover the transverse dimensions of the patient; and 2) large field technique in which a standing patient is treated with a combination of broad beams produced by electron scattering and large SSDs (2–6 m). Salient features of these techniques are discussed below.

A. Translational Technique

This technique has been described by a number of investigators (66, 71, 72). The patient lies on a motor-driven couch and is moved relative to a downward

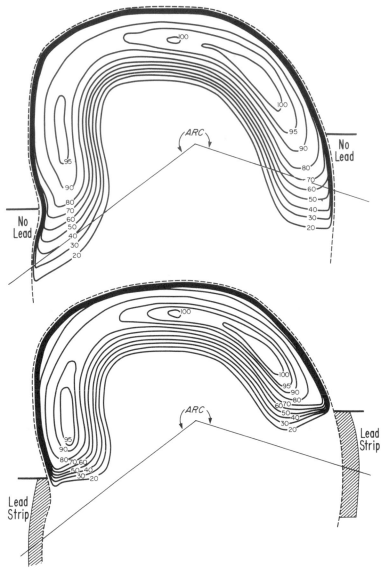

Figure 14.34. Isodose distribution in arc rotation with and without lead strips at the ends of the arc, using a section of an Alderson Rando phantom closely simulating an actual patient cross section. Arc angle = 236°; average radius of curvature = 10 cm; beam energy = 10 MeV; lead strip thickness = 6 mm; field size at the surface = 4.2 × 8.5 cm. [Reprinted with permission from: Khan *et al.* (88).]

directed beam at a suitable velocity. Alternatively, the patient may be stationary and the radiation source translated horizontally. In the latter technique, which has been described by Haybittle (71), a 24-Ci ^{90}Sr β source, in the form of a 60-cm linear array, is used. The source is contained in a shielded source housing and positioned above the couch. The maximum energy of the β particles emitted by ^{90}Sr is 2.25 MeV. However, due to the spectral distribution of β-ray energies, the effective depth of treatment in this case is only a fraction of a millimeter.

The translational technique using a 3-MeV Van de Graaf generator has been described by Wright (72). A well-collimated monoenergetic electron beam is scattered just after leaving the vacuum window to improve uniformity. The beam is then collimated by an aluminum cone with a 5 mm × 45 cm defining slit. The patient is translated under this beam at a suitable speed. Williams *et al.* (73) have described a similar technique with a linear accelerator. No applicator is used in this technique and the x-ray collimators are fully retracted. The patient is treated anteriorly and posteriorly. The dose uniformity along the length of the patient is achieved by moving the patient through a distance sufficient that the areas treated start outside the electron beam, pass through, and finish outside the electron beam. The dose uniformity in the transverse direction is enhanced by suitably combining transversely overlapping fields.

B. Large Field Technique

Large electron fields required for total body skin irradiation can be produced by scattering electrons through wide angles and using large treatment distances. The field is made uniform over the height of the patient by vertically combining multiple fields or vertical arcing. The patient is treated in a standing position with four or six fields directed from equally spaced angles for circumferential coverage of the body surface.

B.1. FIELD FLATNESS

Low energy electron beams are considerably widened by scattering in air. For example, a 6-MeV narrow electron beam, after passing through 4 m of air, achieves a Gaussian intensity distribution with a 50% to 50% width of approximately 1 m (74). This usually gives adequate uniformity over a patient's width. If two such fields are joined together at their 50% lines, the resultant field will be uniform over a height of approximately 1 m. A proper combination of more such fields or a continuous arc can lead to a larger uniform field, sufficient to cover a patient from head to foot (Fig. 14.35, A and B).

The size and shape of an electron beam developed at a distance by air scatter can be estimated by multiple scattering theory. Holt and Perry (74) have used this approach to obtain a uniform field by combining multiple field profiles in proper proportions and angular separation (Fig. 14.35A).

In addition to air, the electron beam is scattered by a scattering foil inside or outside the collimator. However, the x-ray contamination would be increased since unnecessarily wide beams waste electron flux to the sides.

B.2. X-RAY CONTAMINATION

X-ray contamination is present in every therapy electron beam and becomes a limiting factor in total skin irradiation. Ordinarily, these x-rays are contributed by bremsstrahlung interactions produced in the exit window of the

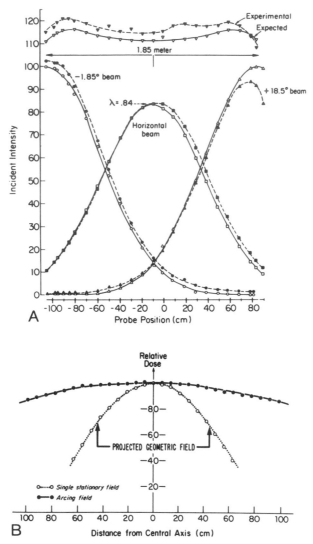

Figure 14.35. A, combination of three beam intensity profiles along the vertical axis to obtain a resultant beam profile. Central beam is directed horizontally while the others are directed at 18.5° from the horizontal. λ is a weighting factor used in an equation developed by Holt and Perry (74). [Reprinted with permission from: Holt and Perry (74).] B, vertical beam profile at the treatment plane for a stationary single field and an arcing field. [Reprinted with permission from: Sewchand *et al.* (78).]

accelerator, scattering foil, ion chambers, beam-defining collimators, air, and the patient. The bremsstrahlung level can be minimized if the electron beam is scattered by air alone before incidence on the patient. This would necessitate some modifications in the accelerator such as removing the scattering foil and other scatterers in the collimation system. Various safety interlocks would be required to make this separation feasible for routine clinical use. Such a system has been developed at Memorial Hospital, New York, on a Varian Clinac-6 (75).

In the Stanford technique, described by Karzmark *et al.* (67, 76, 77), the electron beam, after emerging from the accelerator window, is scattered by a mirror (0.028-inch Al), an aluminum scatterer located externally at the front of the collimator (0.037-inch Al), and about 3 m of air before incidence on the patient. The x-ray contamination incident on the patient is reduced by angling the beam 15° to 10° above and below the horizontal. Since the x-rays produced in the scatterers at the collimators are preferentially directed along the central axes, they largely miss the patient. In addition, this setup provides a large electron field with sufficient dose uniformity in the vertical dimensions of the patient.

B.3. FIELD ARRANGEMENT

In the Stanford technique, the patient is treated with six fields (anterior, posterior, and four obliques) positioned 60° apart around the circumference of the patient. Each field is made up of two component beams, pointing ±15° with respect to the horizontal. The patient treatment positions and the full six-field treatment cycle are illustrated in Fig. 14.36.

The Memorial technique (75) also uses dual fields to obtain field flatness in the vertical direction. The patient is treated from four directions, the anterior, the posterior, and each of the laterals. Holt and Perry (74) reexamined this technique and found that at least six fields are required to achieve adequate uniformity. They recommend eight fields, treating with four fields one day, and rotated four the next.

A multiple field arc technique used at the University of Minnesota has been described by Sewchand *et al.* (78). In this technique, the beam describes an up-and-down arc as the gantry of the linear accelerator rotates in an oscillatory manner analogous to a pendulum. Six fields are used for each cycle of treatment, as in the Stanford technique. The advantage of this technique is that the dose distribution in the vertical plane can be made reproducibly uniform over the height of any patient standing at a distance of about 4 m. However, if the electron beam is scattered by a scattering foil at the position of the collimators, this technique contributes higher x-ray contamination to the patient than does the stationary dual field technique. This problem may be minimized by removing scattering foils and allowing the electron beam to be scattered by air alone, as in the Memorial technique.

B.4. DOSE DISTRIBUTION

The depth-dose distribution in a single large field incident on a patient will depend on the angle of incidence of the beam relative to the surface contour. For an oblique beam, the depth dose curve and its d_{max} shift toward the surface. When multiple large fields are directed at the patient from different angles, the composite distribution shows a net shift with apparent decrease in beam

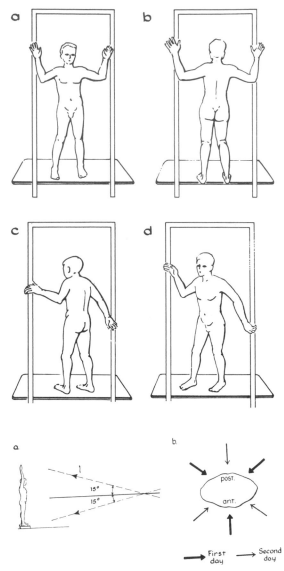

Figure 14.36. Patient positions for the six-field Stanford technique. Patient is treated by two beams at each position, one beam directed 15° below horizontal and the other 15° above horizontal. [Reprinted with permission from: Page *et al.* (95).]

penetration. This shift of the relative depth doses closer to the surface has been explained by Bjarngard *et al.* (79) as being due to greater path lengths taken by the obliquely incident electrons in reaching a point.

Although a dose uniformity of ±10% can be achieved over most of the body surface using the six-field technique, areas adjacent to surface irregularities vary substantially due to local scattering. Areas such as inner thighs and axillae, which are obstructed by adjacent body structures, require supplementary irradiation.

The total bremsstrahlung dose in the midline of the patient for the multiple field technique is approximately twice the level of a single field. This factor of 2 has been experimentally observed by a number of investigators (74, 78, 80).

References

1. Fletcher GH: Introduction. In Tapley N (ed): *Clinical Applications of the Electron Beam.* New York, John Wiley and Sons, 1976, p1.
2. Evans RD: *The Atomic Nucleus,* Chap 18. New York, McGraw-Hill Book Company, Inc, 1955.
3. Johns HE, Laughlin JS: Interaction of radiation with matter. In Hine G, Brownell G (eds): *Radiation Dosimetry.* New York, Academic Press, 1956, p 49.
4. National Council on Radiation Protection and Measurements (NCRP) Report No. 27: *Stopping Powers for Use with Cavity Ionization Chambers,* Handbook 79. Washington, DC, National Bureau of Standards, 1961.
5. Sternheimer RM: The density effect for the ionization loss in various materials. *Phys Rev* 88:851, 1952.
6. ICRU Report No. 33: *Radiation Quantities and Units.* Washington, DC, International Commission on Radiation Units and Measurements, 1980.
7. Berger MJ, Seltzer SM: *Tables of Energy Losses and Ranges of Electrons and Positrons,* NASA SP-3012. Washington, DC, National Aeronautics and Space Administration, 1964.
8. Berger MJ, Seltzer SM: *Additional Stopping Power and Range Tables for Protons, Mesons and Electrons,* NASA SP-3036. Washington, DC, National Aeronautics and Space Administration, 1966.
9. ICRU Report No. 21: *Radiation Dosimetry: Electrons with Initial Energies between 1 and 50 MeV.* Washington, DC, International Commission for Radiation Units and Measurements, 1972.
10. Rossi BB: *High Energy Particles.* Englewood Cliffs, NJ, Prentice-Hall, Inc, 1956.
11. Svensson H, Hettinger G: Dosimetric measurements at the nordic medical accelerators. I. Characteristics of the radiation beam. *Acta Radiol* 10:369, 1971.
12. American Association of Physicists in Medicine (AAPM): Protocol for the dosimetry of high energy electrons. *Phys Med Biol* 11:505, 1966.
13. Nordic Association of Clinical Physics (NACP): Procedures in external radiation therapy dosimetry with electron and photon beams with maximum energies between 1 and 50 MeV. *Acta Radiol* 19:55, 1980.
14. Markus B: Beitrage zur Entwicklung der Dosimetrie schneller Elektronen. *Strahlentherapie* 123:350 and 508; 124:33, 1964.
15. Nusse M: Factors affecting the energy-range relation of fast electrons in aluminum. *Phys Med Biol* 14:315, 1969.
16. Harder D, Schulz HJ: Some new physical data for electron beam dosimetry. In *Proceedings of the European Congress of Radiology.* Amsterdam, Excerpta Medica, 1971.
17. Brahme A, Svensson H: Specification of Electron Beam Quality from the Central-Axis Depth Absorbed-Dose Distribution. *Med Phys* 3:95, 1976.
18. Harder D: Energiespectren Schneller Elecktronen in Verschiedenen Tiefen. In Montreux, Zuppinger A, Poretti G (eds): *Symposium on High-Energy Electrons.* Berlin, Springer Verlag, 1965, p 260.
19. Hospital Physicists' Association: *A Practical Guide to Electron Dosimetry,* HPA Report Series No. 4. London, Hospital Physicists' Association, 1971.
20. American Association of Physicists in Medicine (AAPM), RTC Task Group 21: A protocol for the determination of absorbed dose from high energy photons and electrons. *Med Phys* 10:741, 1983.
21. Boag JW, Currant J: Current collection and ionic recombination in small cylindrical ionization chambers exposed to pulsed radiation. *Br J Radiol* 53:471, 1980.
22. International Council on Radiation Protection and Measurements (ICRU): *Physical Aspects of Irradiation,* NBS Handbook 85. Washington, DC, National Bureau of Standards, 1964.

23. Harder D: The effect of multiple electron scattering on the ionization in gas-filled cavities. *Biophysik* 5:157, 1968.
24. Dutreix J, Dutreix A: Etude compree d'une serie de chambers d'ionization dans des fairceaux d'electrons de 20 et 10 MeV. *Biophysik* 3:249, 1966.
25. Weatherburn H, Stedeford B: Effective measuring position for cylindrical ionization chambers when used for electron beam dosimetry. *Br J Radiol* 50:921, 1977.
26. Johansson KA, Mattsson LO, Lindborg L, Svensson H: Absorbed dose determination with ionization chambers in electron and photon beams with energies between 1 and 50 MeV. In *International Symposium on National and International Standardization of Radiation Dosimetry IAEA-SM-222/35) vol II. International Atomic Energy Agency, Vienna*, 1978, p 243.
27. Loevinger R, Karzmark CJ, Weissbluth M: Radiation dosimetry with high energy electrons. *Radiology* 77:906, 1961.
28. Dutreix J, Dutreix A: Film dosimetry of high energy electrons. *Ann NY Acad Sci* 161:33, 1969.
29. Hettinger G, Svensson H: Photographic film for determination of isodose from betatron electron radiation. *Acta Radiol* 5:74, 1967.
30. NACP: Recommendations of the Nordic Association of Clinical Physics. Procedures in radiation therapy dosimetry with 5 to 50 MeV electrons and roentgen and gamma rays with maximum photon energies between 1 MeV and 50 MeV. *Acta Radiol* 11:603, 1972.
31. Mandour MA, Harder D: Systematic Optimization of the Double-Scatterer System for Electron Beam Field Flattening. *Strahlentherapie* 154:328, 1978.
32. Werner BL, Khan FM, Deibel FC: Model for calculating depth dose distributions for broad electron beam. *Med Phys* 10:582, 1983.
33. Biggs PJ, Boyer AL, Doppke KP: Electron dosimetry of irregular fields on the Clinac-18. *Int J Radiat Oncol Biol Phys* 5:433, 1979.
34. Berger MJ, Seltzer SM: *Tables of Energy-Deposition Distributions in Water Phantoms Irradiated by Point-Monodirectional Electron Beams with Energies from 1 to 60 MeV, and Applications to Broad Beams*, Publication NBSIR 82-2451. Washington, DC, National Bureau of Standards, 1982.
35. Tapley N (ed): *Clinical Applications of the Electron Beam*. New York, John Wiley and Sons, 1976.
36. Laughlin JS: High energy electron treatment planning for inhomogeneities. *Br J Radiol* 38:143, 1965.
37. Laughlin JS, Lundy A, Phillips R, Chu F, Sattar A: Electron-beam treatment planning in inhomogeneous tissue. *Radiology* 85:524, 1965.
38. Okumura Y: Correction of dose distribution for air space in high energy electron therapy. *Radiology* 103:183, 1972.
39. Pohlit W: *Dosimetrie Zur Betatrontherapie*. Stuttgart, Georg Thieme Verlag, 1965.
40. Almond PR: Radiation physics of electron beams. In Tapley N (ed): *Clinical Applications of the Electron Beam*. New York, John Wiley and Sons, 1976, p 7.
41. Khan FM, Sewchand W, Levitt SH: Effect of air space on depth dose in electron beam therapy. *Radiology* 126:249, 1978.
42. Deibel FC, Khan FM, Werner BL: Electron beam treatment planning with measured strip beams. Presented at the 25th Annual Meeting of the American Association of Physicists in Medicine, New York, 1983.
43. Almond PR, Wright AE, Boone ML: High-energy electron dose perturbations in regions of tissue heterogeneity. *Radiology* 88:1146, 1967.
44. Dahler A, Baker AS, Laughlin JS: Comprehensive electron-beam treatment planning. *Ann NY Acad Sci* 161:189, 1969.
45. Boone MLM, Almond PR, Wright AE: High energy electron dose perturbation in regions of tissue heterogeneity. *Ann NY Acad Sci* 161:214, 1969.
46. Prasad SC, Bedwinek JM, Gerber RL: Lung dose in electron beam therapy of chest wall. *Acta Radiol* 22:91, 1983.
47. Dutreix J: Dosimetry. In Gil y Gil and Gil Gayarre (eds): *Symposium on High-Energy Electrons*, Madrid, General Directorate of Health, 1970, p 113.
48. Pohlit W, Manegold KH: Electron-beam dose distribution in inhomogeneous media. In Kramer S, Suntharalingam N, Zinninger GF (eds): *High Energy Photons and Electrons*. New York, John Wiley and Sons, 1976, p 243.
49. Bagne F, Tulloh ME: Low energy electrons. In Orton CG, Bagne F (eds): *Practical Aspects*

of Electron Beam Treatment Planning, AAPM Publication. New York, American Institute of Physics, 1978, p 80.

50. Sharma SC, Deibel FC, Khan FM: Tissue equivalence of bolus materials for electron beams. *Radiology* 146:854, 1983.

51. Goitein M: A technique for calculating the influence of thin inhomogeneities on charged particle beams. *Med Phys* 5:258, 1978.

52. Perry DJ, Holt JG: A model for calculating the effects of small inhomogeneities on electron beam dose distributions. *Med Phys* 7:207, 1980.

53. Giarratano JC, Duerkes RJ, Almond PR: Lead shielding thickness for dose reduction of 7- to 28-MeV electrons. *Med Phys* 2:336, 1975.

54. Khan FM, Moore VC, Levitt SH: Field shaping in electron beam therapy. *Br J Radiol* 49:883, 1976.

55. Goede MR, Gooden DS, Ellis RG, Brickner TJ: A versatile electron collimation system to be used with electron cones supplied with Varian's Clinac 18. *Int J Radiat Oncol Biol Phys* 2:791, 1977.

56. Choi MC, Purdy JA, Gerbi BJ, Abrath FG, Glasgow GP: Variation in output factor caused by secondary blocking for 7-16 MeV electron beams. *Med Phys* 6:137, 1979.

57. Purdy JA, Choi MC, Feldman A: Lipowitz metal shielding thickness for dose reduction of 6-20 MeV electrons. *Med Phys* 7:251, 1980.

58. Asbell SO, Sill J, Lightfoot DA, Brady NL: Individualized eye shields for use in electron beam therapy as well as low-energy photon irradiation. *Int J Radiat Oncol Biol Phys* 6:519, 1980.

59. Khan FM, Werner BL, Deibel FC: Lead shielding for electrons. *Med Phys* 8:712, 1981.

60. Okumura Y, Mori T, Kitagawa T: Modification of dose distribution in high energy electron beam treatment. *Radiology* 99:683, 1971.

61. Weatherburn H, McMillan KTP, Stedford B, Durrant KR: Physical measurements and clinical observations on the backscatter of 10 MeV electrons from lead shielding (correspondence). *Br J Radiol* 48:229, 1975.

62. Saunders JE, Peters VG: Backscattering from metals in superficial therapy with high energy electrons. *Br J Radiol* 47:467, 1974.

63. Nusslin F: Electron back-scattering from lead in a Perspex phantom (correspondence). *Br J Radiol* 48:467, 1974.

64. Gagnon WF, Cundiff JH: Dose enhancement from backscattered radiation at tissue-metal interfaces irradiated with high energy electrons. *Br J Radiol* 53:466, 1980.

65. Klevenhagen SC, Lambert GD, Arbari A: Backscattering in electron beam therapy for energies between 3 and 35 MeV. *Phys Med Biol* 27:363, 1982.

66. Trump JG, Wright KA, Evans WW, Anson JH, Hare HF, Fromer JL, Jacque G, Horne KW: High energy electrons for the treatment of extensive superficial malignant lesions. *Am J Roentgenol* 69:623, 1953.

67. Karzmark CJ, Loevinger R, Steel RE: A technique for large-field, superficial electron therapy. *Radiology* 74:633, 1960.

68. Szur L, Silvester JA, Bewley DK: Treatment of the whole body surface with electrons. *Lancet* 1:1373, 1962.

69. Fuks Z, Bagshaw MA: Total-skin electron treatment of mycosis fungoides. *Radiology* 100:145, 1971.

70. Heller EH: The management of cutaneous manifestations of lymphoma by means of electron beam. *Australas J Dermatol* 13:11, 1972.

71. Haybittle JL: A 24 curie strontium 90 unit for whole-body superficial irradiation with beta rays. *Br J Radiol* 37:297, 1964.

72. Wright KA, Granke RC, Trump JG: Physical aspects of megavoltage electron therapy. *Radiology* 67:533, 1956.

73. Williams PC, Hunter RD, Jackson SM: Whole body electron therapy in mycosis fungoides—successful translational technique achieved by modification of an established linear accelerator. *Br J Radiol* 52:302, 1979.

74. Holt JG, Perry DJ: Some physical considerations in whole skin electron beam therapy. *Med Phys* 9:769, 1982.

75. Edelstein GR, Clark T, Holt JG: Dosimetry for total-body electron-beam therapy in the treatment of mycosis fungoides. *Radiology* 108:691, 1973.

76. Karzmark CJ: Large-field superficial electron therapy with linear accelerators. *Br J Radiol* 37:302, 1964.

77. Karzmark CJ: Physical aspects of whole-body superficial therapy with electrons. *Frontiers Radiat Ther Oncol* 2:36, 1968.
78. Sewchand W, Khan FM, Williamson J: Total-body superficial electron-beam therapy using a multiple-field pendulum-arc technique. *Radiology* 130:493, 1979.
79. Bjarngard BE, Chen GTY, Piontek RN, Svensson GK: Analysis of dose distributions in whole body superficial electron therapy. *Int J Radiat Oncol Biol Phys* 2:319, 1977.
80. Tetenes PJ, Goodwin PN: Comparative study of superficial whole-body radiotherapeutic techniques using a 4-MeV nonangulated electron beam. *Radiology* 122:219, 1977.
81. Hogstrom KR, Mills MD, Almond PR: Electron beam dose calculations. *Phys Med Biol* 26:445, 1981.
82. Mills MD, Hogstrom KR, Almond PR: Prediction of electron beam output factors. *Med Phys* 9:60, 1982.
83. Almond PR: Characteristics of current medical electron accelerator beams. In Chu F (ed): *Proceedings of the Symposium on Electron Beam Therapy.* New York, Memorial Sloan-Kettering Cancer Center, 1979, p 43.
84. Khan FM, Lee JMF: Computer algorithm for electron beam treatment planning. *Med Phys* 6:142, 1979.
85. Becker J, Weitzel G: Neue Formen der Bewegungstrahlung beim 15 MeV-Betatron der Siemens-Reinger-Werke. *Strahlentherapie* 101:180, 1956.
86. Benedetti GR, Dobry H, Traumann L: Computer programme for determination of isodose curves for electron energies from 5–42 MeV. *Electromedica (Siemens)* 39:57, 1971.
87. Rassow J: On the telecentric small-angle pendulum therapy with high electron energies. *Electromedica (Siemens)* 40:1, 1972.
88. Khan FM, Fullerton GD, Lee JM, Moore VC, Levitt SH: Physical aspects of electron-beam arc therapy. *Radiology* 124:497, 1977.
89. Ruegsegger DR, Lerude SD, Lyle D: Electron beam arc therapy using a high energy betatron. *Radiology* 133:483, 1979.
90. Kase KR, Bjarngard BE: Bremsstrahlung dose to patients in rotational electron therapy. *Radiology* 133:531, 1979.
91. Leavitt DD: A technique for optimization of dose distributions in electron rotational therapy (abstr). *Med Phys* 5:347, 1978.
92. Blackburn BE: A practical system for electron arc therapy. In Paliwal B (ed): *Proceedings of the Symposium on Electron Dosimetry and Arc Therapy.* New York, AAPM/American Institute of Physics, 1982, p 295.
93. Thomadsen B: Tertiary collimation of moving electron beams. In Paliwal B (ed): *Proceedings of the Symposium on Electron Dosimetry and Arc Therapy.* New York, AAPM/American Institute of Physics, 1982, p 315.
94. Paliwal B (ed): *Proceedings of the Symposium on Electron Dosimetry and Arc Therapy.* New York, AAPM/American Institute of Physics, 1982.
95. Page V, Gardner A, Karzmark CJ: Patient dosimetry in the treatment of large superficial lesions. *Radiology* 94:635, 1970.
96. Holt JG, Mohan R, Caley R, Buffa A, Reid A, Simpson LD, Laughlin JS: Memorial electron beam AET treatment planning system. In Orton CG, Bagne F (eds): *Practical Aspects of Electron Beam Treatment Planning.* New York, American Institute of Physics, 1978.
97. Ekstrand KE, Dixon RL: Obliquely incident electron beams. *Med Phys* 9:276, 1982.
98. McKenzie AL: Air-gap correction in electron treatment planning. *Phys Med Biol* 24:628, 1979.
99. Deibel FC, Khan FM, Werner BL: Electron beam treatment planning with strip beams. *Med Phys* 10:527 (abstr), 1983.
100. Berger MJ, Seltzer SM: *Stopping Powers and Ranges of Electrons and Positrons,* 2nd ed. Washington, DC, US Department of Commerce, National Bureau of Standards, 1983.
101. Boyer AL, Fullerton GD, Mira MD, Mok EC: An electron beam pseudoarc technique. In Paliwal B (ed): *Proceedings of the Symposium on Electron Dosimetry and Arc Therapy.* New York, AAPM/American Institute of Physics 1982, p 267.
102. Khan FM: Calibration and treatment planning of electron beam arc therapy. In Paliwal B (ed): *Proceedings of the Symposium on Electron Dosimetry and Arc Therapy.* New York, AAPM/American Institute of Physics, 1982, p 249.
103. Werner BL, Khan FM, Deibel FC: Model for calculating electron beam scattering in treatment planning. *Med Phys* 9:180, 1982.

CHAPTER 15

Brachytherapy

Brachytherapy is a method of treatment in which sealed radioactive sources are used to deliver radiation at a short distance by interstitial, intracavitary, or surface application. With this mode of therapy, a high radiation dose can be delivered locally to the tumor with rapid dose fall-off in the surrounding normal tissue. In the past, brachytherapy was carried out mostly with radium or radon sources. Currently, use of artificially produced radionuclides such as ^{137}Cs, ^{192}Ir, ^{198}Au, and ^{125}I is rapidly increasing.

New technical developments have stimulated increased interest in brachytherapy: the introduction of artificial isotopes, afterloading devices to reduce personnel exposure, and automatic devices with remote control to deliver controlled radiation exposure from high activity sources. Although electrons are being increasingly used as an alternative to interstial implants, brachytherapy continues to remain an important mode of therapy, either alone or combined with external beam.

15.1 RADIOACTIVE SOURCES

From the time of its discovery, radium has been the most commonly used isotope in brachytherapy. However, artificial radioisotopes offer special advantages in some situations because of their γ ray energy, source flexibility, source size, and half-life. Table 15.1 lists the most commonly used sources for brachytherapy with their relevant physical properties.

A. Radium

A.1. DECAY

Radium is the sixth member of the uranium series which starts with $^{238}_{92}$U and ends with stable $^{206}_{82}$Pb (Fig. 2.3). Radium disintegrates with a half-life of about 1600 years to form radon.

$$^{226}_{88}\text{Ra} \xrightarrow[\sim 1600 \text{ years}]{} {}^{222}_{86}\text{Rn} + {}^{4}_{2}\text{He}$$

The product nucleus radon is a heavy inert gas which in turn disintegrates into its daughter products as shown in Fig. 2.3. As a result of the decay process from radium to stable lead, at least 49 γ rays are produced with energies ranging from 0.184 to 2.45 MeV. The average energy of the γ rays from radium

Table 15.1.
Physical characteristics of radionuclides used in brachytherapy

Radionuclide	Half-life	Photon energy (MeV)	Half-value layer (mm lead)	Exposure rate constant R/cm²/mCi-h
^{226}Ra	1600 years	0.047–2.45 (0.83 avg)	8.0	8.25*† (R/cm²/mg-h)
^{222}Rn	3.83 days	0.047–2.45 (0.83 avg)	8.0	10.15*‡
^{60}Co	5.26 years	1.17, 1.33	11.0	13.07‡
^{137}Cs	30.0 years	0.662	5.5	3.26‡
^{192}Ir	74.2 days	0.136–1.06 (0.38 avg)	2.5	4.69‡
^{198}Au	2.7 days	0.412	2.5	2.38‡
^{125}I	60.2 days	0.028 avg	0.025	1.46‡

* In equilibrium with daughter products.
† Filtered by 0.5 mm Pt.
‡ Unfiltered.

in equilibrium with its daughter products and filtered by 0.5 mm of platinum is 0.83 MeV (1). A filtration of at least 0.5 mm platinum provided by the source case is sufficient to absorb all the α particles and most of the β particles emitted by radium and its daughter products. Only γ rays are used for therapy.

Since the half-life for radioactive decay is much greater for ^{226}Ra than for any of its daughter products, radium, when placed in a sealed container, achieves a secular equilibrium with its daughters (Fig. 2.5). The period of time required to establish equilibrium is about 1 month from the time of encapsulation.

A.2. SOURCE CONSTRUCTION

The radium is supplied mostly in the form of radium sulfate or radium chloride which is mixed with an inert filler and loaded into cells about 1 cm long and 1 mm in diameter. These cells are made of 0.1–0.2-mm thick gold foil and are sealed to prevent leakage of radon gas. The sealed cells are then loaded into the platinum sheath which in turn is sealed. A radium source contains 1 to 3 cells depending upon the source length. Radium sources are manufactured as needles or tubes in a variety of lengths and activities (Fig. 15.1).

A.3. SOURCE SPECIFICATION

Radium sources are specified by: (i) active length, the distance between the ends of the radioactive material; (ii) physical length, the distance between the actual ends of the source; (iii) activity or strength of source, milligrams of radium content; and (iv) filtration, transverse thickness of the capsule wall, usually expressed in terms of millimeters of platinum.

Linear activity of a source can be determined by dividing the activity by the active length. Figure 15.1 illustrates three types of radium needles used for

RADIUM NEEDLES

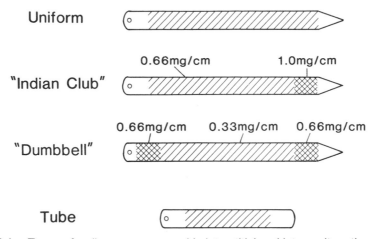

Figure 15.1.   Types of radium sources used in interstitial and intracavitary therapy.

implants: needles of uniform linear activity, needles with higher activity at one end (Indian club), and needles with high activity at both ends (dumbbell). Uniform linear activity needles may be "full intensity" (0.66 mg/cm) or "half intensity" (0.33 mg/cm). Needles are also constructed with linear activities of 0.5 and 0.25 mg/cm. Tubes for intracavitary and mold therapy are usually furnished in multiples of 5 mg of radium filtered by 1 mm platinum.

In order to test the uniformity of activity distribution, an autoradiograph is obtained by placing the source on an unexposed x-ray film for a period of time long enough to obtain reasonable darkening of the film. The source may be radiographed at the same time to show physical dimensions of the source superimposed on the autoradiograph. Figure 15.2 shows an autoradiograph obtained in this manner. The exposed film may be scanned with a densitometer to obtain optical density distribution. Uniformity of activity distribution can thus be assessed from such a distribution.

A.4. EXPOSURE RATE CONSTANT[1]

The activity of a radioactive nuclide emitting photons is related to the exposure rate by the exposure rate constant, Γ_δ (see Section 8.5 for derivation).

---

[1] ICRU (5) defines the exposure rate constant as:

$$\Gamma_\delta = \frac{l^2}{A} \left(\frac{dx}{dt}\right)_\delta$$

where $\left(\dfrac{dx}{dt}\right)_\delta$ is the exposure rate due to photons of energy greater than δ, at a distance l from a point source of activity A. Special units of Γ_δ are R/m² h⁻¹ Ci⁻¹ or any convenient multiple of these.

This quantity replaces, but is not identical to, the specific γ ray constant. The latter applied

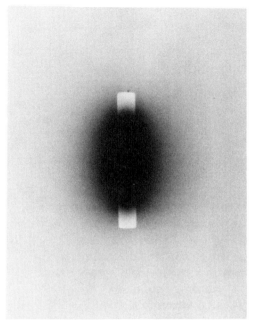

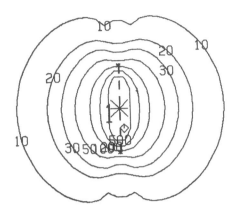

Figure 15.2. An autoradiograph of a cesium-137 tube. Isodose curves are shown for the same source in the diagram on the right.

In brachytherapy, this constant is usually expressed as numerically equal to the exposure rate in R/h at a point 1 cm from a 1-mCi *point* source. In the case of radium, the source strength is specified in terms of mg of radium instead of mCi.

ICRU (2) has recommended that Γ_δ for radium filtered by 0.5 mm platinum be taken as 8.25 R/cm^{2}h^{-1} mg^{-1}. Table 15.2 gives Γ_δ factors for radium with other filtrations. These values are based on relative transmission measurements *vs.* platinum thickness (3) and normalized to $\Gamma_\delta = 8.25$ for 0.5 mm platinum.

A.5. RADON HAZARD

Leakage of radon gas from a radium source represents a significant hazard if the source is broken. The sources are, however, doubly encapsulated to

---

to γ rays only and did not include the exposure rate of emitted x-rays such as characteristic x-rays and internal bremsstrahlung.

A further change has been made by the ICRU (6). A new quantity, called *air kerma rate constant*, has been recommended to replace the exposure rate cosntant. This quantity is still named Γ_δ, but is now defined as

$$\Gamma_\delta = \frac{l^2}{A}\left(\frac{dk_{\mathrm{air}}}{dt}\right)_\delta$$

where k_{air} is the air kerma. The SI unit for this quantity is m^{2}J kg^{-1}. When the special names, gray (Gy) and bequerel (Bq) are used, the unit becomes m^{2}Gy Bq^{-1} sec^{-1}.

Table 15.2.
Exposure rate constant for radium point source filtered by various thicknesses of platinum

Filtration (mm Pt)	Γ_δ (R/cm^2 h^{-1} mg^{-1})
0	9.09
0.5	8.25
0.6	8.14
0.7	8.01
0.8	7.90
0.9	7.81
1.0	7.71
1.5	7.25
2.0	6.84

From Shalek and Sotvall (1)

prevent such an occurrence. Spontaneous rupture of a sealed radium source due to pressure buildup of helium gas (from α particle disintegrations) is considered unlikely. Van Roosenbeek *et al.* (4) have calculated that sources encapsulated in platinum may remain safely sealed for more than 400 years.

B. Cesium-137

Cesium-137 is a γ ray-emitting radioisotope which is used as a radium substitute in both interstitial and intracavitary brachytherapy. It is supplied in the form of insoluble powders or ceramic microspheres, labeled with ^{137}Cs, and doubly encapsulated in stainless steel needles and tubes. The advantages of ^{137}Cs over radium are that it requires less shielding (compare half-value layers in Table 15.1) and is less hazardous in the microsphere form. With a long half-life of about 30 years, these sources can be used clinically for about 7 years without replacement, although the treatment times have to be adjusted to allow for radioactive decay (2% per year).

^{137}Cs emits γ rays of energy 0.662 MeV. The decay scheme shows that ^{137}Cs transforms to ^{137}Ba by the process of β^- decay but 93.5% of the disintegrations are followed by γ rays from the ^{137}Ba metastable state. The β particles and low energy characteristic x-rays are absorbed by the stainless steel material, so that the clinical source is a pure γ emitter.

It should be emphasized that Γ_δ is defined in terms of an ideal point source. Any practical source will have a finite size and would necessitate corrections for photon attenuation and scattering.

The γ rays from cesium have nearly the same penetrating power as radium γ rays in tissue. Meisberger *et al.* (7) have compared the measured and calculated depth dose values along the transverse axes of the sources and showed that the exposure in water to exposure in air ratio is the same for radium and cesium for depths up to 10 cm. Significant differences, however, exist between radium and cesium doses at points along oblique angles (near the longitudinal axis) due to the filtration effect (8, 9). Not only is the attenuation of γ rays in steel and platinum quite different, but also cesium emits monoenergetic γ rays while radium emits γ rays of wide energy range.

The exposure rate constant Γ_δ for unfiltered ^{137}Cs is 3.26 R/cm^2 mCi^{-1} h^{-1} (10). Comparing this with the Γ_δ of 8.25 R/cm^2 mg^{-1}h^{-1} for radium filtered by 0.5 mm Pt, the conversion factor is $\dfrac{8.25}{3.26} = 2.53$ mCi of ^{137}Cs/mg of ^{226}Ra. However, along the transverse axes of clinical sources (cesium with 0.5 mm steel and radium with 0.5 mm Pt filtration), the mean conversion factor has been calculated to be 2.55 for cesium needles and 2.59 for cesium tubes (9).

C. Cobalt-60

^{60}Co has been used for brachytherapy but is rarely used now. The main advantage of ^{60}Co is its high specific activity which allows fabrication of small sources required for some special applicators. However, it is more expensive than ^{137}Cs and has a short half-life (5.26 years) necessitating more frequent replacement and a complex inventory system.

Cobalt brachytherapy sources are usually fabricated in the form of a wire which is encapsulated in a sheath of platinum iridium or stainless steel. The sources can be used to replace ^{226}Ra in intracavitary applications. Curie-sized cobalt sources have also been used in a unit called the Cathetron (30–32). This is a remote-loading device and provides high dose rates for intracavitary therapy, *e.g.* 250–300 cGy/min at point "A." (See Section 15.6C.1 for definition of point "A.")

D. Iridium-192

Iridium-192 (alloy of 30% Ir and 70% Pt) sources are fabricated in the form of thin flexible wires which can be cut to desired lengths. Nylon ribbons containing iridium seeds 3 mm long and 0.5 mm in diameter, spaced with their centers 1 cm apart, are also commonly used. Both the wires and the seed ribbons are quite suitable for the afterloading technique (11, 12) (see Section 15.6B).

^{192}Ir has a complicated γ ray spectrum with an average energy of 0.38 MeV. Because of the lower energy, these sources require less shielding for personnel protection (compare half-value layers in Table 15.1). ^{192}Ir has the disadvantage of a short half-life (74.2 days). However, the half-life is long compared to the average treatment time so that the sources can be used in nonpermanent implants similar to radium and cesium. The activity varies by only a few percent during an average implant duration.

Many values have been cited in the literature for Γ_δ for ^{192}Ir. The differences in the calculated values arise because different spectroscopic data were used by each investigator. This problem has been discussed in detail by Glasgow and Dillman (13). Basing their calculations on the most recent nuclear spectroscopy data for ^{192}Ir, they recommend a value of 4.69 R/cm^2 h^{-1} mCi^{-1}.

E. Gold-198

Seeds or "grains" consisting of a radioactive isotope of gold, ^{198}Au, are used for interstitial implants. They are used in the same way as radon seeds have been used for permanent implants. ^{198}Au has a half-life of 2.7 days and emits a monoenergetic γ ray of energy 0.412 MeV. Beta rays of maximum energy 0.96 MeV are also emitted but are absorbed by the 0.1-mm thick platinum wall surrounding the seed. A gold seed is typically 2.5 mm long with an outer diameter of 0.8 mm.

Because of its lower γ ray energy, personnel protection problems with gold are easier to manage than those of radon. Moreover, radon seeds continue to exhibit low level γ activity for many years due to bremsstrahlung arising from high energy β particles emitted by its long-lived daughter products. It is suspected that this chronic irradiation may be carcinogenic (14). For these reasons and because ^{198}Au is a suitable substitute for radium biologically, gold seeds have replaced radon seeds for the most part.

F. Iodine-125

^{125}I is gaining a wide use for permanent implants in radiotherapy (15, 16). The advantages of this isotope over radon and gold-198 are its long half-life (60.2 day), which is convenient for storage, and its low photon energy which requires less shielding. However, the dosimetry of ^{125}I is much more complex than the conventional interstitial sources.

The ^{125}I seed consists of a titanium tube containing two ion exchange resin spheres, separated by a radioopaque gold marker. The ion exchange resin beads are impregnated with ^{125}I in the form of the iodide ion. The titanium tube is welded at both ends to form a cylindrical capsule of dimensions 4.5 × 0.8 mm.

^{125}I decays exclusively by electron capture to an excited state of ^{125}Te, which spontaneously decays to the ground state with the emission of a 35.5-keV γ photon. Characteristic x-rays in the range of 27–35 keV are also produced due to the electron capture and internal conversion processes. Titanium encapsulation serves to absorb liberated electrons and x-rays with energies less than 5 keV.

Significant differences exist in the published values of exposure rate constant for ^{125}I. Recently, Schulz *et al.* (80) have reported a calculated value of 1.464 R/cm^2 mCi^{-1} h^{-1} for an unfiltered point source. The average exposure rate for an actual ^{125}I seed (manufactured by 3M Company, St. Paul, Minnesota) was estimated to be 1.089 R/cm^2 mCi^{-1} h^{-1}.

15.2 CALIBRATION OF BRACHYTHERAPY SOURCES

A. Specification of Source Strength

The strength of a brachytherapy source may be specified in three ways.

A.1. ACTIVITY

The source strength for any radionuclide may be specified in terms of millicuries (mCi). The exposure rate at any particular point is proportional to the product of activity and its exposure rate constant. Errors, however, may be introduced in this method from the fact that corrections must be applied for the source and wall filtration and that the exposure rate constant may not be known accurately. It should be recalled that the accuracy of the exposure rate constant depends critically on the accurate knowledge of the spectroscopic data and the relevant absorption coefficients.

A.2. EQUIVALENT MASS OF RADIUM

This system specifies the strength of a source in terms of milligram-radium equivalent (mg-Ra eq). This equivalence is usually obtained by comparing exposure rates at a particular point from the given source and a radium source placed at the same distance. While this specification can be used for computation of dose to tissue, it is unsatisfactory in the sense that it does not represent a real physical quantity. Moreover, the method assumes that the measuring device is energy independent, which is a rather demanding requirement due to the wide range of photon energies and filtrations encountered in brachytherapy sources.

A.3. EXPOSURE RATE AT A SPECIFIED DISTANCE

The National Council on Radiation Protection and Measurements (NCRP) (29) recommends that the strength of any γ emitter should be specified directly in terms of exposure rate in air at a specified distance such as 1 m. This specification can be carried out simply by measuring exposure rate in free air at a distance sufficiently large that the given source can be treated as a point. A long distance measurement geometry minimizes the dependence of the calibration upon the construction of the source and the detector since both can be treated as points. In addition, the effect of oblique transmission of γ rays through the source capsule becomes negligible.

Loevinger (17) has recommended calibration of brachytherapy sources in terms of absorbed dose in water, close to the source. However, such calibrations are not routinely available. So, until these are available, the exposure rate calibration, far from the source, remains the most appropriate method.

There are historical reasons that make it convenient to specify brachytherapy sources in terms of the equivalent mass of radium. However, such a specification is indirect and is prone to errors, as pointed out earlier. Since some users, especially the physicians who are accustomed to radium sources, continue to use mg-Ra eq, it has been suggested (29) that the exposure rate could be expressed in terms of "effective" equivalent mass of radium. This conversion is simply made by dividing the exposure rate at 1 m by the exposure rate constant of radium (encapsulated in a container with a specified wall thickness) at 1 m. It should, however, be emphasized that the best way to calibrate and specify brachytherapy sources is still in terms of exposure rate at a distance of 1 m. The effective mg-Ra eq should be used only to provide an approximate output comparison with radium sources.

Example. An iridium-192 source has been calibrated and its strength is specified as 0.495 mR/h at 1 m. What is the strength of this source in terms of effective mg-Ra eq?

Exposure rate constant of radium filtered by 0.5 mm Pt = 8.25 R·cm²/h·mg = 0.825 mR·m²/h·mg

$$\text{Effective mg-Ra eq} = \frac{0.495}{0.825} = 0.600 \text{ mg}$$

Note that such a conversion of units must explicitly specify the radium source in terms of a point source and its filtration.

B. Exposure Rate Calibration

The National Bureau of Standards (NBS) has established exposure rate calibration standards for some of the brachytherapy sources, *e.g.* ^{226}Ra, ^{60}Co, ^{137}Cs, and ^{192}Ir. The NBS method consists of calibrating a working standard of each type using open-air geometry and a series of spherical graphite cavity chambers (18, 19). A given source is then calibrated by intercomparison with the working standard using a 2.5-liter spherical aluminum ionization chamber, positioned at a distance of about 1 m. A similar procedure is used for calibrating a radium source except that the working standards of radium have been calibrated in terms of actual mass of radium.

Calibration of clinical sources should be directly traceable to NBS. This means that the sources should be calibrated by direct comparison with an NBS-calibrated source of the same kind, *i.e.* the same radionuclide, with the same encapsulation, size, and shape. If a well-type ionization chamber is used, it should bear a calibration factor determined with an NBS-calibrated source of the same kind.

B.1. OPEN-AIR MEASUREMENTS

Figure 15.3 is a schematic representation of an open-air measurement geometry for the calibration of brachytherapy sources. The arrangement consists of a large source to ion chamber distance relative to source and detector dimensions. The apparatus is set up as far away as possible from potential scattering surfaces. Since the output from brachytherapy sources is low at large distances, the chamber volume should be large, *e.g.* 100 ml or larger. A signal-to-noise ratio greater than 100:1 should be achievable.

Because of the difficulty in obtaining "good geometry" conditions, the open-air method is a time-consuming measurement. It is not suitable for routine calibration checks required in a busy department. A well-type ionization chamber is more suited to routine measurements.

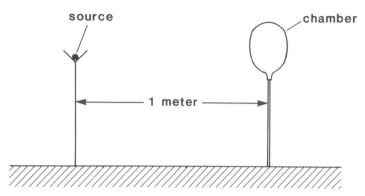

Figure 15.3. Schematic drawing of open air geometry for exposure rate calibration of brachytherapy sources.

B.2. WELL-TYPE ION CHAMBERS

Routine calibration of brachytherapy sources is usually carried out with a "re-entrant"-type ion chamber in which the walls of the chamber surround the source, approximating a 4π measurement geometry. Examples of such chambers are those designed by the British National Physics Laboratory (20), a re-entrant chamber designed by Radiological Physics Center (21), a spherical aluminum chamber designed by NBS (22), and commercially available dose calibrators (23–25).

Figure 15.4 is a chematic drawing of a dose calibrator, Capintec Model CRC-10. This unit consists of an aluminum wall ion chamber filled with argon gas under high pressure. The collection potential applied to the chamber is about 150 V. A source holder is devised to reproduce the source geometry in relation to the surrounding chamber walls.

The dose calibrator is traditionally used for assay of radiopharmaceuticals in which the instrument response is interpreted as activity in units of mCi. These activity calibrations of various isotopes are based on relative chamber response measured by intercomparison with the respective standards calibrated by NBS directly in terms of activity (26). However, these standards are usually in the form of an aqueous suspension of the isotope sealed in a glass ampule. These vendor calibrations of the instrument are, therefore, not valid for brachytherapy sources because of differences in construction between brachytherapy and standard sources. Even the practice of using a radium standard for calibrating different sources is prone to significant errors due to energy dependence of the instrument (24, 25, 27). In addition, the response of well chambers is known to depend on the source position in the well and on the length of the source (21). Correction factors must be determined for these effects for a given instrument and the type of sources to be calibrated.

The energy dependence of the chamber arises from absorption and scattering of photons and secondary electrons in the chamber walls and the gas. Besides this intrinsic energy dependence, oblique filtration through the source encap-

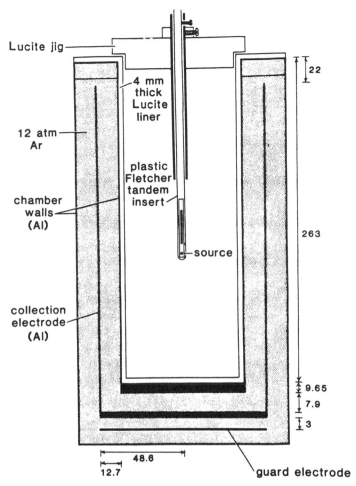

Figure 15.4. Schematic drawing of a dose calibrator, Capintec Model CRC-10 [Reprinted with permission from: Williamson *et al.* (23).]

sulation affects the chamber response both by photon absorption and by producing changes in the energy spectrum. This effect of source construction on the chamber response has been studied in detail by Williamson *et al.* (23, 28), for commonly used brachytherapy sources. These authors conclude: "In these apparatuses, all one can count on is a linear response with respect to exposure rate given fixed energy, filtration, and source position. For each isotope, an exposure calibrated standard is needed" (23). These studies support the recommendations that the brachytherapy sources should be calibrated in terms of exposure rate using exposure calibrated standards of the same kind (17, 29).

15.3 CALCULATION OF DOSE DISTRIBUTIONS

A. Exposure Rate

Exposure rate distribution around a linear brachytherapy source can be calculated using the Sievert integral, introduced by Rolf Sievert (33) in 1921. The method (1, 34) consists of dividing the line source into small elementary sources and applying inverse square law and filtration corrections to each. Consider a source of active length L and filtration t (Fig. 15.5). The exposure rate dI at a point $P(x, y)$ contributed by the source element of length dx is given by

$$dI(x, y) = \frac{A}{L} \cdot \Gamma \cdot dx \cdot \frac{1}{r^2} \cdot e^{-\mu' \cdot t \cdot \sec\theta} \qquad (15.1)$$

where A and Γ are the activity and exposure rate constant of the unfiltered source and μ' is the effective attenuation coefficient for the filter. Other variables are defined by Fig. 15.5. Making use of the following relationships:

$$r = y \sec \theta$$

$$x = y \tan \theta$$

$$dx = y \sec^2\theta \; d\theta$$

and integrating Equation 15.1, we obtain the exposure rate $I(x, y)$ for the whole source.

$$I(x, y) = \frac{A\Gamma}{Ly} \int_{\theta_1}^{\theta_2} e^{-\mu' \cdot t \cdot \sec\theta} \; d\theta \qquad (15.2)$$

The above Sievert integral can be evaluated by numerical methods (1).

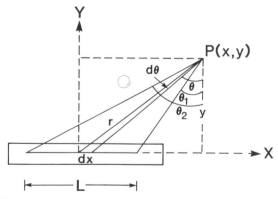

Figure 15.5. Diagram illustrating geometrical relationships used in calculation of exposure at point P, from a linear source.

If the source intensity is specified in terms of exposure rate $\dot{X}_s$ at a specified distance s far from the source, *i.e.* $s \gg L$, then the Sievert integral can be written as:

$$I(x, y) = \frac{\dot{X}_s \cdot s^2}{Ly} \cdot e^{\mu' t} \int_{\theta_1}^{\theta_2} e^{-\mu' \cdot t \cdot \sec\theta} d\theta \qquad (15.3)$$

Alternatively, if the source strength is specified in terms of equivalent mass of radium, m_{eq}, such that $\dot{X}_s = m_{eq} \cdot \Gamma_{Ra} \cdot s^{-2}$, then

$$I(x, y) = \frac{m_{eq} \cdot \Gamma_{Ra}}{Ly} \cdot e^{\mu' t} \int_{\theta_1}^{\theta_2} e^{-\mu' \cdot t \cdot \sec\theta} d\theta \qquad (15.4)$$

Several additional corrections are applied to accurately compute the exposure rate using the Sievert integral. A correction for self-absorption in the source material, although small for clinical sources, has been used by Shalek and Stovall (1). Wall thickness, t, should be corrected for the internal radius of the source since some photons traverse a thickness of filter greater than the radial thickness of the wall (35, 36). Depending upon the type of source and filtration, the energy spectrum may be significantly altered by the filter. Not only is an "effective attenuation coefficient" needed, this coefficient varies with filter thickness (36, 37). This problem becomes more severe when the effects of oblique filtration are considered (38).

In the case of ^{226}Ra encapsulated in platinum, measured values of μ' [Whyte (37) and Keyser (36)] may be used (see Fig. 15.6). However, if such data are not available for a given source-filter combination, calculated values have to be used. Williamson *et al.* (38) give the following expression for μ' as a function of filter thickness d:

$$\mu'(d) = -\left(\frac{1}{t}\right) \ln \left[\frac{\sum_i p_i E_i (\mu_{en}/\rho)_i^{air} e^{-\mu_{en}^i \cdot d}}{\sum_i p_i E_i (\mu_{en}/\rho)_i^{air}} \right] \qquad (15.5)$$

where p_i denotes the number of photons with energy E_i emitted per disintegration, and $(\mu_{en}/\rho)_i^{air}$ is the mass energy absorption coefficient in air for photon of energy E_i.

Since the Sievert integral uses the energy absorption coefficient, the underlying assumption is that the emitted energy fluence is exponentially attenuated by the filter thickness traversed by the photons. This is an approximation which has been shown to work well for ^{226}Ra and ^{192}Ir seeds in the region bounded by the active source ends (1, 38). However, Monte Carlo simulations (38) have shown that beyond the end of the active source region, the Sievert approach introduces significant errors and practically breaks down in the extreme oblique directions.

Figure 15.7 compares the radial exposure rate distribution of a line source of radium with that of a point source of radium, both filtered by 1 mm Pt.

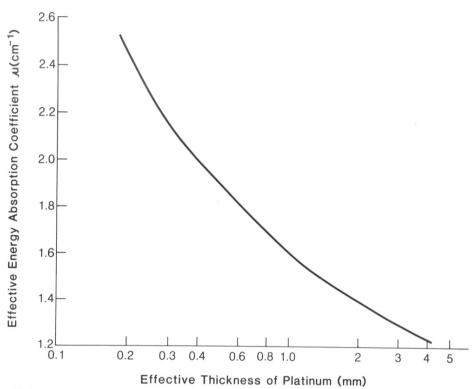

Figure 15.6. Effective energy absorption coefficients of radium gamma rays in platinum. Data are from Whyte (37) and Keyser (36).

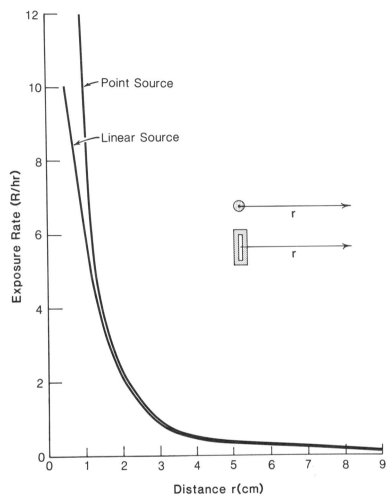

Figure 15.7.   Plot of exposure rate from 1-mg ^{226}Ra source as a function of radial distance. Point source with 1.0 mm Pt filtration. Linear source with 1.0 mm Pt filtration, 1.5 cm active length.

Whereas the curve for the point source represents an inverse square law function, the linear source curve was obtained using the Sievert integral. The exposure rate constant for ^{226}Ra with 1 mm Pt filter was assumed to be 7.71 R/cm^2 mg^{-1} h^{-1}. It is evident from the figure that for the linear source, the exposure rate is less than that predicted by the inverse square law, especially at points close to the source. This is as expected since the photons reaching these points from the source extremities travel larger distances and suffer oblique filtration which is greater than the radial wall thickness. As the distance is increased, however, these effects of the linear source approach those of the point source and, therefore, its exposure rate curve approaches inverse square law.

B. Absorbed Dose in Tissue

The Sievert integral gives the exposure rate distribution in air and considers only the inverse square law and filtration effects. When a source is implanted in the tissue, one needs to consider, in addition, attenuation as well as scattering in the surrounding tissue. The exposure rate calculated at a point in tissue can then be converted into absorbed dose rate by using the appropriate roentgen-to-rad factor (see Chapter 8).

Several investigators have experimentally determined the ratio of exposure in water to exposure in air as a function of distance for a number of isotopes. Because of the large discrepancies between various sets of experimental data, Meisberger *et al.* (45) formulated a third order polynomial to fit the average of their theoretical and all available experimental data (39–45). This polynomial is commonly used for routine calculation of absorbed dose in tissue in various comptuer programs.

More recently, Webb and Fox (46) calculated the dose distribution around point γ ray emitters in water by the Monte Carlo method. Their results agree very well with Meisberger's average or "selected" curve.

The radial dependence of dose in a water medium, with the inverse square law removed can also be represented by $D_r = B_r e^{-\mu r}$ where μ denotes the linear attenuation coefficient and B_r is a buildup factor at distance r from the source. This expression is similar to the ratio of exposure in water to exposure in air. Evans (47) has suggested that B_r may be represented by

$$B_r = 1 + k_a \, (\mu r)^{k_b} \tag{15.6}$$

where k_a and k_b are constants. Kornelsen and Young (48) have fitted the Monte Carlo data of Webb and Fox (46) to determine the constants k_a and k_b. These are given in Table 15.3. Figure 15.8 shows the curves calculated by these authors.[2]

Figure 15.8 shows that at short distances, the attenuation of the primary photons is very much compensated for by the contribution of scattered photons with the result that the exposure in water is almost equal to the exposure in air at the same point. However, tissue attenuation overtakes scattering at larger distances. For radium sources, the net reduction is about 1% per cm of intervening tissue up to 5 cm.

It is instructive to study the dose fall-off with distance in tissue. Fig. 15.9 is a plot of percent dose as a function of distance in water for point sources of ^{60}Co, ^{226}Ra, ^{137}Cs, ^{198}Au, ^{192}Ir, and ^{125}I. These plots are also compared with the inverse square law function $\left(\dfrac{1}{r^2}\right)$. These data show that over a distance of about 5 cm the percent dose rates for ^{226}Ra, ^{60}Co, and ^{137}Cs are about equal

---

[2] The authors appear to have normalized the dose values to unity at $r = 1$ cm. Spot checks of Fig. 15.8 revealed that the tissue attenuation correction factor is given by D_r/D_1, where D_1 is the dose at 1 cm.

Table 15.3.
Constants k_a and k_b determined by use of Monte Carlo data

Isotope	μ (cm²/g)	k_a	k_b
⁶⁰Co	0.0632	0.896	1.063
²²⁶Ra	0.0811	1.17	1.19
¹³⁷Cs	0.0858	1.14	1.20
¹⁹⁸Au	0.105	1.48	1.32
¹⁹²Ir	0.113	1.59	1.36

Data from Kornelsen and Young (48).

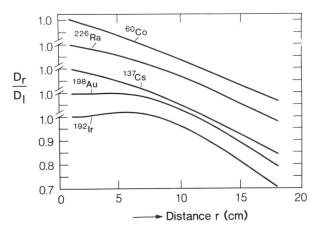

Figure 15.8. Attenuation correction factor in water as a function of distance for a point source. Curves are calculated by Equation 15.6 [Kornelsen and Young (48)] and fitted to Monte Carlo data of Webb and Fox (46).

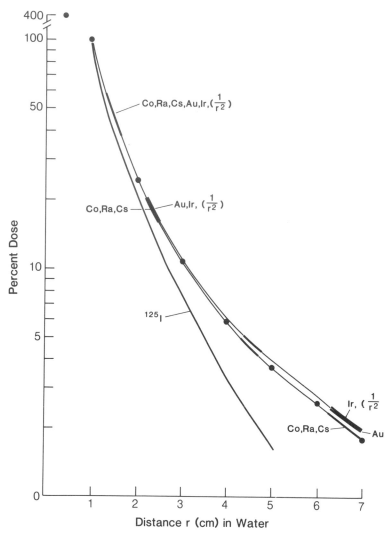

Figure 15.9. Percent dose variation with distance in water for point sources of ^{60}Co, ^{226}Ra, ^{137}Cs, ^{198}Au, ^{192}Ir, and ^{125}I. Function $\left(\dfrac{1}{r^2}\right)$ represents inverse square fall-off. ^{125}I data are from Krishnaswamy (52) and the other isotope data were calculated from Fig. 15.8 in addition to the inverse square law.

and show a slight decrease below inverse square law due to tissue attenuation. The curves for ^{192}Ir and ^{198}Au, on the other hand, are practically indistinguishable from the inverse square law curve up to about 5 cm. The dose distribution for ^{125}I progressively deviates from the inverse square law due to increased tissue attenuation for this isotope. However, up to about 1 cm, all the curves are indistinguishable due to the severity of the inverse square law effect at such short distances.

Absorbed dose rate tables for linear radium sources have been published by Shalek and Stovall (1) which take into acocunt attenuation and scattering in tissue. Similar data are also available for ^{137}Cs and ^{125}I (9, 52). Such tables are useful for manual calculations as well as for checking the accuracy of computer calculations.

C. Isodose Curves

The above methods can be used to calculate absorbed dose to a matrix of points around a source. The isodose curves are then constructed by interpolation between points, connecting those points receiving the same dose. Because of the complex and time-consuming calculations required to generate isodose curves, the job is ideally suited for computers. Presently, almost all commercial treatment planning computers offer brachytherapy software which can perform sophisticated treatment planning involving three-dimensional distribution of multiple sources.

Experimental determination of isodose curves is sometimes necessary to check new calculation algorithms. Film and TLD (see Chapter 8) require the least apparatus for such measurements. Film offers a high resolution but has a serious limitation of energy dependence, *i.e.* increased sensitivity to low energy photons present in the nuclides' γ ray spectrum and the scattered radiation. TLD shows energy dependence (49) also but to a lesser degree than the film.

Automatic isodose plotters (50, 51) have also been used to measure isodose curves. The γ ray detector used in these instruments is a small scintillation detector. The scintillation counter is connected to an automatic isodose recording device. The output of the scintillation counter is independently calibrated by comparison with a calibrated source of the same kind.

Figure 15.10 shows an example of isodose curves around a radium needle. Examination of the curves indicates that close to the source they are more or less elliptical. At large distances, the isodose curves become circles, since the source behaves as a point source. The dip in the curves close to the source axis is due to the effect of oblique filtration.

15.4 SYSTEMS OF IMPLANT DOSIMETRY

The objectives of treatment planning are: (a) to determine the distribution and type of radiation sources to provide optimum dose distribution, and (b) to provide a complete dose distribution in the irradiated volume. Numerous systems of dosimetric planning have been devised over the past 50 years. Of these the Paterson-Parker system (53) and the Quimby system (54) have received the most widespread use. These and other systems were designed during the times when computers were not available for routine treatment planning. Extensive tables and elaborate rules of source distribution were devised to facilitate the process of manual treatment planning. Then a more significant development occurred: the use of digital computers to calculate isodose distributions for individual patients (55–57). This gave the radiother-

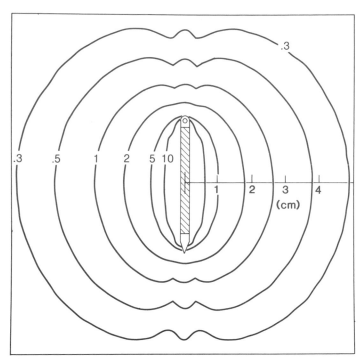

Figure 15.10. Isodose curves in terms of rad/h around a 1-mg radium source. Active length = 3.0 cm; filtration = 0.5 mm Pt.

apist freedom to deviate from the established system. Although, the old systems with their rules and tables are still being used, the computer treatment planning is fast replacing the traditional systems. Some of these methods will be reviewed here to illustrate the basic problems and concepts of brachytherapy planning.

A. The Paterson-Parker System

The Paterson-Parker or Manchester system (53) was developed to deliver uniform dose (within ±10%) to a plane or volume. The system specified rules of source distribution to achieve the dose uniformity and provided dosage tables for these idealized implants.

A.1. PLANAR IMPLANT

In the case of planar implants the uniformity of dose is achieved in parallel plane at 0.5 cm from the implanted plane and within the area bounded by the projection of the peripheral needles upon that plane. The "stated" dose, determined from the Paterson-Parker tables, is 10% higher than the minimum dose. The maximum dose should not exceed 10% above the stated dose to satisfy the uniformity criterion. The dose is, however, much more nonuniform within the plane of implant. For example, the dose at the surface of the needles is about five times the stated dose.

The distribution rules for the planar implants are: 1) the ratio between the amount of radium in the periphery and the amount of radium over the area itself depends on the size of the implant. *e.g.*

Area	Fraction used in periphery
Less than 25 cm^2	⅔
25–100 cm^2	½
Over 100 cm^2	⅓

2) The spacing of the needles should not be more than 1 cm from each other or from the crossing ends.

3) If the ends of the implant are uncrossed (Fig. 15.11, B or C), the effective area of dose uniformity is reduced.[3] The area is therefore reduced by 10% for each uncrossed end for table reading purposes.

4) In the case of multiple implant planes, the radium should be arranged as in 1), 2), and 3), and the planes should be parallel to each other.

A.2. VOLUME IMPLANTS

Some tumors are better implanted using three-dimensional shapes such as cylinders, spheres, or cuboids.

1) The total amount of radium is divided into eight parts and distributed as follows for the various shapes. The cylinder is composed of: belt, four parts; core, two parts; each end, one part (see Fig. 15.12): sphere: shell, six parts; core, two parts; and cuboid: each side, one part; each end, one part; core, two parts.

2) The needles should be spaced as uniformly as possible, not more than 1 cm apart. There should be at least eight needles in the belt and four in the core.

3) If the ends of the volume implant are uncrossed, 7.5% is deducted from the volume for uncrossed end for table reading purposes.

A.3. PATERSON-PARKER TABLES

The Paterson-Parker tables (53) are designed to give milligram hours/1000 roentgens (mg-h/1000 R) for implants of various sizes, both for planar and volume implants. In order to convert Paterson-Parker roentgens to rads in tissue, one needs to make the following corrections: (i) exposure rate constant (Γ): the tables assume $\Gamma = 8.4$ R/cm^2/mg-h instead of the current value of 8.25 R/cm^2/mg-h. (ii) a roentgen-to-rad factor of 0.957 should be used to

---

[3] If it is not possible to cross an end, one can increase the size of the implant by using longer needles so that the effective area of dose uniformity adequately covers the tumor. Again, 10% is deducted from the implant area for each uncrossed end for table reading purposes.

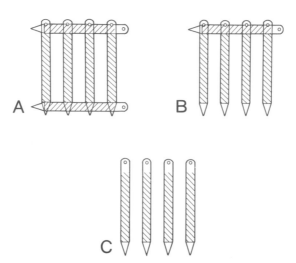

Figure 15.11. Examples of three planar implants: (a) both ends crossed; (b) one end uncrossed; (c) both ends uncrossed.

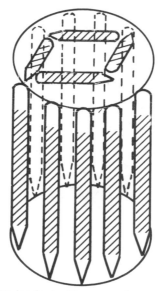

Figure 15.12. Example of a volume implant with one end uncrossed. The implant has 8 needles in the belt, 4 in the core (not shown), and 4 at one end. Whereas the needles in the belt and core are 1 mg each, the crossing needles at the end are 0.5 mg each, thus satisfying the Paterson-Parker rule of radium distribution.

convert exposure into dose in muscle. (iii) oblique filtration: Paterson-Parker tables do not take into account increased attenuation by oblique filtration by the platinum capsule, giving rise to a 2–4% error for typical implants. (iv) Paterson-Parker tables are based on exposure in air. Corrections are needed for tissue attenuation and scattering (Section 15.3B).

Stovall and Shalek (58) have demonstrated that, for typical planar and volume implants, a combined factor of 0.90 selects an isodose curve approximately equivalent to the Paterson-Parker dosage. Thus, the mg-h/1000 R in the original Paterson-Parker tables should be considered equivalent to mg-h/900 rad.

A.4. DETERMINATION OF IMPLANT AREA OR VOLUME

Dosage tables for interstitial implants require the knowledge of area or volume of implant. If the needles are close to the surface, one can determine the size of the implant directly. If not, it has to be determined radiographically.

Orthogonal Radiographs. Three-dimensional localization of individual sources can be obtained by orthogonal (perpendicular) radiographs, such as anteroposterior (AP) and lateral (Lat) views. It is important that the central axes of the AP and Lat x-ray beams meet at a point, approximately in the middle of the implant. This can be easily achieved by an isocentric radiographic unit, such as a treatment simulator. For the above isocentric geometry, the film magnification factor is given by SFD/SAD, where SFD is source-film distance and SAD is source-axis distance. Alternatively, a circular object such as a metallic ring, may be taped to the patient at the level of the implant. The ratio of the largest outside diameter of the ring image to the actual outside diameter of the ring gives the magnification factor.

In order to determine the width or length of an implant, one needs to determine the distance between two points, three dimensionally. Figure 15.13 illustrates the principle of deriving this information from orthogonal radiographs. Let $A(x_1,y_1,z_1)$ and $B(x_2,y_2,z_2)$ be the two points in question. Then by the application of the Pythagorean theorem, it can be shown that

$$AB = (x_2 - x_1)^2 + (y_2 - y_1)^2 + (z_2 - z_1)^2 \qquad (15.7)$$

a) Lateral Radiograph   b) Anteriorposterior Radiograph

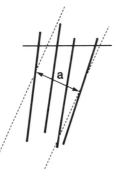
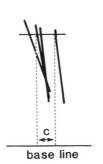

base line

Figure 15.13.   Orthogonal radiographs of an implant. Baseline is parallel to the edge of the film.

Equation 15.7 can also be written as:

$$AB = \sqrt{a^2 + c^2} \tag{15.8}$$

where a is the length of the image of AB on one of the radiographs and c is the projection of the image of AB to the baseline in the other radiograph (the baseline is a line perpendicular to the intersection of the radiographs, usually parallel to the edges of the films). Figure 15.13 assumes a magnification factor of unity. However, in actual practice, a and c will have to be corrected for film magnification.

Thus, by determining the width of the implant image on one film and its width projected to the baseline on the other, one can calculate the actual width of the implant. The length of the implant can also be determined the same way but is usually given by the known active length of the needles.

Example—Figure 15.13, a and b, shows the AP and lateral radiographs of a planar implant which was planned according to the Paterson-Parker system. Assume a magnification factor of 1.4 for both films. Determine the time to deliver 6500 rad at 0.5 cm from the plane of implant.

Given width of the implant image on the lateral radiograph $= a = 3.8$ cm:

Projection of AP image on baseline $= c = 0.9$ cm

$$\text{Peripheral needles} = 3 \times 2 \text{ mg}$$

$$\text{Central needles} = 2 \times 1 \text{ mg}$$

All needles have active length of 3 cm and 0.5 mm Pt filtration.

Treatment distance $= 0.5$ cm from the plane of implant

$$\text{Width of implant} = \sqrt{\left(\frac{3.8}{1.4}\right)^2 + \left(\frac{0.9}{1.4}\right)^2} = 2.79 \text{ cm}$$

$$\text{Length of implant} = 3 \text{ cm}$$

$$\text{Area of implant} = 2.79 \times 3 = 8.4 \text{ cm}^2$$

Since one end is uncrossed, the area for table reading purposes $= 8.4 - 10\%$ $(8.4) = 7.6$ cm^2. From Paterson-Parker tables, the mg-h/1000 R or mg-h/900 rad required $= 200$.

$$\text{mg-h required to deliver 6500 rad} = 200 \times \frac{6500}{900} = 1444$$

$$\text{time required} = \frac{1444 \text{ mg-h}}{8 \text{ mg}} = 181 \text{ h}$$

$$\text{dose rate} = \frac{6500}{181} = 36 \text{ rad/h}$$

B. The Quimby System

The Quimby system (54) of interstitial implantation is characterized by a uniform distribution of sources of equal linear activity. Consequently, this arrangement of sources results in a nonuniform dose distribution, higher in the central region of treatment. For planar implants, the Quimby table gives the milligram-hours required to produce 1000 R in the center of the treatment planes, up to 3-cm distance from the plane of implant. The stated dose is thus the maximum dose in the plane of treatment. For volume implants, the stated dose is the minimum dose within the implanted volume.

The original Quimby tables, like the Manchester tables, are based on an exposure rate constant of 8.4 $R/cm^2/mg$-h instead of the currently accepted value of 8.25 $R/cm^2/mg$-h. Also, other corrections, namely roentgen-to-rad factor, oblique filtration, and tissue attenuation, have to be applied as in the case of the Paterson-Parker tables.

Shalek and Stovall compared the Quimby and the Paterson-Parker systems for selected idealized cases and found that fundamental differences exist between the two systems. They caution against the use of these systems interchangeably. "It is imperative that a radiotherapist use one radium system to the exclusion of the other" (1).

C. The Memorial System

The Memorial system, as described by Laughlin *et al.* (56) in 1963, is an extension of the Quimby system and is characterized by complete dose distributions around lattices of point sources of uniform strength spaced 1 cm apart. Based on computer-generated dose distributions, tables were constructed which gave milligram-hours to deliver 1000 rads at designated points, *e.g.* "minimum peripheral" and "reference maximum dose" points in the plane 0.5 cm from the source plane for the planar implants. For volume implants, similar data points within the implanted volume as well as "central line peripheral dose" points were chosen. These tables use proper exposure rate constant and include the effects of oblique filtration and tissue attenuation.

Another method, known as the "dimension averaging" technique has also been used at Memorial Hospital for permanent implants (59, 60). The method is based on the rationale that radiation tolerance of tissue depends on the size of the implant and the smaller volumes could be intentionally given larger doses. According to this method, the total activity required for an implant is directly proportional to the average of the three dimensions of the implant region.

Mathematically,

$$A = K \cdot \bar{d} \tag{15.9}$$

where A is the activity in mCi and d is the averaged dimension, *i.e.* $\bar{d} = (a + b + c)/3$, where a, b, and c are the three mutually perpendicular dimensions. The constant K of proportionality is based on clinical experience: $K = 10$ for ^{222}Rn and $K = 5$ for ^{125}I.

In addition to the total activity required for an implant, one needs to know the number of seeds and the spacing between seeds. Anderson (60) has described a nomogram for ^{125}I seed spacing which takes into account the elongation factor for the implant shape, *e.g.* spheroid or cylinder.

D. The Paris System

The Paris system (61) of dosimetry is intended primarily for removable implants of long line sources, such as ^{192}Ir wires. The system prescribes wider spacing for longer sources and relates it also to the treatment volume. The dose is prescribed in terms of the "reference isodose" which is usually taken to be 85% of the "basal dose": the average of the minimum doses between sources. Since ^{192}Ir is used in conjunction with afterloading techniques (discussed in Section 15.6B), the sources can be withdrawn at different times to optimize dose distributions.

15.5 COMPUTER DOSIMETRY SYSTEM

The older dosimetry systems are based on idealized implants conforming to certain distribution rules. In actual practice, however, such ideal distributions are seldom realized. With a computer, it is possible not only to preplan implants, but a complete isodose distribution corresponding to the final source distribution is possible as well. The rapid turnaround time with the modern computer systems allows the therapist to modify the implant, if necessary, on the basis of three-dimensional dose distribution.

Computer calculation of a brachytherapy dose distribution consists basically of repeated calculation of dose at a point for each of the implant sources. The total dose at a given point is determined by summing the individual source contributions. Point dose rates are computed for each of a grid of points arranged in a cubic lattice so that isodose curves may be generated in any arbitrary plane. The isodose patterns can also be magnified and superimposed on an implant radiograph for viewing the distribution in relation to the patient's anatomy.

A. Localization of Sources

Dose calculation algorithms require spatial coordinates for each radioactive source. Three-dimensional reconstruction of the source geometry is usually accomplished by using a set of two radiographs, exposed with either orthogonal or "stereo-shift" geometry. Most programs allow input of the film coordinates using a digitizer.

A.1. ORTHOGONAL IMAGING METHOD

As discussed in Section 15.4A.4, the orthogonal radiographs are taken at right angles, with the central axes of the x-ray beams meeting approximately in the middle of the implant. Usually, AP film and lateral film, exposed isocentrically, provide such a geometry. The coordinate system is conventionally established with the X axis from the right to the left of the patient, the Y axis from inferior to superior, and the Z axis from posterior to anterior. The AP film represents a magnified view of the implant image projected onto the X-Y plane while the lateral film presents the image projected on to the Z-Y plane. The origin of the coordinate system is chosen to be a point identified to be the same on both films such as one end of a source. The sources can be identified by comparing the y coordinates of the ends on both films. For example, a source end having the smallest y coordinate on one film will have the smallest y coordinate on the other film also, since the Y axis is common to both films. After all the sources have been identified, the tip and end of each linear source image are sampled with a digitizer, sampling each end sequentially from one film to the other. The source coordinates on each film are corrected for magnification and stored in the computer as x, y, and z coordinates of each source end. The program also determines errors in source localization by comparing the y coordinates (which should be the same) of a source end on both films and comparing the calculated physical length with the actual physical length of the source. If (x_1,y_1,z_1) and (x_2,y_2,z_2) are the coordinates of the two ends of the source, then the length L of the source is given by:

$$L = \sqrt{(x_2 - x_1)^2 + (y_2 - y_1)^2 + (z_2 - z_1)^2} \qquad (15.10)$$

A.2. STEREO-SHIFT METHOD

The stereo-shift method of source localization consists of taking two radiographs of the same view but the patient or the x-ray tube is shifted a certain distance (*e.g.* 20 cm) between the two exposures. The principle of the method is illustrated in Fig. 15.14. Suppose both films are AP, parallel to the X-Y plane of the patient as the tube is shifted in the Y direction between films. A tabletop fiducial marker is used to serve as origin at O. Since the x,y coordinates of a point source or a source end can be obtained from either of the films, the z coordinates can be derived as follows.

Let

P = point to be localized three dimensionally

y_1 = distance between images of P and O on the first film

y_2 = distance between images of P and O on the second film

s = film shift in the origin O due to tube shift

d = tube shift distance

F = target-to-film distance

f = table-to-film distance

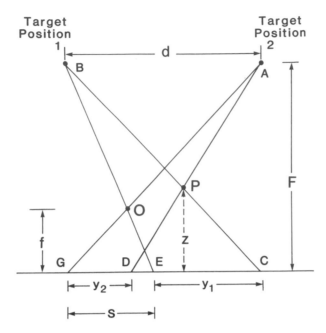

Figure 15.14. Diagram illustrating- stereo-shift method of source localization. Drawing is modified from Anderson (60).

From similar triangles APB and CPD

$$\frac{d}{y_1 + s - y_2} = \frac{F - z}{z} \tag{15.11}$$

Also, from similar triangles AOB and EOG

$$\frac{d}{s} = \frac{F - f}{f} \tag{15.12}$$

From Equations 15.11 and 15.12, we get

$$z = F \frac{(F - f)(y_2 - y_1) - d \cdot f}{(F - f)(y_2 - y_1) - d \cdot F} \tag{15.13}$$

The accuracy of the orthogonal film method is generally better than that of the stereo-shift method (62). For example, small errors in the measurement of y coordinates produces a large error in the z values. However, the stereo-shift method is more suitable for cases where sources cannot be easily identified by orthogonal films such as a large number of seeds or some sources being masked by overlying bone.

B. Dose Computation

Earlier computer programs were used mostly to obtain linear source tables, buildup factors, and scatter factors. Later, programs became available (55–57) to calculate isodose distributions for individual patients. Currently, almost all treatment planning software packages provide brachytherapy dosimetry. Most of these programs use either the Sievert integral directly or precalculated dose tables for different types of sources. Some, but not all, use tissue attenuation corrections, discussed earlier in Section 15.3B.

For radium and other long-lived isotopes, the dose rates, presented in the form of isodose curves, can be directly used to calculate implant duration. In the case of temporary implants of relatively short-lived isotopes such as ^{192}Ir, the computer calculates cumulated dose, using decay correction for the implant duration. An approximate time for the implant duration can first be determined from dose rate $\dot{D}_0$ without decay correction and the total dose to be delivered. The cumulated dose D_c is then given by:

$$D_c = D_0 \cdot T_{av}(1 - e^{-\frac{t}{T_{av}}}) \tag{15.14}$$

where T_{av} is the average life and t is the implant duration.

For permanent implants such as ^{125}I or ^{198}Au, cumulated dose (to complete decay) is given by

$$D_c = \dot{D}_0 \cdot T_{av} = 1.44 \cdot \dot{D}_0 \cdot T_{1/2} \tag{15.15}$$

C. Dose Specification

The problem of dose specification in brachytherapy is made difficult by the inability in most cases to localize the target volume, the severe dose gradients within the treatment volume, and intense hot spots in the implanted region. Although the computer gives complete dose distributions in any plane, this does not simplify the problem of specifying the dose by a single value, the target dose. However, when brachytherapy is used as a method of boost therapy, the overall uncertainty in dose prescription is reduced.

In general, dose specification should be based on clinical experience with careful analysis of the irradiation technique and dosimetry. Existing systems such as Manchester, Quimby, Memorial, and Paris all provide guidelines for dose specification but, as discussed earlier, these systems are not equivalent. Since the computer gives dose distributions three dimensionally, most clinicians tend to prescribe by a minimum dose by selecting an isodose surface which adequately covers the target volume. In practice, the volume coverage of a selected isodose curve is viewed in several planes and correlated with the size and location of the target area.

It should be pointed out that the selection of an isodose curve for dose specification involves other important considerations besides minimum, maximum, or average dose. The success or failure of a treatment depends not only on the dose distribution but also on the dose, time, and volume of implant.

15.6 IMPLANTATION TECHNIQUES

Brachytherapy sources are applied in three ways: external applicators or molds, interstitial implantation, and intracavitary therapy. A choice of one technique or the other is dictated primarily by the size and location of the tumor. For example, surface molds are used to treat small superficial areas, such as the ear or the lip; interstitial therapy is indicated when the tumor is well localized and can be implanted directly according to accepted rules of distribution; intracavitary therapy is used when applicators containing radioactive sources can be introduced into body cavities. In all these cases, owing to the short treatment distance, the geometry of source distribution is critical.

A. Surface Molds

Plastic molds are prepared (63) to conform to the surface to be treated and the sources are securely positioned on the outer surface of the mold. The distance between the plane of the sources to the skin surface is chosen to give a treatment distance of usually 0.5 to 1.0 cm. The dosimetry and source distribution rules are the same for external molds as for interstitial sources (53).

B. Interstitial Therapy

In interstitial therapy, the radioactive sources are fabricated in the form of needles, wires, or seeds, which can be inserted directly into the tissue. There are basically two types of interstitial implants: temporary and permanent. In a temporary implant, the sources are removed after the desired dose has been delivered (*e.g.* radium needles, iridium wires, or iridium seeds). In a permanent implant, the sources are left permanently in the implanted tissues (*e.g.* ^{222}Rn, ^{198}Au, ^{125}I seeds). In general, a temporary implant provides better control of source distribution and dosimetry than a permanent implant. However, the permanent implant is a one-time procedure and is a preferred method for some tumors such as those in the abdominal and thoracic cavities.

A major improvement in temporary implant technique occurred with the introduction of "afterloading" techniques (64, 65) in which the sources are loaded into tubes previously implanted in the tissues. This procedure eliminates exposure in the operating room, x-ray room, and the areas through which the patient is transported. "Dummy" sources are used for radiographic localization and dosimetry. The radioactive sources are loaded after the patient is returned to his room and the implant has been evaluated.

Figure 15.15 illustrates the basic principles of the afterloading technique described by Henschke *et al.* (64). Stainless steel needles (*e.g.* 17 gauge) are first implanted in and around the tumor. The nylon tubes are threaded through

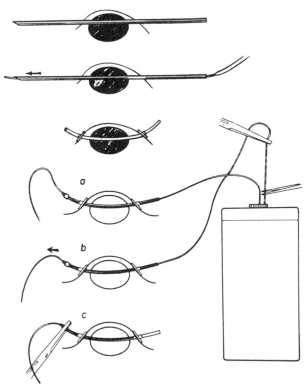

Figure 15.15.   Illustration of an afterloading technique for ^{192}Ir seeds. [Reprinted with permission from: Hilaris (66).]

the needles and the needles are then withdrawn, leaving the nylon tubes in place. The nylon tubes are secured in position by buttons on the skin surface. The tube ends are then usually cut off a few centimeters beyond the buttons.

Many variations of the above procedure have been published in the literature. Further details can be obtained from the book by Hilaris (66).

The simplest device for permanent implants is a single-seed inserter consisting of a stainless steel needle. Each seed is individually loaded into the tip of this needle and, after insertion into the tissue, the seed is pushed out by a stylet. This technique, however, is unsatisfactory for the implantation of deep-seated tumors and volume implants requiring many seeds.

An afterloading technique has also been adopted for the permanent implants (67). The first step in this technique consists of inserting unloaded 17-gauge stainless steel needles into the tumor. The needles are spaced 1 to 2 cm apart depending upon the size of the tumor. The needles are then afterloaded with radioactive seeds, using a special implantation instrument which allows insertion of several seeds at different depths, determined by a gauge as the needle is withdrawn.

Seed-introducing guns (66, 68) have been devised which allow preloading of radioactive seeds into a magazine from which they are pushed into the needle, and then into the tissue. These instruments are convenient to use and can provide greater precision than possible with single seed inserters.

C. Intracavitary Therapy: Uterine Cervix

Intracavitary therapy is mostly used for cancers of the uterine cervix, uterine body, and vagina. A variety of applicators have been designed to hold the sources in a fixed configuration. A cervix applicator basically consists of a central tube, called the tandem, and lateral capsules or "ovoids." The ovoids are separated from each other by spacers.

Since the first application of radium in the treatment of cancer of the uterus in 1908, several techniques have evolved, most of which are modifications of the Stockholm technique (69) and the Paris technique (70). The Manchester system which evolved from the Paris technique, uses a rubber uterine tandem to hold one to three radium tubes and rubber ovoids, separated by a rubber spacer, to each hold a radium tube. The radiation is delivered in at least two applications. In the Fletcher-Suit applicator (65, 71) (Fig. 15.16) the tandem and the ovoids (or the colpostats) are made of stainless steel and then secured to hollow handles to permit afterloading of the sources. Tables have been devised with various combinations of external beam therapy and intracavitary radium using standard loadings (72).

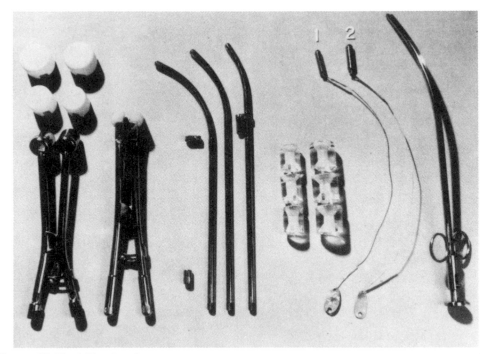

Figure 15.16. A Fletcher-Suite applicator set. [Reprinted with permission from: Fletcher (72).]

C.1. DOSE SPECIFICATION

Despite extensive experience with the treatment of carcinoma of the cervix, the problem of dose specification continues to be an elusive one. Two major systems have emerged over the past several decades: milligram-hours of radium and the dose to points A and B. Papers have been written to correlate the two systems (73, 74) but recent analysis has demonstrated that such correlations are fraught with large uncertainties in dose prescription (75).

Point A was originally defined as 2 cm superior to the lateral vaginal fornix and 2 cm lateral to the cervical canal (76). Later, it was redefined to be 2 cm superior to the external cervical os (or cervical end of the tandem), and 2 cm lateral to the cervical canal (77). Point B is defined 3 cm lateral to point A.

Ideally, a point A represents the location where the uterine vessels cross the ureter. It is believed that the tolerance of these structures is the main limiting factor in the irradiation of the uterine cervix. However, the anatomic relationship of point A varies from patient to patient (78). Point B, on the other hand, is a more stable point and represents dose to the lateral structures in the pelvis such as the obturator nodes.

Computers permit routine calculation of intracavitary dose distribution. Figure 15.17 shows an intracavitary cesium application using three sources in the tandem, approximately 15-10-10 mg Ra eq; and ovoids each containing 15 mg Ra eq. Isodose distribution for this application is shown in Fig. 15.18. Dose to point A and B for individual patients can be easily derived from these distributions. However, the dose to point A is markedly affected by the position

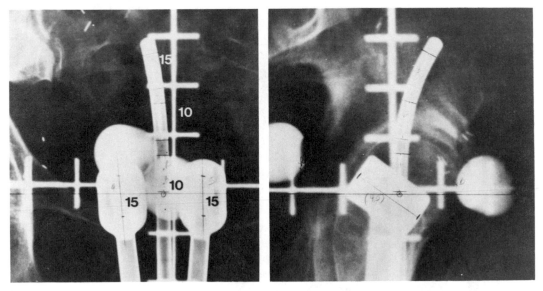

Figure 15.17. AP and lateral views of an intracavitary cesium application. Rectum and bladder are localized with a contrast material.

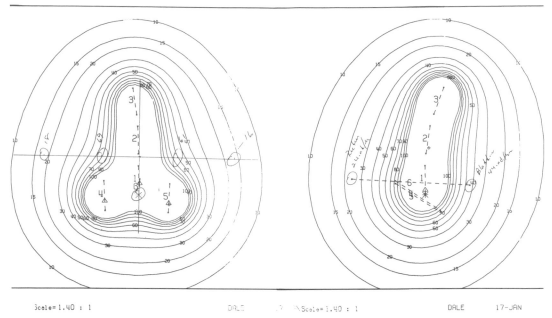

Scale=1.40 : 1   DALE   Scale=1.40 : 1   DALE   17-JAN

Figure 15.18.   Isodose distributions in planes containing the initial part of the tandem. Left, AP view; right, lateral view.

of the colpostats and tandem (75), thus making it difficult to interpret the significance of dose to point *A*.

Although the quest continues for a better system of dose specification, it seems appropriate to examine all the variables individually for each patient, *i.e.* milligram-hours, dose to points *A* and *B*, and the isodose distribution in several planes of interest. The duration of intracavitary treatment should still be based on dose to point *A*, provided the overall isodose distribution is acceptable.

C.2. DOSE TO BLADDER AND RECTUM

The colpostats in the Fletcher-Suit applicator are partially shielded at the top and the bottom to provide some protection to bladder and rectum. However, dosimetrically it is difficult to demonstrate the extent of protection actually provided by these shields.

The dose to bladder and rectum depends on the distribution of sources in a given application. If this dose is assessed to be too high either by measurement or calculation, one has the option of altering the geometry of the sources. Although various instruments, including intracavitary ionization chambers, are available for such measurements, the calculation method has been found to be more reliable in this case. The localization of bladder and rectum can be performed using radiographs taken with contrast media in the bladder and rectum. The maximum dose to bladder and rectum should be, as far as possible, less than the dose to point A (*e.g.* 80% or less of the dose to point A).

C.3. TREATMENT OF UTERINE CORPUS

Cancer of the uterine body can be treated with radium or cesium sources using Heyman capsules (79). These capsules are available in different sizes, each containing 5 to 10 mg Ra eq source. The Heyman technique consists of packing the uterine cavity with multiple sources. Tables have been published which specify dose to the inside surface of the uterine cavity in terms of milligram-hours (79). These dosages have been established on the basis of various measurements and, therefore, individual patient calculations are usually not required.

References

1. Shalek RJ, Stovall M: Dosimetry in implant therapy. In Attix FH, Roesch WC (eds): *Radiation Dosimetry*, Vol. III. New York, Academic Press, 1969, Chap 31.
2. ICRU Report No. 10C: *Radioactivity.* Washington, DC, International Commission on Radiation Units and Measurements, 1963.
3. Whyte GN: Attenuation of radium gamma radiation in cylindrical geometry. *Br J Radiol* 28:635, 1955.
4. Van Roosenbeek E, Shalek RJ, Moore EB: Safe encapsulation period for sealed medical radium sources. *Am J Roentgenol* 102:697, 1968.
5. ICRU Report No. 19: *Radiation Quantities and Units.* Washington, DC, International Commission on Radiation Units and Measurements, 1971.
6. ICRU Report No. 33: *Radiation Quantities and Units.* Washington, DC, International Commission on Radiation Units and Measurements, 1980.
7. Meisberger LL, Keller RJ, Shalek RJ: The effective attenuation in water of gamma rays of gold 198, iridium 192, cesium 137, radium 226, and cobalt 60. *Radiology* 90:953, 1968.
8. Horsler AFC, Jones JC, Stacey AJ: Cesium 137 sources for use in intracavitary and interstitial radiotherapy. *Br J Radiol* 37:385, 1964.
9. Krishnaswamy V: Dose distribution about ^{137}Cs sources in tissue. *Radiology* 105:181, 1972.
10. Attix FH: Computed values of specific gamma ray constant for ^{137}Cs and ^{60}Co. *Phys Med Biol* 13:119, 1968.
11. Henschke UK, Hilaris BS, Mahan GD: Afterloading in interstitial and intracavitary radiation therapy. *Am J Roentgenol* 90:386, 1963.
12. Pierquin B, Chassagne D, Baillet F, Raynol M: L'endocurietherapie des Cancers de la Langue Mobile et due Plancher buccal par l'iridium-192. *Rev Med* 31:1947, 1971.
13. Glasgow GP, Dillman LT: Specific γ-ray constant and exposure rate constant of ^{192}Ir. *Med Phys* 6:49, 1979.
14. Boggs RF, Williams KD, Schmidt GD: Radiological health aspects of spent radon seeds. *Radiat Health Data Rep* 10:185, 1969.
15. Hilaris BS (ed): *Handbook of Interstitial Brachytherapy.* Acton, MA, Publishing Science Group, 1975.
16. Kim JH, Hilaris BS: Iodine 125 source in interstitial tumor therapy. *Am J Roentgenol* 123:163, 1975.
17. Loevinger R: The role of standards laboratory in brachytherapy. In Shearer DR (ed): *Recent Advances in Brachytherapy Physics*, AAPM Med. Phys. Monograph No. 7. New York, American Institute of Physics, 1981.
18. Loftus TP: Standardization of cesium-137 gamma-ray sources in terms of exposure units (roentgens). *J Res Natl. Bur Stand (US)* 74A:1–6, 1970.
19. Loftus TP: Standarization of iridium-192 gamma-ray sources in terms of exposure. *J Res Natl. Bur Stand (US)* 85:19–25, 1980.
20. Dale JWG, Perry WE, Pulfer RF: A beta-gamma ionization chamber for substandards of radioactivity. I and II. *Int J Radiat Isotopes* 10:65, 1961.
21. Berkley LW, Hanson WF, Shalek RJ: Discussion of the characteristics and results of measurements with a portable well ionization chamber for calibration of brachytherapy

sources. In Shearer DR (ed): *Recent Advances in Brachytherapy Physics.* New York, American Institute of Physics, 1981.

22. Loftus TP: Standardization of iridium-192 gamma ray sources in terms of exposure. *J Res Natl. Bur Stand (US)* 80:19, 1979.
23. Williamson JF, Khan FM, Sharma SC, Fullerton GD: Methods for routine calibration of brachytherapy sources. *Radiology* 142:511, 1982.
24. Kubiatowciz DO: Calibration of cesium-137 brachytherapy sources. In Shearer DR (ed): *Recent Advances in Brachytherapy Physics.* New York, American Institute of Physics, 1981.
25. Cobb PD, Chen TS, Kase KR: Calibration of brachytherapy iridium-192 sources. *Int J Radiat Oncol Biol Phys* 7:259, 1981.
26. Suzuki A, Suzuki MN, Weis AM: Analysis of a radioisotope calibration. *J Nucl Med Technol* 4:193, 1976.
27. Boyer AL, Cobb PD, Kase KR, Chen TS: In Shearer DR (ed): *Recent Advances in Brachytherapy Physics.* New York, American Institute of Physics, 1981.
28. Williamson JF, Morin RL, Khan FM: Dose calibrator response to brachytherapy sources: a Monte Carlo and analytic evaluation. *Med Phys* 10:135, 1983.
29. National Council on Radiation Protection and Measurements (NCRP): Specification of Gamma-Ray Brachytherapy Ssources, NCRP Report No. 41. Washington, DC, US Government Printing Office, 1974.
30. O'Connell D, Joslin CA, Howard N, Ramsey NW, Liversage WE: The treatment of uterine carcinoma using the cathetron. *Br J Radiol* 40:882, 1967.
31. Joslin CAF, Smith CW: The use of high activity ⁶⁰Co sources for intracavitary and surface mould therapy. *Proc R Soc Med* 63:1029, 1970.
32. Snelling MD, Lambert HE, Yarnold JR: The treatment of carcinoma of the cervix and endometrium at the Middlesex Hospital. *Clin Radiol* 30:253, 1979.
33. Sievert RM: Die Intensitätsverteilung der Primären γ-Strahlung in der Nähe medizinischer Radiumpräparate. *Acta Radiol* 1:89, 1921.
34. Young MEJ, Batho HF: Dose tables for linear radium sources calculated by an electronic computer. *Br J Radiol* 37:38, 1964.
35. Evans RD, Evans RO: Studies of self absorption in gamma-ray sources. *Rev Mod Phys* 20:305, 1948.
36. Keyser GM: Absorption correction for radium standarization. *Can J Phys* 29:301 1951.
37. Whyte GN: Attenuation of radium gamma radiation in cylindrical geometry. *Br J Radiol* 28:635, 1955.
38. Williamson JF, Morin RL, Khan FM: Monte Carlo evaluation of the Sievert integral for brachytherapy dosimetry. *Phys Med Biol* 28:1021, 1983.
39. Van Dilla MA, Hine GJ: Gamma-ray diffusion experiments in water. *Nucleonics* 10:54, 1952.
40. Ter-Pogossian M, Ittner WB, III, Aly SM: Comparison of air and tissue doses for radium gamma rays. *Nucleonics* 10:50, 1952.
41. Wooton P, Shalek RJ, Fletcher GH: Investigation of the effective absorption of radium and cobalt gamma radiation in water and its clinical significance. *Am J Roentgenol* 71:683, 1954.
42. Reuss A, Brunner F: Phantommessungen mit den Mikroionisationskammern des Bomke-Dosimeters an Radium and Kobalt 6. *Stahlentherapie* 103:279, 1957.
43. Kenney GN, Kartha KIP, Cameron JR: Measurement of the absorption and build-up factor for radium, cobalt 60 and cesium 137. *Phys Med Biol* 11:145, 1966.
44. Meredith WJ, Greene D, Kawashima K: The Attenuation and Scattering in a Phantom of Gamma Rays from Some Radionuclides Used in Mould and Interstitial Gamma-Ray Therapy. *Br J Radiol* 39:280, 1966.
45. Meisberger LL, Keller R, Shalek RJ: The effective attenuation in water of the gamma rays of gold-198, iridium-192, cesium-137, radium-226 and cobalt-60. *Radiology* 90:953, 1968.
46. Webb S, Fox RA: The dose in water surrounding point isotropic gamma-ray emitters. *Br J Radiol* 52:482, 1979.
47. Evans RD: *The Atomic Nucleus.* New York, McGraw-Hill, 1955, p 732. Also in Attix FH, Roesch WC (eds): *Radiation Dosimetry*, Vol. I. New York, Academic Press, 1967, p 151.
48. Kornelsen RO, Young MEJ: Brachytherapy build-up factors. *Br J Radiol* 54:136, 1981.
49. Cameron JR, Suntharalingam N, Kenney GN: *Thermoluminescence Dosimetry.* Madison, University of Wisconsin Press, 1968.
50. Hine GJ, Friedman M: Isodose measurements of linear radium sources in air and water by means of an automatic isodose recorder. *Am J Roentgenol* 64:989, 1950.
51. Cole A, Moore EB, Shalek RJ: A simplified automatic isodose recorder. *Nucleonics* 11:46, 1953.

52. Krishnaswamy V: Dose distribution around an ^{125}I seed source in tissue. *Radiology* 126:489, 1978.
53. Merredith WJ (ed): *Radium Dosage. The Manchester System.* Edinburgh, Livingstone, Ltd, 1967.
54. Glasser O, Quimby EH, Taylor LS, Weatherwax JL, Morgan RH: *Physical Foundations of Radiolgoy*, 3rd ed. New York, Harper and Row, 1961.
55. Stovall M, Shalek RJ: A Study of the explicit distribution of radiation in interstitial implantation. I. A method of calculation with an automatic digital computer. *Radiology* 78:950, 1962.
56. Laughlin, JS, Siler WM, Holodny EI, Ritter FW: A dose description system for interstitital radiation therapy. *Am J Roentgenol* 89:470, 1963.
57. Powers WE, Bogardus CR, White W, Gallagher T: Computer estimation of dosage of interstitial and intracavitary implants. *Radiology* 85:135, 1965.
58. Stovall M, Shalek RJ: The M. D. Anderson method for the computation of isodose curves around interstitial and intracavitary radiation sources. III. Roentgenograms for input data and the relation of isodose calculations to the Paterson Parker system. *Am J Roentgenol* 102:677, 1968.
59. Henschke UK, Cevc P: Dimension averaging—a simple method for dosimetry of interstitial implants. *Radiat Biol Ther* 9:287, 1968.
60. Anderson LL: Dosimetry of interstitial radiation therapy. In Hilaris BS (ed): *Handbook of Interstitial Brachytherapy.* Acton, MA, Publishing Sciences Group, 1975, p 87.
61. Pierquin B, Dutreix A, Paine C: The Paris system in interstitial radiation therapy. *Acta Radiol Oncol* 17:33, 1978.
62. Sharma SC, Williamson JF, Cytacki E: Dosimetric analysis of stereo and orthogonal reconstruction of interstitial implants. *Int J Radiat Oncol Biol Phys* 8:1803, 1982.
63. Paterson R: *The Treatment of Malignant Disease by Radiotherapy.* Baltimore, The Williams and Wilkins Co, 1963.
64. Henschke UK, Hilaris BS, Mahan GD: Afterloading in interstitial and intracavitary radiation therapy. *Am J Roentgenol* 90:386, 1963.
65. Suit HD, Moore EB, Fletcher GH, Worsnop B: Modifications of Fletcher ovoid system for afterloading using standard-size radium tubes (milligram and microgram). *Radiology* 81:126, 1963.
66. Hilaris BS (ed): *Handbook of Interstitial Brachytherapy.* Acton, MA, Publishing Science Group, 1975.
67. Henschke UK: Interstitial implantation with radioisotopes. In Hahn PF (ed): *Therapeutic Use of Artificial Radioisotopes.* New York, John Wiley and Sons, 1956, p 375.
68. Jones CH, Taylor KW, Stedeford JBH: Modification to the Royal Marsden Hospital gold grain implantation gun. *Br J Radiol* 38:672, 1965.
69. Heyman J: The technique in the treatment of cancer uteri at radium-hemmet. *Acta Radiol* 10:49, 1929.
70. Regaud C: Radium therapy of cancer at the radium institute of Paris. *Am J Roentgenol* 21:1, 1929.
71. Fletcher GH, Shalek RJ, Cole A: Cervical radium applicators with screening in the direction of bladder and rectum. *Radiology* 60:77, 1953.
72. Fletcher GH: *Textbook of Radiotherapy*, 2nd ed. Philadelphia, Lea and Febiger, 1973, p 620.
73. Cunningham DE, Stryker JA, Velkley DE, Chung CK: Intracavitary dosimetry: a comparison of MGHR prescription to doses at points A and B in cervical cancer. *Int J Radiat Oncol Biol Phys* 7:121, 1981.
74. Bhatnagar JP, Kaplan C, Specht R: A rule of thumb for dose rate at point A for the Fletcher-Suit applicator. *Br J Radiol* 53:511, 1980.
75. Potish RA, Deibel FC, Khan FM: The relationship between milligram-hours and dose to point A in carcinoma of the cervix. *Radiology* 145:479, 1982.
76. Tod MC, Meredith WJ: A dosage system for use in the treatment of cancer of the uterine cervix. *Br J Radiol* 11:809, 1938.
77. Tod M, Meredith WJ: Treatment of cancer of the cervix uteri—a revised "Manchester Method." *Br J Radiol* 26:252, 1953.
78. Schwaz G: An evaluation of the Manchester system of treatment of carcinoma of the cervix. *Am J Roentgenol* 105:579, 1969.
79. Heyman J, Reuterwall O, Benner S: The radiumhemmet experience with radiotherapy in cancer of the corpus of the uterus. *Acta Radiol* 22:11, 1941.
80. Schulz RJ, Chandra P, Nath R: Determination of the exposure rate constant for ^{125}I using a scintillation detector. *Med Phys* 7:355, 1980.

CHAPTER 16

Radiation Protection

Radiation exposure limits or standards were introduced as early as the start of this century when the potential hazards of radiation were realized. One of the first standard setting bodies was the International Commission on Radiological Protection (ICRP) which continues its function through its series of publications. These reports form the basis for many national protection guidelines. In the United States, the National Council on Radiation Protection and Measurements (NCRP) has functioned as a primary standard-setting body through its separate publications. One of the agencies with regulatory powers in this country is the Nuclear Regulatory Commission (NRC) which has control over the use of all reactor-produced materials (*e.g.* ^{60}Co, ^{192}Ir). The naturally occurring radioactive materials (*e.g.* radium, radon) and x-ray machines are regulated by individual states.

16.1 DOSE EQUIVALENT

Since the biological effects of radiation depend not only on dose but also on the type of radiation, the dosimetric quantity relevant to radiation protection is the dose equivalent (H). It is defined as:

$$H = D \cdot Q \cdot N \tag{16.1}$$

where D is the absorbed dose, Q is the quality factor for the radiation, and N is the product of all other modifying factors.

The SI unit for both dose and dose equivalent is joules per kilogram, but the special name for the SI unit of dose equivalent is sievert (Sv).

$$1 \text{ Sv} = 1 \text{ J/kg}$$

If dose is expressed in units of rad, the special unit for dose equivalent is called the rem.

$$H \text{ (rem)} = D \text{ (rad)} \cdot Q \cdot N$$

Since Q and N are factors and have no units,

$$1 \text{ rem} = 10^{-2} \text{ J/kg}$$

The use of quality factor in radiation protection is analogous to the use of RBE (relative biological effectiveness) in radiobiology. However, the quality factor is a somewhat arbitrarily chosen conservative value based on a range of RBEs related to the linear energy transfer (LET) of the radiation. Thus, the Q factor encompasses RBEs in a very broad sense, independent of the organ, or tissue or of the biological end point under consideration.

The factor N is used to express the modification of biological effect due to nonuniform distribution of internally deposited radionuclides.

Although the dose equivalent for particular situations can be calculated (1), it is convenient for quick and rough calculations to have a table of practical quality factors available. Table 16.1 gives these approximate factors for a variety of radiations used in radiotherapy.

16.2 BACKGROUND RADIATION

Radiation is a part of man's natural environment. The average exposure to natural background radiation in the United States is estimated at about 100 millirems/year. This background radiation is contributed principally by three sources: terrestrial radiation, cosmic radiation, and radiation from radioactive elements in our bodies. Table 16.2 gives average values of background radiation to which the body is exposed annually.

The terrestrial radiation varies over the earth because of differences in the amount of naturally occurring elements in the earth's surface. Similarly, cosmic radiation levels change with elevation. For example, air travel exposes individuals to increased radiation exposure. It has been estimated that at 30,000 feet the dose equivalent is about 0.5 millirem/h (4).

The internal irradiation arises mainly from ^{40}K in our body which emits β and γ rays and decays with a half-life of 1.3×10^9 years. Lungs are exposed to radiation from inhaled air which contains minute amount of ^{222}Rn.

Table 16.1.
Approximate quality factors

Radiation	Quality factor
X-rays, γ rays, and electrons	1
Neutrons	3–10, depending on energy
Heavy particles	1–20

Data are from NCRP Report No. 39 (2).

Table 16.2.
Natural background radiation in the United States*

Radiation source	Millirems/year†
Cosmic rays	28
Terrestrial	26
Radionuclides in the body	27
Total (rounded)	80

* Data are from NCRP Report No. 45 (3).
† Dose equivalent for whole body exposure.

In addition to the background radiation, the population is exposed to radiation from various medical procedures—the planned exposure of patients, as distinct from occupational exposures received by health personnel. It was estimated by the U. S. Public Health Service that the average annual genetically significant dose equivalent[1] in 1970 was about 20 millirems/year from radiologic procedures.

Under ordinary circumstances, exposures from natural background radiation and medical procedures are not included in the occupational exposure controls for the individual cases.

16.3 LOW LEVEL RADIATION EFFECTS

A vast literature exists on the biological effects of radiation. Discussions pertinent to radiation protection can be found in reports of the United Nations Scientific Committee on the Effects of Atomic Radiation (5).

Whereas large doses of radiation produce identifiable effects within a relatively short period, the effects are difficult to ascertain at low doses (*e.g.* less than 10 rad). The difficulty is due mainly to the extremely low frequency with which these effects might occur. The statistical problems are enormous in identifying small effects in the constant presence of spontaneously occurring effects. However, certain effects have been demonstrated in man and other mammals at doses lower than those required to produce acute radiation syndrome but greatly in excess of dose limits recommended by the standard settings bodies. Thus, appropriate exposures to low level radiation may produce: (a) genetic effects—radiation-induced gene mutations, chromosome breaks and anomalies; (b) neoplastic diseases—incidence of leukemia, thyroid tumors, skin lesions; (c) effect on growth and development—adverse effects on fetus and young children; (d) effect on life span—diminishing of life span or premature aging; and (e) cataracts—opacification of the eye lens.

The dose-response curve for the above effects, however, has not been established at low dose levels. A linear dose-response curve has been assumed by the standard setting bodies for regulatory purposes. In addition, it is assumed that there is no threshold. In other words, there is no minimum dose below which the radiation effects can be considered absent.

Many analysts believe that these two assumptions may overestimate the biological effects at low dose levels. Some have proposed a linear quadratic dose-response curve which assigns relatively reduced effects to low doses. However, in the absence of more reliable data it seems prudent to adopt a conservative model, the nonthreshold linear response, for predicting low dose effects. For further discussion of dose-response models, the reader is referred to References 6–9.

---

[1] The genetically significant dose equivalent is the per capita dose equivalent when the long-term genetic effects of radiation are averaged over the whole population. This dose is expected to produce the same total genetic injury to the population as do the actual doses received by the various individuals (2).

16.4 MAXIMUM PERMISSIBLE DOSE EQUIVALENT (MPDE)

Maximum limits on dose equivalent have been proposed for persons whose occupation centers around radiation as well as for the general population. These standards have been set with the belief that at these dose levels there is a negligible probability of any demonstrable bodily injury to the individual. However, the NCRP cautions against the view that any dose below the MPDE is "safe" and any dose above it is "unsafe." The choice of MPDE is rather based on the interpretation of what is considered to be an acceptable risk for the applied conditions. The risk-benefit criteria have been discussed in the NCRP Report No. 39 (2).

A. Age-Proration Formula

The NCRP (10) introduced a formula for maximum accumulated dose for whole body exposure to occupational persons:

$$\text{Maximum accumulated dose equivalent} = (N - 18) \times 5 \text{ rems} \qquad (16.2)$$

where N is the number of years of age.

Although this formula gives an annual limit of 5 rems/year, it deemphasizes the "sanctity" of a firm annual limit. In other words, the limit may be exceeded in any given year as long as the accumulated exposures remain within the formula limits. Administratively, however, it is prudent to maintain compliance with the formula on a yearly basis. In many institutions, the dose limits are monitored on a monthly basis.

B. Occupational *vs.* Nonoccupational Exposure Limits

The maximum permissible dose equivalents for radiation workers have been set higher than those for members of the general public. For example, the whole body MPDE for occupationally exposed persons is recommended at 5 rems in any one year compared to 0.5 rem in any one year for the public. This 10:1 ratio of occupational limits has been decided because of several reasons (2). The population limits have been derived from the occupational limits by accounting additionally, in the case of general public, for (a) difficulty or lack of monitoring exposures; (b) absence of periodic medical examination; (c) greater diversity of age including fetuses and young children; and (d) lack of free choice that is implied in occupational exposures.

A still lower limit has been recommended for the genetically significant dose equivalent (GSDE). The concept of GSDE implies that the long-term genetic effects of radiation can be averaged over the whole population. The average MPDE to the gonads for the population as a whole has been set at 0.17 rem/year per person. Similarly, average MPDE to the whole body for the population as a whole is also 0.17 rem/year per person. Thus, the average population limits for both the genetic and somatic effects are about one-third of the MPDE for an individual member of the public.

C. Critical Organs

Radiation protection guidelines take into account the susceptibility of certain organs and tissues to radiation injury. Although such a compartmentalization is complex especially for the somatic effects because of the general interplay between various tissues, it is sometimes important to consider specific tissues or structures which are considered critical for potential late effects.

For general irradiation of the whole body, the critical organs are: (a) gonads, for genetic effects; (b) bone marrow, for induction of leukemia; (c) lens of the eye, for cataracts; and (d) skin, for skin cancer. Other limiting organs have been determined for internally deposited radionuclides such as thyroid, gastrointestinal tract, lung, bone, and kidney. For more extensive discussions on the choice of limiting organs, the reader should consult NCRP Report No. 39 (2).

D. MPDE Levels

Table 16.3 summarizes the dose-limiting recommendations. The rationale and criteria for these limits is provided in NCRP Report No. 39 (2). It should be realized, however, that the MPDE values represent maximum limits and that the actual exposures should be kept "as low as praticable."

Table 16.3.
Maximum permissible dose equivalent recommendations

Occupational	
Whole body exposure	
Prospective annual limit	5 rems in any one year
Long term accumulation to age N years	$(N - 18) \times 5$ rems
Skin	15 rems in any one year
Hands	75 rems in any one year
Forearms	30 rems in any one year
Other organs	15 rems in any one year
Pregnant women	0.5 rem in gestation period
Public	
Individuals	0.5 rem in any one year
Students	0.1 rem in any one year
Population	
Genetic	0.17 rem average per year
Somatic	0.17 rem average per year
Family of radioactive patient	
Individual under age 45	0.5 rem in any one year
Individual over age 45	5 rems in any one year

From NCRP Report No. 39 (2).

16.5 STRUCTURAL SHIELDING DESIGN

Radiation protection guidelines for the design of structural shielding for radiation installations are discussed in the NCRP reports (11–13). These reports contain the necessary technical information as well as recommendations for planning new facilities and remodeling existing facilities. The reader is referred to these reports for comprehensive details on this subject. This section will discuss only some of the basic factors which are considered in the calculation of barrier thicknesses.

Protective barriers are designed to ensure that the dose equivalent received by any individual does not exceed the applicable maximum permissible value. The areas surrounding the room are designated as *controlled* or *noncontrolled* depending on whether or not the exposure of persons in the area is under the supervision of a Radiation Protection Supervisor. For protection calculations, the MPDE is assumed to be 0.1 rem/week for the controlled areas and 0.01 rem/week for the noncontrolled areas. These values approximately correspond to the annual limits of 5 rems/year and 0.5 rem/year, respectively.

Protection is required against three types of radiation: the primary radiation, the scattered radiation, and the leakage radiation through the source housing. A barrier sufficient to attenuate the useful beam to the required degree is called the *primary barrier*. The required barrier against stray radiation (leakage and scatter) is called the *secondary barrier*. The following factors enter into the calculation of barrier thicknesses.

1) *Workload* (*W*): for x-ray equipment operating below 500 kVp, the workload is usually expressed in milliampere minutes per week, which can be computed by multiplying the maximum mA with approximate minutes/week of beam "on" time. For megavoltage machines, the workload is usually stated in terms of weekly dose delivered at 1 m from the source. This can be estimated by multiplying the number of patients treated per week with the dose delivered per patient at 1 m. *W* is expressed in rad/week at 1 m.

2) *Use Factor* (*U*): fraction of the operating time during which the radiation under consideration is directed toward a particular barrier. Although the use factors vary depending upon the techniques used in a given facility, typical values are given in Table 16.4.

3) *Occupancy Factor* (*T*): fraction of the operating time during which the area of interest is occupied by the individual. If more realistic occupancy factors are not available, values given in Table 16.5 may be used.

4) *Distance* (*d*): distance in meters from the radiation source to the area to

Table 16.4.
Typical use factor for primary protective barriers

Location	Use factor
Floor	1
Walls	¼
Ceiling	¼–½, depending on equipment and techniques

Table 16.5.
Typical occupancy factors

Full occupancy ($T = 1$)
Work areas, offices, nurses' stations
Partial occupancy ($T = \frac{1}{4}$)
Corridors, rest rooms, elevators with operators
Occasional occupancy ($T = \frac{1}{8}-\frac{1}{16}$)
Waiting rooms, toilets, stairways, unattended elevators, outside areas used only for pedestrians or vehicular traffic

be protected. Inverse square law is assumed for both the primary and stray radiation.

A. Primary Radiation Barrier

Suppose the maximum permissible dose equivalent for the area to be protected is P (*e.g.* 0.1 rad/week for controlled and 0.01 rad/week for noncontrolled area).[2] If B is the transmission factor for the barrier to reduce the primary beam dose to P in the area of interest, then

$$P = \frac{WUT}{d^2} \cdot B \tag{16.3}$$

Therefore, the required transmission factor B is given by

$$B = \frac{P \cdot d^2}{WUT} \tag{16.4}$$

By consulting broad beam attenuation curves (Figs. 16.1 and 16.2) for the given energy beam, one can determine the barrier thickness required. More data on beam attenuation are available in the NCRP handbooks (12, 13).

The choice of barrier material, *e.g.* concrete, lead, or steel, depends on structural and spatial considerations. Since concrete is relatively cheap, the walls and roof barriers are usually constructed out of concrete. Lead or steel can be used where space is at a premium. For megavoltage x and γ radiation, equivalent thickness of various materials can be calculated by comparing tenth value layers (TVL) for the given beam energy. If such information is not available specifically for a given material, density ratio can be used in most cases. Densities and TVLs for different materials and beam energies are given in the NCRP publications (12, 13).

B. Secondary Barrier for Scattered Radiation

Radiation is scattered from the patient in all directions. The amount of scattered radiation depends on the beam intensity incident on the scatterer,

---

[2] For x and γ radiations, one can assume 1 rad = 1 rem.

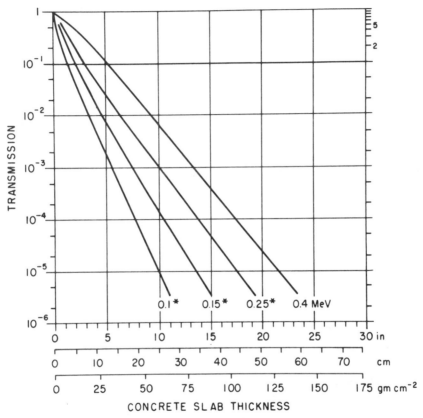

Figure 16.1. Transmission through concrete (density 2.35 g cm^{-3}) of x-rays produced by 0.1- to 0.4-MeV electrons, under broad-beam conditions. Electron energies designated by an asterisk were accelerated by voltages with pulsed wave form; unmarked electron energies were accelerated by a constant potential generator. Curves represent transmission in dose-equivalent index ratio. [Reprinted with permission from: NCRP Report No. 51 (13).]

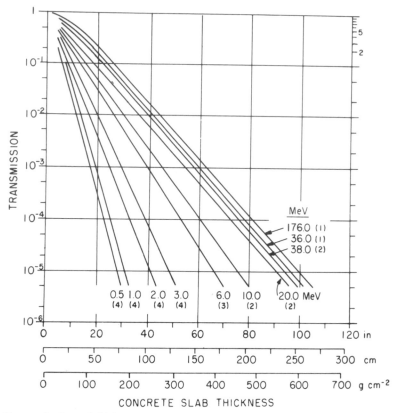

Figure 16.2. Transmission of thick-target x-rays through ordinary concrete (density 2.35 g cm⁻³), under broad-beam conditions. Energy designations on each curve (0.5 to 176 MeV) refer to the monoenergetic electron energy incident on the thick x-ray production target. Curves represent transmission to dose-equivalent index ratio. (Reprinted with permission from: NCRP Report No. 51 (13).]

the quality of radiation, the area of the beam at the scatterer, and the scattering angle. The ratio of scattered dose to the incident dose may be denoted by α. Table 16.6 gives values of α for various angles and beam qualities. For megavoltage beams, α is usually assumed to be 0.1% for 90° scatter.

The scattered radiation, in general, has lower energy compared to the incident energy. However, the softening of the beam due to Compton scatter depends on the incident energy and the direction of scatter. For orthovoltage radiation, the quality of scattered radiation is usually assumed to be the same as that of the incident beam. For megavoltage beams, on the other hand, the maximum energy of the 90° scattered radiation is 500 keV. Therefore, the transmission of this scattered radiation through a barrier is estimated to be approximately the same as that for a 500-kVp useful beam. At smaller scattering angles, however, the scattered beam has greater penetrating power

Table 16.6.
Ratio, α, of scattered to incident exposure

Scattering angle (from central ray)	γ rays	X-rays	
	^{60}Co	4 MV	6 MV
15			9×10^{-3}
30	6.0×10^{-3}		7×10^{-3}
45	3.6×10^{-3}	2.7×10^{-3}	1.8×10^{-3}
60	2.3×10^{-3}		1.1×10^{-3}
90	0.9×10^{-3}		0.6×10^{-3}
135	0.6×10^{-3}		0.4×10^{-3}

From NCRP Report No. 34 (12). Scattered radiation measured at 1 m from phantom when field area is 400 cm^2 at the phantom surface; incident exposure measured at center of field but without phantom.

(14). In addition, a greater fraction of the incident beam is scattered at smaller angles (12, 14).

Suppose a transmission factor of B_s is required to reduce the scattered dose to an acceptable level P in the area of interest; then

$$P = \frac{\alpha \cdot WT}{d^2 \cdot d'^2} \cdot \frac{F}{400} \cdot B_s \tag{16.5}$$

where α is the fractional scatter at 1 m from the scatterer, for beam area of 400 cm^2 incident at the scatterer, d is the distance from source to the scatterer, d' is the distance from the scatterer to the area of interest, and F is the area of the beam incident at the scatterer. The use factor for the secondary barrier is considered unity.

Thus, the barrier transmission B_s is given by

$$B_s = \frac{P}{\alpha WT} \cdot \frac{400}{F} \cdot d^2 \cdot d'^2 \tag{16.6}$$

The required thickness of concrete or lead can be determined for appropriate transmission curves given in the NCRP reports (12, 13) or Figs. 16.1 and 16.2.

C. Secondary Barrier for Leakage Radiation

For therapy units below 500 kVp, the maximum leakage allowed from the tube housing is 1 R/h at a distance of 1 m from the source. The leakage limit for the megavoltage therapy units is 0.1% of the primary beam dose at 1 m. The same limit applies to teletherapy units such as ^{60}Co with the source in the beam "ON" position.

Since leakage radiation is present whenever the machine is operated, the use factor for leakage is unity. Suppose the required secondary barrier for leakage radiation has a transmission factor of B_L to reduce the leakage dose to the maximum permissible level P (R/week).

For therapy units below 500 kVp

$$P = \frac{WT}{d^2 \cdot 60I} \cdot B_L \qquad (16.7)$$

where I is the maximum tube current. The number 60 is used to convert leakage limit of 1 R/h to 1/60 R/min since the workload W is expressed in terms of mA-min/week.

For a megavoltage therapy unit,

$$P = \frac{0.001 \; WT}{d^2} \cdot B_L \qquad (16.8)$$

The factor 0.001 is the 0.1% leakage limit through the source housing.

Thus, the transmission factor B_L for the leakage barrier is given by

$$B_L = \frac{P \cdot d^2 \cdot 60I}{WT} \quad \text{[Therapy below 500 kVp]} \qquad (16.9)$$

and

$$B_L = \frac{P \cdot d^2}{0.001 \; WT} \quad \text{[Therapy above 500 kVp]} \qquad (16.10)$$

The quality of leakage radiation is approximately the same as that of the primary beam. Therefore, the transmission curve for the primary beam should be used to determine the leakage barrier thickness (Figs. 16.1 and 16.2).

For megavoltage therapy installations, the leakage barrier usually far exceeds that required for the scattered radiation because the leakage radiation is more penetrating than the scattered radiation. For the lower energy x-ray beams, however, the difference between the barrier thickness for the leakage and for the scattered radiation is relatively less.

A barrier designed for primary radiation provides adequate protection against leakage and scattered radiation. If a barrier is designed for stray radiation only, the thickness is computed for leakage and scattered radiations separately. If the thicknesses of the two barriers differ by at least three HVLs, the thicker of the two will be adequate. If the difference is less than three HVLs, one HVL should be added to the larger one to obtain the required secondary barrier.

D. Door Shielding

Unless a maze entranceway is provided, the door must provide shielding equivalent to the wall surrounding the door. For megavoltage installations, a door which provides direct access to the treatment room will have to be extremely heavy. It will require a motor drive as well as a means of manual operation in case of emergency. A maze arrangement, on the other hand, drastically reduces the shielding requirements for the door. The function of the maze is to prevent direct incidence of radiation at the door. With a proper maze design, the door is exposed only to the multiply scattered radiation of significantly reduced intensity and energy. For example, in Fig. 16.3, radiation is scattered at least twice before incidence on the door. Each Compton scatter at 90° or greater will reduce the energy to 500 keV or less. The intensity will also be greatly reduced at each large angle scatter. The door shielding in this case can be calculated by tracing the path of the scattered radiation from the patient to the door and repeatedly applying Equation 16.6. For megavoltage units, the attenuation curves for the 500-kVp x-rays may be used to determine the door shielding from multiply scattered x-rays. In most cases, the required shielding turns out to be less than 6 mm of lead.

E. Protection against Neutrons

High energy x-ray beams (*e.g.* >10 MV) are contaminated with neutrons. These are produced by high energy photons and electrons incident on the various materials of target, flattening filter, collimators, and other shielding components. The cross sections for (e,n) reactions are smaller by a factor of about 10 than those for (γ,n) reactions. Because of this, the neutron production during electron beam therapy mode is quite small compared to that during the x-ray mode.

The neutron contamination increases rapidly as the energy of the beam is

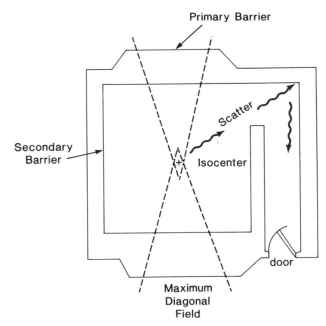

Figure 16.3. Schematic diagram of a megavoltage x-ray therapy installation (drawing not to scale). Radiation scatter from patient can reach the door, as shown.

increased from 10 to 20 MV, and then remains approximately constant above this. Measurements have shown (16–18) that in the 16 to 25 MV x-ray therapy mode the neutron dose equivalent along central axis is approximately 0.5% of the x-ray dose and falls off to about 0.1% outside the field. Sohrabi and Morgan (17) have listed a wide range of neutron contamination values which have been reported in the literature for some medical accelerators.

The energy spectrum (19) of emitted neutrons within the x-ray beam is similar to the uranium fission spectrum, showing a broad maximum in the range of 1 MeV. The neutron energy is considerably degraded after multiple scattering from walls, roof, and floor and consequently the proportion of the fast neutron (>0.1 MeV) reaching the inside of the maze is usually small.

Concrete barriers designed for x-ray shielding are sufficient for protection against neutrons. However, the door has to be protected against neutrons that diffuse into the maze and reach the door. Reflections from the walls cause a reduction in the neutron fluence and, depending upon the accelerator configuration, a decrease in neutron fluence of two orders of magnitude (10^{-2}) from machine location to the inside of the maze can be expected (20). The shielding required for the door can be further reduced by the maze design. In general, a longer maze (>5 m) is desirable in reducing the neutron fluence at the door. Finally, a few inches of a hydrogenous material such as polyethylene can be added to the door to thermalize the neutrons and reduce the neutron dose further. A steel or lead sheet may be added to the door to protect against scattered x-rays, as discussed above.

When thermal neutrons are absorbed by the nuclei of atoms within the shielding door, energetic γ radiations (called the neutron-capture γ rays) are produced. These radiations have a spectrum of energies ranging up to 8 MeV, but most have energies in the region of 1 MeV. Unless the neutron fluence at the door is high such as in the case of a short maze, the intensity of capture γ rays generated within the shielding door is usually low. Since the capture γ rays have high energy, thick sheets of lead are required to provide effective attenuation. Thus, it is more desirable to reduce the neutron fluence incident at the door such as by designing a longer maze than to have a high neutron fluence at the door and add prohibitive amounts of lead shielding to the door to attenuate the capture γ rays.

Computation of shielding requirements for a high energy installation requires many considerations which cannot be discussed in adequate detail in this text. The reader is referred to the literature for further guidance (13, 19, 21, 22).

16.6 PROTECTION AGAINST RADIATION FROM BRACHYTHERAPY SOURCES

This subject has been dealt with in detail in NCRP Report No. 40 (15). In this section, only a brief review will be given of some practical guidelines that have been developed for safe handling and use of brachytherapy sources.

A. Storage

Lead-lined safes with lead-filled drawers are commercially available for storing brachytherapy sources. In choosing a particular safe, consideration should be given to the adequacy of shielding, distribution of sources, and time required for personnel to remove sources from, and return sources to, the safe.

The storage area for radium should be ventilated by a direct filtered exhaust to the outdoors, because of the possibility of radon leaks. Similar arrangement is also recommended for encapsulated powdered sources or sources containing microspheres. This precaution is taken so that if a source ruptures, the radionuclide is not drawn into the general ventilation system of the building.

The storage rooms are usually provided with a sink for cleaning source applicators. The sink should be provided with a filter or trap to prevent loss of source.

B. Source Preparation

A source preparation bench should be provided close to the safe. The preparation and dismantling of source applicators should be carried out behind a suitable barrier to adequately shield the operator. Many facilities are equipped with a protective "L-block," usually constructed of lead. A lead glass viewing window provides some protection by providing shielding as well as a suitable distance between the face of the operator and the sources.

Brachytherapy sources must never be touched with the hands. Suitably long forceps should be used to provide as much distance as practical between sources and the operator.

Besides various kinds of protective shielding available for brachytherapy applications, the operator must be aware of the effectiveness of time and distance in radiation protection. Exposures of individuals can be greatly reduced if, as far as practical, the time spent in the vicinity of the sources is minimized and the distance from the sources is maximized.

Certain brachytherapy techniques have the advantages of giving reduced exposure to personnel. For example, afterloading techniques involve no exposure to operating room personnel or x-ray technologists. Some exposure is received during the loading and removal of sources but even these exposures can be reduced by using mobile protective shields. The use of low energy sources in place of radium or radon is another example in which personnel exposure can be minimized.

C. Source Transportation

The sources can be transported in lead containers or leaded carts. The thickness of lead required will depend on the type of source and the amount of radioactive material to be transported. A table of required thickness for various conditions is given in NCRP Report No. 40 (15).

D. Leak Testing

Various methods of leak testing of a sealed source are available (15). A radium source can be checked for radon leaks by placing it in a small test tube with some activated carbon or a ball of cotton. After 24 h, the carbon or the cotton ball can be counted in a scintillation-well counter. It is sometimes convenient to leak test the entire stock of radium by pumping the air from the safe and passing it through on an activated charcoal filter. The filter is counted for α activity. If a leak is detected, then individual sources will have to be tested to isolate the defective source.

Periodic leak testing of radium is usually specified by state regulations. A source is considered to be leaking if a presence of 0.005 μCi or more of removable contamination is measured. The leaking source should be returned to a suitable agency which is authorized for the disposal of radioactive materials.

16.7 RADIATION PROTECTION SURVEYS

After the installation of radiation equipment, a qualified expert must carry out a radiation protection survey of the installation. The survey includes checking equipment specifications and interlocks related to radiation safety and evaluation of potential radiation exposure to individuals in the surrounding environment.

A. Radiation Monitoring Instruments

The choice of a particular radiation detector or dosimeter depends on the type of measurement required. In radiation protection surveys, low levels of radiation are measured and, therefore, the instrument must be sensitive enough to measure such low levels. The detectors most often used for x-ray measurements are the ionization chambers, Geiger counters, thermoluminescent dosimeters (TLD), and photographic film. The TLD and film dosimetry has been discussed in Chapter 8. In this section, the Geiger counter and an ionization chamber suitable for low level radiation measurements will be briefly described.

A.1. IONIZATION CHAMBER

An ionization chamber used for low level x-ray measurements (of the order of milliroentgens per hour) has a large volume (~600 cc) to obtain high sensitivity (Fig. 16.4). A DC voltage is applied between the outer shell and the central electrode to collect ionization charge produced by radiation in the internal air volume when the chamber is exposed to radiation. This causes an ion current to flow in the external circuit. These currents are extremely small, however, and special electrometer circuitry including a current amplifier is required to measure them. The output current is directly proportional to the exposure rate.

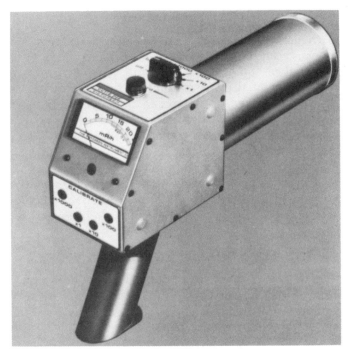

Figure 16.4. A Cutie Pie survey meter. (Courtesy of the Victoreen Instrument Division, Cleveland, OH.)

An ion chamber survey meter is usually calibrated for exposure in a γ ray beam from a cesium or a radium brachytherapy source using an open-air measurement geometry (see Section 15.2B.1). For accurate usage at middle and high energies, the energy response curve for the chamber should be used to correct the exposure. Additional corrections for temperature and pressure and angular dependence may also be necessary.

A.2. GEIGER-MÜLLER COUNTERS

The Geiger-Müller counter (or G-M tube for short) consists essentially of a cylindrical cathode with a fine wire stretched along the axis of the cylinder. The tube is filled with a special mixture of gases at a pressure of about 100 mm Hg. The voltage applied to the electrodes is much higher than the saturation voltage applied to an ionization chamber. Potential is so high that the particles from the original ionization become energetic enough to produce further secondary ionization giving rise to "gas amplification." If the voltage is high enough that an "avalanche" of charge is generated by the original ionizing event, independent of its size, the detector is called a Geiger-Müller counter.

The G-M tube is much more sensitive than the ionization chamber. For example, the Geiger counter can detect individual photons or individual particles which could never be observed in a ionization chamber. However, this detector is not a dose-measuring device. Although a Geiger counter is useful for preliminary surveys to detect the presence of radiation, ionization chambers are recommended for quantitative measurement. Because of their inherently slow recovery time (~50–300 μs), they can never record more than 1 count/machine pulse. Thus, a G-M counter could significantly underestimate radiation levels when used to count radiation around pulsed machines such as accelerators.

A.3. NEUTRON DETECTORS

Neutrons can be detected with the aid of their various interactions. In a hydrogenous material, neutrons produce hydrogen recoils or protons which can be detected by ionization measurements, proportional counters, scintillation counters, cloud chambers, or photographic emulsions. Neutrons can also be detected by their induced nuclear reactions. Certain materials, called activation detectors, become radioactive when exposed to neutrons. The detector, after exposure to the neutron field, is counted for β or γ ray activity.

Neutron measurements in or near the primary x-ray beam can be made with passive detectors such as activation detectors, without being adversely affected by pulsed radiation. An activation detector can be used either as a bare threshold detector or inside a moderator such as polyethylene. An example of bare threshold detector is phosphorus (in the form of phosphorus pentoxide) which has been successfully used by several investigators to measure neutrons in as well as outside the primary beam (18, 24). A phosphorus detector can monitor both fast and slow or thermal neutrons utilizing $^{31}P(n,p)^{31}Si$ and $^{31}P(n,\gamma)^{32}P$ reactions. The activation products ^{31}Si and ^{32}P are essentially pure β emitters and are counted using a calibrated liquid scintillation spectrometer. The problem of photon interference (activation of the detector by photons) is minimal with this detector.

Moderated activation systems suffer from photoneutron production in the moderator itself. Therefore, these detectors are primarily useful outside the primary beam. Examples of the moderated activation detectors are activation remmeters and moderated foil detectors. A gold foil placed in a polyethylene cylinder (24 cm long and 22 cm in diameter) has been used by Rogers and Van Dyk (25) for measurements outside the primary photon beam. McCall *et al.* (26) have developed a system in which a gold foil is surrounded by a polyethylene cylinder covered by a layer of cadmium and boron to absorb thermal neutrons. The activity induced in the gold foil is measured by using a calibrated Ge(Li) detector system.

Outside the treatment room, it is a common practice to use two detectors which respond predominantly to one or the other radiation. For example, a conventional air-filled ionization chamber with nonhydrogenous walls (carbon) predominantly measures photons and its response to neutrons can be negligible since n/γ ratio outside the shield is usually small and the neutrons are low energy. An ion chamber with hydrogenous walls, on the other hand, can detect both neutrons and x-rays. An ion chamber which can be filled with either argon or propane to obtain a predominantly photon or photon plus neutron response, respectively, has also been used to estimate photon and neutron exposure rates outside the shield of a medical accelerator (23). Also, proportional counters, with filling gases such as BF_3, are often used inside moderators to detect thermalized neutrons with good discrimination against signals produced by photons. Such a gas proportional counter, used either in the counting mode or current measurement, may be regarded as an ionization chamber with internal gas multiplication. The voltage is high enough so that ionization by collision occurs and, as a result, the current due to primary ionization is increased manyfold. The basis of the detection system is the reaction $^{10}B(n,\alpha)^{7}Li$, whereby the α particles can be counted or the ionization current caused by them is measured. A moderated BF_3 counter will also count proton recoil particles produced by neutrons in the hydrogenous material.

Figure 16.5 shows one of the commercially available neutron survey meters, the Eberline Neutron Rem Counter. The instrument consists of a BF_3 propor-

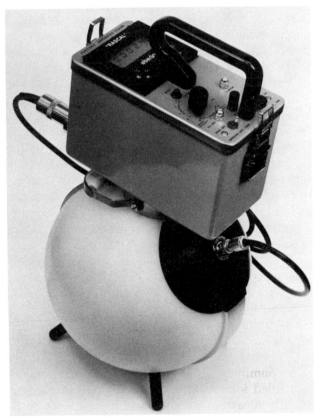

Figure 16.5.   A portable neutron rem counter, "Rascal". (Courtesy of Eberline, Santa Fe, NM.)

tional counter surrounded by a 9-inch cadmium-loaded polyethylene sphere to moderate the neutrons. The counter operates typically at 1600 to 2000 V and can be used for measuring neutrons from thermal to approximately 10-MeV energy. The response is displayed in terms of count rate, mR/hr, and millirems/h. The survey meter is calibrated using an NBS calibrated Pu-Be neutron source.

B. Equipment Survey

Some of the design specifications (NCRP Report No. 33, Sections 3.4.1 and 4.2.2) related to patient and personnel safety can be determined by visual inspection. Various operational and beam-limiting interlocks are checked out as part of the field testing of the machine. The leakage radiation through the source housing may be measured as follows.

1) The collimator opening is blocked with at least 10 half-value layers of lead. 2) Sheets of prepacked film may be wrapped around the source housing to locate areas of high radiation leakage. 3) Using an ionization chamber of appropriate volume or sensitivity, the dose rate is determined at a distance of 1 m from the source, as a function of the primary beam dose rate at 1 m. These measurements should be made in selected directions in which leakage is expected to be maximum.

4) In the case of ^{60}Co teletherapy, the leakage radiation through the source housing with the beam "ON" position are determined in the same manner as above. In the beam "OFF" condition, however, measurements are made in 14 different directions to determine the average and maximum leakage dose rate (11). A calibrated ionization chamber such as a Cutie Pie is a suitable instrument for these measurements.

The following limits apply to the leakage radiation through the source housing.

1) For therapy unit below 500 kVp, the exposure rate should not exceed 1 R/h at a distance of 1 m from the source. 2) For therapy units above 500 kVp, the leakage dose rate at 1 m from the source should not exceed 0.1% of the primary beam dose rate at that distance. This limit also applies to radioisotopes units (*e.g.* ^{60}Co) with the beam in the "ON" position. 3) The leakage exposure rate for the γ beam teletherapy equipment with the beam in the "OFF" position must not exceed 2 mR/h on the average and 10 mR/h in any one direction, both measured at 1 m from the source. 4) If a unit is equipped with a beam interceptor to reduce structural shielding requirements, the radiation transmitted through the interceptor must not exceed 0.1% of the useful beam. It should also reduce by the same factor the radiation scattered by the patient through an angle of up to 30° from the central ray.

C. Area Survey

Areas outside the treatment room which are accessible to any individual should be designated as controlled or noncontrolled, depending upon whether the exposure of persons in the area is monitored or not. Exposure levels in these areas should be measured with the beam oriented in various possible directions. The transmitted radiation through the primary barrier should be measured with the beam of maximum size directly incident at the barrier. Measurements outside the secondary barriers should be made with a phantom at the treatment position. Other operational conditions such as total body irradiation may present special treatment conditions which should be considered in the area survey.

The results of the survey should be evaluated by taking into account the actual operating conditions, including workload, use factor, occupancy factor, and attenuation and scattering of the useful beam by the patient. The environmental safety will be considered acceptable if no person is likely to receive more than the applicable MPDE.

The survey data based on instantaneous dose rate measurements should be supplemented with cumulative radiation measurements and personnel monitoring over appropriate time periods.

If, as a result of a radiation survey, supplementary shielding is added to the protective barriers, a survey should be made to evaluate the adequacy of the shielding after the modification.

16.8 PERSONNEL MONITORING

Personnel monitoring must be used in controlled areas for occupationally exposed individuals. Cumulative radiation monitoring is mostly performed with film badges, although TLD badges are also used in some cases. Since the badge is mostly used to monitor whole body exposure, it should be worn on the chest or abdomen. Special badges may also be used to measure exposure to specific parts of the body (*e.g.* hands) if higher exposures are expected there during particular procedures.

Although film monitoring is a simple and convenient method of personnel monitoring, it has certain drawbacks. The energy dependence poses a major problem, especially when an individual is exposed to both soft and high energy radiation. However, some information is obtained concerning beam quality by placing filters of different materials and thickness to partly cover the film. By comparing the film darkening under the filter with that of the part without filter gives some indication of the penetration ability of the radiation.

Radiation monitoring during a particular procedure may also be performed with pocket dosimeters. These instruments are useful where exposure needs to be monitored more frequently than possible with the regular film badge service.

References

1. Relative Biological Effectiveness (RBE) Committee of the ICRP and ICRU: Report of the RBE Committee to the International Commission on Radiological Protection and on Radiological Units and Measurements. *Health Phys* 9:357, 1963.
2. NCRP Report No. 39: *Basic Radiation Protection Criteria.* Washington, DC, National Council on Radiation Protection and Measurements, 1971.

3. NCRP Report No. 45: *Natural Background Radiation in the United States.* Washington, DC, National Council on Radiation Protection and Measurements, 1975.

4. Friedell HL: Radiation protection—concepts and trade-offs. In *Perception of Risk, Proceedings of the National Council on Radiation Protection and Measurements.* Washington, DC, 1980.

5. United States Scientific Committee on the Effects of Atomic Radiation: *Report of the United Nations Scientific Committee on the Effects of Atomic Radiation.* United Nations, New York, General Assembly, Official Records: 13th Session, Suppl No. 17 (A/3838) (1958); 17th Session, Suppl. No. 16 (A/5216) (1962); 21st Session, Suppl No. 14 (A/6314) (1966); 24th Session, Suppl No. 13 (A/7613) (1969).

6. Elkind MM: The initial part of the survival curve: implication for low-dose-rate radiation responses. *Radiat Res* 71:1, 1977.

7. Withers HR: Response of tissues to multiple small dose fractions. *Radiat Res* 71:24, 1977.

8. Brown MM: The shape of the dose-response curve for radiation carcinogenesis: extrapolation to low doses. *Radiat Res* 71:34, 1977.

9. Upton AC: Radiological effects of low doses: implications for radiological protection. *Radiat Res* 71:51, 1977.

10. National Committee on Radiation Protection and Measurements: Maximum permissible radiation exposures to man, a preliminary statement of the National Committee on Radiation Protection and Measurement. *Radiology* 6:260, 1957.

11. NCRP Report No. 33: *Medical X-ray and Gamma-ray Protection for Energies up to 10 MeV. Equipment Design and Use.* Washington, DC, National Council of Radiation Protection and Measurements, 1968.

12. NCRP Report No. 34: *Medical X-ray and Gamma-ray Protection for Energies up to 10 MeV. Structural Shielding Design and Evaluation.* Washington, DC, National Council on Radiation Protection and Measurements, 1970.

13. NCRP Report No. 51: *Radiation Protection Design Guidelines for 0.1–100 MeV Particle Accelerator Facilities.* Washington, DC, National Council on Radiation Protection and Measurements, 1977.

14. Karzmark CJ, Capone T: Measurements of 6 MV x-rays. II. Characteristics of secondary radiation. *Br J Radiol* 41:224, 1968.

15. NCRP Report No. 40: *Protection against Radiation from Brachytherapy Sources.* Washington, DC, National Council on Radiation Protection and Measurements, 1972.

16. Axton E, Bardell A: Neutron production from electron accelerators used for medical purposes. *Phys Med Biol* 17:293, 1972.

17. Sohrabi M, Morgan KZ: Neutron dosimetry in high energy x-ray beams of medical accelerators. *Phys Med Biol* 24:756, 1979.

18. Price KW, Nath R, Holeman GR: Fast and thermal neutron profiles for a 25-MV x-ray beam. *Med Phys* 5:285, 1978.

19. NCRP Report No. 31: *Shielding for High-Energy Electron Accelerator Installations.* Washington, DC, National Committee on Radiation Protection and Measurements, 1964.

20. Deye JA, Young FC: Neutron production from a 10 MV medical linac. *Phys Med Biol* 22:90, 1977.

21. ICRP Report No. 4: *Protection against elecromagnetic radiation above 3 MeV and Electrons, Neutrons and Protons.* New York, International Commission on Radiological Protection, Pergamon Press, 1964.

22. Kersey R: Estimation of neutron and gamma radiation doses in the entrance mazes of SL 75-20 linear accelerator treatment rooms. *Medicamundi* 24:151, 1979 (Published by Philips Medical Systems, Inc, Shelton, CT).

23. Schulz RJ: Argon/propane ionization—chamber dosimetry for mixed x-ray/neutron fields. *Med Phys* 5:525, 1978.

24. Bading JR, Zeitz L, Laughlin JS: Phosphorus activation neutron dosimetry and its application to an 18-MV radiotherapy accelerator. *Med Phys* 9:835, 1982.

25. Rogers DWO, Van Dyk G: Use of a neutron remmeter to measure leakage neutrons from medical electron accelerators. *Med Phys* 8:163, 1981.

26. McCall RC, Jenkins TM, Shore RA: Transport of accelerator produced neutrons in a concrete room. *IEEE Trans Nucl Sci* NS-26:1593, 1979.

Appendix

Table A.1.

Ratios of average, restricted stopping powers for photon beams, $\Delta = 10$ keV

Nominal accelerating potential (MV)	$(\bar{L}/\rho)_{air}^{med}$							
	Water	Polystyrene	Acrylic	Graphite	A-150	C-552	Bakelite	Nylon
2	1.135	1.114	1.104	1.015	1.154	1.003	1.084	1.146
^{60}Co	1.134	1.113	1.103	1.012	1.151	1.000	1.081	1.142
4	1.131	1.108	1.099	1.007	1.146	0.996	1.075	1.136
6	1.127	1.103	1.093	1.002	1.141	0.992	1.070	1.129
8	1.121	1.097	1.088	0.995	1.135	0.987	1.063	1.120
10	1.117	1.094	1.085	0.992	1.130	0.983	1.060	1.114
15	1.106	1.083	1.074	0.982	1.119	0.972	1.051	1.097
20	1.096	1.074	1.065	0.977	1.109	0.963	1.042	1.087
25	1.093	1.071	1.062	0.968	1.106	0.960	1.038	1.084
35	1.084	1.062	1.053	0.958	1.098	0.952	1.027	1.074
45	1.071	1.048	1.041	0.939	1.087	0.942	1.006	1.061

Data are from J. R. Cunningham and R. J. Schulz, as published in Reference 1.

Table A.2.

Ratios of mass stopping powers and mass energy absorption coefficients for cobalt-60 γ rays

Chamber wall or buildup cap	$(\bar{L}/\rho)_{air}^{wall}$ ($\Delta = 10$ keV)	$(\bar{\mu}_{en}/\rho)_{wall}^{air}$
Polystyrene	1.112	0.928
Acrylic	1.103	0.925
Graphite	1.010	0.999
Water	1.133	0.899
A-150	1.145	0.906
Nylon	1.141	0.910
C-552	1.000	1.000
Bakelite	1.080	0.945

These data apply to ion chambers exposed in air and are from Johns and Cunningham (2).

Table A.3.

Stopping power ratios, $\left(\dfrac{L}{\rho}\right)_{air}^{water}$, for electron beams ($\Delta$ = 10 keV)

Depth (g/cm²)	Electron beam energy (MeV)																			
	60.0	50.0	40.0	30.0	25.0	20.0	18.0	16.0	14.0	12.0	10.0	9.0	8.0	7.0	6.0	5.0	4.0	3.0	2.0	1.0
0.0	0.902	0.904	0.912	0.928	0.940	0.955	0.961	0.969	0.977	0.986	0.997	1.003	1.011	1.019	1.029	1.040	1.059	1.078	1.097	1.116
0.1	0.902	0.905	0.913	0.929	0.941	0.955	0.962	0.969	0.978	0.987	0.998	1.005	1.012	1.020	1.030	1.042	1.061	1.081	1.101	1.124
0.2	0.903	0.906	0.914	0.930	0.942	0.956	0.963	0.970	0.978	0.988	0.999	1.006	1.013	1.022	1.032	1.044	1.064	1.084	1.106	1.131
0.3	0.904	0.907	0.915	0.931	0.943	0.957	0.964	0.971	0.979	0.989	1.000	1.007	1.015	1.024	1.034	1.046	1.067	1.089	1.112	1.135
0.4	0.904	0.908	0.916	0.932	0.944	0.958	0.965	0.972	0.980	0.990	1.002	1.009	1.017	1.026	1.036	1.050	1.071	1.093	1.117	1.136
0.5	0.905	0.909	0.917	0.933	0.945	0.959	0.966	0.973	0.982	0.991	1.003	1.010	1.019	1.028	1.039	1.054	1.076	1.098	1.122	
0.6	0.906	0.909	0.918	0.934	0.946	0.960	0.967	0.974	0.983	0.993	1.005	1.012	1.021	1.031	1.043	1.058	1.080	1.103	1.126	
0.8	0.907	0.911	0.920	0.936	0.948	0.962	0.969	0.976	0.985	0.996	1.009	1.016	1.026	1.037	1.050	1.067	1.090	1.113	1.133	
1.0	0.908	0.913	0.922	0.938	0.950	0.964	0.971	0.979	0.988	0.999	1.013	1.021	1.031	1.043	1.058	1.076	1.099	1.121		
1.2	0.909	0.914	0.924	0.940	0.952	0.966	0.973	0.981	0.991	1.002	1.017	1.026	1.037	1.050	1.066	1.085	1.108	1.129		
1.4	0.910	0.916	0.925	0.942	0.954	0.968	0.976	0.984	0.994	1.006	1.022	1.032	1.044	1.058	1.075	1.095	1.117	1.133		
1.6	0.912	0.917	0.927	0.944	0.956	0.971	0.978	0.987	0.997	1.010	1.027	1.038	1.050	1.066	1.084	1.104	1.124			
1.8	0.913	0.918	0.929	0.945	0.957	0.973	0.981	0.990	1.001	1.014	1.032	1.044	1.057	1.074	1.093	1.112	1.130			
2.0	0.914	0.920	0.930	0.947	0.959	0.975	0.983	0.993	1.004	1.018	1.038	1.050	1.065	1.082	1.101	1.120	1.133			
2.5	0.917	0.923	0.934	0.952	0.964	0.981	0.990	1.000	1.013	1.030	1.053	1.067	1.083	1.102	1.120	1.131				
3.0	0.919	0.926	0.938	0.956	0.969	0.987	0.997	1.008	1.023	1.042	1.069	1.084	1.102	1.119	1.129					
3.5	0.922	0.929	0.941	0.960	0.974	0.994	1.004	1.017	1.034	1.056	1.085	1.102	1.118	1.128						
4.0	0.924	0.932	0.944	0.964	0.979	1.001	1.012	1.027	1.046	1.071	1.101	1.116	1.126							
4.5	0.927	0.935	0.948	0.969	0.985	1.008	1.021	1.037	1.059	1.086	1.115	1.125	1.127							
5.0	0.929	0.938	0.951	0.973	0.990	1.016	1.030	1.049	1.072	1.101	1.123	1.126								
5.5	0.931	0.940	0.954	0.978	0.996	1.024	1.040	1.061	1.086	1.113	1.125									
6.0	0.934	0.943	0.958	0.983	1.002	1.033	1.051	1.074	1.100	1.121										
7.0	0.938	0.948	0.965	0.993	1.017	1.054	1.075	1.099	1.118	1.122										
8.0	0.943	0.954	0.972	1.005	1.032	1.076	1.098	1.116	1.120											
9.0	0.947	0.960	0.981	1.018	1.049	1.098	1.114	1.118												
10.0	0.952	0.966	0.990	1.032	1.068	1.112	1.116													
12.0	0.962	0.980	1.009	1.062	1.103															
14.0	0.973	0.996	1.031	1.095	1.107															
16.0	0.986	1.013	1.056	1.103																
18.0	1.000	1.031	1.080																	
20.0	1.016	1.051	1.094																	
22.0	1.032	1.070																		
24.0	1.048	1.082																		
26.0	1.062	1.085																		
28.0	1.071																			
30.0	1.075																			

Table is from Reference 1 which is based on data by M. Berger, Radiation Physics Division, Center for Radiation Research, National Bureau of Standards, Washington, D. C. 20234.

Table A.4.

Stopping power ratios, $\left(\dfrac{\bar{L}}{\rho}\right)_{air}^{polystyrene}$, for electron beams ($\Delta = 10$ keV)

Depth (g/cm²)	\multicolumn{20}{c}{Electron beam energy (MeV)}																			
	60.0	50.0	40.0	30.0	25.0	20.0	18.0	16.0	14.0	12.0	10.0	9.0	8.0	7.0	6.0	5.0	4.0	3.0	2.0	1.0
0.0	0.875	0.878	0.887	0.903	0.915	0.929	0.936	0.943	0.950	0.959	0.970	0.975	0.982	0.990	0.999	1.010	1.030	1.049	1.069	1.089
0.1	0.876	0.879	0.888	0.904	0.916	0.930	0.936	0.943	0.951	0.960	0.970	0.977	0.983	0.991	1.000	1.011	1.032	1.052	1.074	1.100
0.2	0.876	0.880	0.889	0.905	0.917	0.931	0.937	0.944	0.952	0.961	0.972	0.978	0.985	0.993	1.002	1.013	1.034	1.056	1.080	1.109
0.3	0.877	0.881	0.890	0.906	0.917	0.931	0.938	0.945	0.953	0.962	0.973	0.979	0.986	0.994	1.004	1.016	1.038	1.061	1.086	1.114
0.4	0.878	0.882	0.891	0.907	0.918	0.932	0.939	0.946	0.954	0.963	0.974	0.980	0.988	0.996	1.007	1.019	1.042	1.066	1.092	1.116
0.5	0.878	0.883	0.892	0.908	0.919	0.933	0.940	0.947	0.955	0.964	0.975	0.982	0.990	0.999	1.009	1.023	1.046	1.071	1.098	
0.6	0.879	0.883	0.893	0.909	0.920	0.934	0.941	0.948	0.956	0.965	0.977	0.984	0.992	1.001	1.012	1.027	1.051	1.076	1.103	
0.8	0.881	0.885	0.894	0.911	0.922	0.936	0.943	0.950	0.959	0.968	0.980	0.988	0.996	1.006	1.019	1.035	1.060	1.087	1.111	
1.0	0.882	0.887	0.896	0.912	0.924	0.938	0.945	0.952	0.961	0.971	0.984	0.992	1.001	1.012	1.026	1.044	1.070	1.096		
1.2	0.883	0.888	0.898	0.914	0.926	0.940	0.947	0.955	0.963	0.974	0.988	0.996	1.006	1.019	1.034	1.054	1.080	1.105		
1.4	0.884	0.889	0.900	0.916	0.927	0.942	0.949	0.957	0.966	0.978	0.992	1.001	1.012	1.026	1.043	1.064	1.089	1.111		
1.6	0.886	0.891	0.901	0.918	0.929	0.944	0.951	0.959	0.969	0.981	0.997	1.007	1.019	1.033	1.052	1.073	1.098			
1.8	0.887	0.892	0.903	0.919	0.931	0.946	0.954	0.962	0.972	0.985	1.002	1.012	1.025	1.041	1.060	1.083	1.106			
2.0	0.888	0.894	0.904	0.921	0.933	0.948	0.956	0.965	0.975	0.989	1.007	1.018	1.032	1.049	1.069	1.092	1.110			
2.5	0.891	0.897	0.908	0.925	0.937	0.954	0.962	0.972	0.984	0.999	1.020	1.034	1.050	1.070	1.091	1.108				
3.0	0.893	0.900	0.911	0.929	0.942	0.959	0.969	0.979	0.992	1.010	1.035	1.051	1.069	1.090	1.105					
3.5	0.896	0.903	0.914	0.933	0.947	0.965	0.975	0.987	1.002	1.023	1.051	1.069	1.088	1.103						
4.0	0.898	0.905	0.917	0.937	0.951	0.971	0.982	0.995	1.013	1.036	1.068	1.086	1.101							
4.5	0.900	0.908	0.920	0.941	0.956	0.978	0.990	1.005	1.024	1.051	1.085	1.099	1.105							
5.0	0.902	0.910	0.923	0.945	0.961	0.985	0.998	1.015	1.037	1.067	1.097	1.103								
5.5	0.904	0.913	0.927	0.949	0.966	0.992	1.008	1.026	1.051	1.081	1.102									
6.0	0.906	0.915	0.930	0.954	0.972	1.000	1.017	1.038	1.065	1.093										
7.0	0.910	0.920	0.936	0.963	0.984	1.018	1.040	1.063	1.089	1.100										
8.0	0.914	0.925	0.943	0.973	0.998	1.039	1.063	1.086	1.098											
9.0	0.918	0.930	0.950	0.985	1.013	1.061	1.084	1.095												
10.0	0.922	0.936	0.958	0.997	1.030	1.081	1.093													
12.0	0.931	0.949	0.976	1.024	1.067															
14.0	0.942	0.963	0.995	1.056	1.085															
16.0	0.953	0.978	1.016	1.078																
18.0	0.966	0.994	1.041																	
20.0	0.979	1.011	1.061																	
22.0	0.994	1.030																		
24.0	1.008	1.047																		
26.0	1.023	1.057																		
28.0	1.036																			
30.0	1.045																			

Table is from Reference 1 which is based on data by M. Berger, Radiation Physics Division, Center for Radiation Research, National Bureau of Standards, Washington, D. C. 20234.

Table A.5.

Stopping power ratios, $\left(\dfrac{L}{\rho}\right)^{acrylic}_{air}$, for electron beams ($\Delta$ = 10 keV)

Depth (g/cm²)	Electron beam energy (MeV)																			
	60.0	50.0	40.0	30.0	25.0	20.0	18.0	16.0	14.0	12.0	10.0	9.0	8.0	7.0	6.0	5.0	4.0	3.0	2.0	1.0
0.0	0.870	0.874	0.882	0.898	0.909	0.923	0.929	0.936	0.944	0.953	0.963	0.969	0.975	0.983	0.992	1.003	1.023	1.043	1.063	1.083
0.1	0.871	0.875	0.883	0.899	0.910	0.924	0.930	0.937	0.945	0.953	0.964	0.970	0.976	0.984	0.993	1.005	1.025	1.046	1.068	1.093
0.2	0.872	0.875	0.884	0.900	0.911	0.925	0.931	0.938	0.945	0.954	0.965	0.971	0.978	0.986	0.995	1.007	1.028	1.050	1.073	1.101
0.3	0.872	0.876	0.885	0.901	0.912	0.925	0.932	0.939	0.946	0.955	0.966	0.972	0.979	0.988	0.997	1.010	1.031	1.054	1.079	1.106
0.4	0.873	0.877	0.886	0.902	0.913	0.926	0.933	0.939	0.947	0.956	0.967	0.974	0.981	0.990	1.000	1.013	1.035	1.059	1.085	1.107
0.5	0.874	0.878	0.887	0.902	0.914	0.927	0.933	0.940	0.948	0.958	0.969	0.975	0.983	0.992	1.003	1.016	1.040	1.064	1.091	
0.6	0.875	0.879	0.888	0.903	0.915	0.928	0.934	0.941	0.949	0.959	0.970	0.977	0.985	0.994	1.006	1.020	1.044	1.069	1.095	
0.8	0.876	0.880	0.889	0.905	0.916	0.930	0.936	0.944	0.952	0.962	0.974	0.981	0.989	1.000	1.012	1.029	1.054	1.080	1.103	
1.0	0.877	0.882	0.891	0.907	0.918	0.932	0.938	0.946	0.954	0.964	0.977	0.985	0.994	1.006	1.020	1.038	1.064	1.089		
1.2	0.878	0.883	0.893	0.909	0.920	0.934	0.940	0.948	0.957	0.968	0.981	0.990	1.000	1.012	1.028	1.048	1.073	1.097		
1.4	0.880	0.885	0.894	0.910	0.922	0.936	0.943	0.951	0.960	0.971	0.986	0.995	1.006	1.020	1.037	1.057	1.083	1.103		
1.6	0.881	0.886	0.896	0.912	0.924	0.938	0.945	0.953	0.963	0.975	0.990	1.000	1.012	1.027	1.045	1.067	1.091			
1.8	0.882	0.887	0.897	0.914	0.926	0.940	0.947	0.956	0.966	0.978	0.995	1.006	1.019	1.035	1.054	1.076	1.098			
2.0	0.883	0.889	0.899	0.915	0.927	0.942	0.950	0.958	0.969	0.982	1.000	1.012	1.026	1.043	1.063	1.085	1.103			
2.5	0.886	0.892	0.902	0.919	0.932	0.948	0.956	0.965	0.977	0.992	1.014	1.028	1.044	1.063	1.085	1.101				
3.0	0.888	0.895	0.906	0.923	0.937	0.953	0.962	0.973	0.986	1.004	1.029	1.045	1.063	1.083	1.098					
3.5	0.891	0.898	0.909	0.927	0.941	0.959	0.968	0.980	0.996	1.016	1.045	1.063	1.082	1.096						
4.0	0.893	0.900	0.912	0.931	0.946	0.965	0.975	0.989	1.006	1.030	1.062	1.080	1.094							
4.5	0.895	0.903	0.915	0.935	0.951	0.971	0.983	0.998	1.018	1.045	1.079	1.092	1.097							
5.0	0.897	0.905	0.918	0.939	0.956	0.978	0.991	1.008	1.031	1.061	1.090	1.096								
5.5	0.900	0.908	0.921	0.943	0.962	0.986	1.000	1.020	1.045	1.075	1.095									
6.0	0.902	0.910	0.924	0.947	0.968	0.994	1.010	1.032	1.059	1.086										
7.0	0.905	0.915	0.930	0.957	0.981	1.012	1.033	1.058	1.083	1.092										
8.0	0.909	0.920	0.937	0.967	0.995	1.033	1.056	1.080	1.090											
9.0	0.913	0.925	0.945	0.979	1.011	1.055	1.077	1.088												
10.0	0.917	0.931	0.953	0.991	1.029	1.075	1.086													
12.0	0.926	0.943	0.970	1.018	1.067															
14.0	0.937	0.957	0.989	1.051	1.076															
16.0	0.948	0.973	1.011	1.071																
18.0	0.961	0.989	1.036																	
20.0	0.974	1.006	1.055																	
22.0	0.989	1.025																		
24.0	1.004	1.042																		
26.0	1.019	1.050																		
28.0	1.031																			
30.0	1.039																			

Table is from Reference 1 which is based on data by M. Berger, Radiation Physics Division, Center for Radiation Research, National Bureau of Standards, Washington, D. C. 20234.

Table A.6.

Ratios of mean mass-energy absorption coefficients, $\left(\dfrac{\bar{\mu}_{en}}{\rho}\right)^{med}_{air}$ for various materials

Nominal accelerating potential (MV)	$(\bar{\mu}_{en}/\rho)^{med}_{air}$							
	Water	Polystyrene	Acrylic	Graphite	A-150	C-552	Bakelite	Nylon
2	1.111	1.072	1.078	0.992	1.100	1.000	1.051	1.090
[60]Co-6	1.111	1.072	1.078	0.997	1.099	1.000	1.055	1.092
8	1.109	1.068	1.075	0.997	1.092	0.998	1.052	1.090
10	1.108	1.066	1.072	0.995	1.089	0.997	1.049	1.087
15	1.105	1.053	1.063	0.986	1.078	0.995	1.039	1.075
20	1.094	1.038	1.051	0.975	1.065	0.992	1.027	1.061
25	1.092	1.032	1.047	0.971	1.060	0.991	1.022	1.055
35	1.085	1.016	1.034	0.960	1.044	0.989	1.009	1.039
45	1.074	0.980	1.009	0.937	1.010	0.983	0.982	1.000

The data are applicable to ionization measurements made in phantom. The table is from Reference 1 which is based on data from Johns and Cunningham (2).

Table A.7.
Photon mass attenuation coefficients, μ/ρ, and mass energy-absorption coefficients, μ_{en}/ρ, in m^2/kg for energies 1 keV to 20 MeV (multiply m^2/kg by 10 to convert to cm^2/g). The numbers following the + or − refer to the power of 10. For example, first entry 3.617 + 02 should be read as 3.617×10^2.

Photon energy (eV)	Air, dry $\bar{Z} = 7.78$ $\rho = 1.205$ kg/m³ (20°C) 3.006×10^{26} e/kg		Water $\bar{Z} = 7.51$ $\rho = 1000$ kg/m³ 3.343×10^{26} e/kg		Muscle $\bar{Z} = 7.64$ $\rho = 1040$ kg/m³ 3.312×10^{26} e/kg	
	μ/ρ	μ_{en}/ρ	μ/ρ	μ_{en}/ρ	μ/ρ	μ_{en}/ρ
1.0 + 03	3.617 + 02	3.616 + 02	4.091 + 02	4.089 + 02	3.774 + 02	3.772 + 02
1.5 + 03	1.202 + 02	1.201 + 02	1.390 + 02	1.388 + 02	1.275 + 02	1.273 + 02
2.0 + 03	5.303 + 01	5.291 + 01	6.187 + 01	6.175 + 01	5.663 + 01	5.651 + 01
3.0 + 03	1.617 + 01	1.608 + 01	1.913 + 01	1.903 + 01	1.828 + 01	1.813 + 01
4.0 + 03	7.751 + 00	7.597 + 00	8.174 + 00	8.094 + 00	8.085 + 00	7.963 + 00
5.0 + 03	3.994 + 00	3.896 + 00	4.196 + 00	4.129 + 00	4.174 + 00	4.090 + 00
6.0 + 03	2.312 + 00	2.242 + 00	2.421 + 00	2.363 + 00	2.421 + 00	2.354 + 00
8.0 + 03	9.721 − 01	9.246 − 01	1.018 + 00	9.726 − 01	1.024 + 00	9.770 − 01
1.0 + 04	5.016 − 01	4.640 − 01	5.223 − 01	4.840 − 01	5.284 − 01	4.895 − 01
1.5 + 04	1.581 − 01	1.300 − 01	1.639 − 01	1.340 − 01	1.668 − 01	1.371 − 01
2.0 + 04	7.643 − 02	5.255 − 02	7.958 − 02	5.367 − 02	8.099 − 02	5.531 − 02
3.0 + 04	3.501 − 02	1.501 − 02	3.718 − 02	1.520 − 02	3.754 − 02	1.579 − 02
4.0 + 04	2.471 − 02	6.694 − 03	2.668 − 02	6.803 − 03	2.674 − 02	7.067 − 03
5.0 + 04	2.073 − 02	4.031 − 03	2.262 − 02	4.155 − 03	2.257 − 02	4.288 − 03
6.0 + 04	1.871 − 02	3.004 − 03	2.055 − 02	3.152 − 03	2.045 − 02	3.224 − 03
8.0 + 04	1.661 − 02	2.393 − 03	1.835 − 02	2.583 − 03	1.822 − 02	2.601 − 03
1.0 + 05	1.541 − 02	2.318 − 03	1.707 − 02	2.539 − 03	1.693 − 02	2.538 − 03
1.5 + 05	1.356 − 02	2.494 − 03	1.504 − 02	2.762 − 03	1.491 − 02	2.743 − 03
2.0 + 05	1.234 − 02	2.672 − 03	1.370 − 02	2.966 − 03	1.358 − 02	2.942 − 03
3.0 + 05	1.068 − 02	2.872 − 03	1.187 − 02	3.192 − 03	1.176 − 02	3.164 − 03
4.0 + 05	9.548 − 03	2.949 − 03	1.061 − 02	3.279 − 03	1.052 − 02	3.250 − 03
5.0 + 05	8.712 − 03	2.966 − 03	9.687 − 03	3.299 − 03	9.599 − 03	3.269 − 03
6.0 + 05	8.056 − 03	2.953 − 03	8.957 − 03	3.284 − 03	8.876 − 03	3.254 − 03
8.0 + 05	7.075 − 03	2.882 − 03	7.866 − 03	3.205 − 03	7.795 − 03	3.176 − 03
1.0 + 06	6.359 − 03	2.787 − 03	7.070 − 03	3.100 − 03	7.006 − 03	3.072 − 03
1.5 + 06	5.176 − 03	2.545 − 03	5.755 − 03	2.831 − 03	5.702 − 03	2.805 − 03
2.0 + 06	4.447 − 03	2.342 − 03	4.940 − 03	2.604 − 03	4.895 − 03	2.580 − 03
3.0 + 06	3.581 − 03	2.054 − 03	3.969 − 03	2.278 − 03	3.932 − 03	2.257 − 03
4.0 + 06	3.079 − 03	1.866 − 03	3.403 − 03	2.063 − 03	3.370 − 03	2.043 − 03
5.0 + 06	2.751 − 03	1.737 − 03	3.031 − 03	1.913 − 03	3.001 − 03	1.894 − 03
6.0 + 06	2.523 − 03	1.644 − 03	2.771 − 03	1.804 − 03	2.743 − 03	1.785 − 03
8.0 + 06	2.225 − 03	1.521 − 03	2.429 − 03	1.657 − 03	2.403 − 03	1.639 − 03
1.0 + 07	2.045 − 03	1.446 − 03	2.219 − 03	1.566 − 03	2.195 − 03	1.548 − 03
1.5 + 07	1.810 − 03	1.349 − 03	1.941 − 03	1.442 − 03	1.918 − 03	1.424 − 03
2.0 + 07	1.705 − 03	1.308 − 03	1.813 − 03	1.386 − 03	1.790 − 03	1.367 − 03

Data are from Hubbell (3).

Table A.7 continued

	Fat		Bone		Polystyrene (C_8H_8)	
	$\bar{Z} = 6.46$		$\bar{Z} = 12.31$		$\bar{Z} = 5.74$	
	$\rho = 920$ kg/m^3		$\rho = 1850$ kg/m^3		$\rho = 1046$ kg/m^3	
	3.34×10^{26} e/kg		3.192×10^{26} e/kg		3.238×10^{26} e/kg	
	μ/ρ	μ_{en}/ρ	μ/ρ	μ_{en}/ρ	μ/ρ	μ_{en}/ρ
	2.517 + 02	2.516 + 02	3.394 + 02	3.392 + 02	2.047 + 02	2.046 + 02
	8.066 + 01	8.055 + 01	1.148 + 02	1.146 + 02	6.227 + 01	6.219 + 01
	3.535 + 01	3.526 + 01	5.148 + 01	5.133 + 01	2.692 + 01	2.683 + 01
	1.100 + 01	1.090 + 01	2.347 + 01	2.303 + 01	8.041 + 00	7.976 + 00
	4.691 + 00	4.621 + 00	1.045 + 01	1.025 + 01	3.364 + 00	3.312 + 00
	2.401 + 00	2.345 + 00	1.335 + 01	1.227 + 01	1.704 + 00	1.659 + 00
	1.386 + 00	1.338 + 00	8.129 + 00	7.531 + 00	9.783 − 01	9.375 − 01
	5.853 − 01	5.474 − 01	3.676 + 00	3.435 + 00	4.110 − 01	3.773 − 01
	3.048 − 01	2.716 − 01	1.966 + 00	1.841 + 00	2.150 − 01	1.849 − 01
	1.022 − 01	7.499 − 02	6.243 − 01	5.726 − 01	7.551 − 02	5.014 − 02
	5.437 − 02	3.014 − 02	2.797 − 01	2.450 − 01	4.290 − 02	2.002 − 02
	3.004 − 02	8.881 − 03	9.724 − 02	7.290 − 02	2.621 − 02	6.059 − 03
	2.377 − 02	4.344 − 03	5.168 − 02	3.088 − 02	2.177 − 02	3.191 − 03
	2.118 − 02	2.980 − 03	3.504 − 02	1.625 − 02	1.982 − 02	2.387 − 03
	1.974 − 02	2.514 − 03	2.741 − 02	9.988 − 03	1.868 − 02	2.153 − 03
	1.805 − 02	2.344 − 03	2.083 − 02	5.309 − 03	1.724 − 02	2.152 − 03
	1.694 − 02	2.434 − 03	1.800 − 02	3.838 − 03	1.624 − 02	2.293 − 03
	1.506 − 02	2.747 − 03	1.490 − 02	3.032 − 03	1.448 − 02	2.631 − 03
	1.374 − 02	2.972 − 03	1.332 − 02	2.994 − 03	1.322 − 02	2.856 − 03
	1.192 − 02	3.209 − 03	1.141 − 02	3.095 − 03	1.147 − 02	3.088 − 03
	1.067 − 02	3.298 − 03	1.018 − 02	3.151 − 03	1.027 − 02	3.174 − 03
	9.740 − 03	3.318 − 03	9.274 − 03	3.159 − 03	9.376 − 03	3.194 − 03
	9.008 − 03	3.304 − 03	8.570 − 03	3.140 − 03	8.672 − 03	3.181 − 03
	7.912 − 03	3.226 − 03	7.520 − 03	3.061 − 03	7.617 − 03	3.106 − 03
	7.112 − 03	3.121 − 03	6.758 − 03	2.959 − 03	6.847 − 03	3.005 − 03
	5.787 − 03	2.850 − 03	5.501 − 03	2.700 − 03	5.571 − 03	2.744 − 03
	4.963 − 03	2.619 − 03	4.732 − 03	2.487 − 03	4.778 − 03	2.522 − 03
	3.972 − 03	2.282 − 03	3.826 − 03	2.191 − 03	3.822 − 03	2.196 − 03
	3.390 − 03	2.055 − 03	3.307 − 03	2.002 − 03	3.261 − 03	1.977 − 03
	3.005 − 03	1.894 − 03	2.970 − 03	1.874 − 03	2.889 − 03	1.820 − 03
	2.732 − 03	1.775 − 03	2.738 − 03	1.784 − 03	2.626 − 03	1.706 − 03
	2.371 − 03	1.613 − 03	2.440 − 03	1.667 − 03	2.227 − 03	1.548 − 03
	2.147 − 03	1.508 − 03	2.263 − 03	1.598 − 03	2.060 − 03	1.446 − 03
	1.840 − 03	1.361 − 03	2.040 − 03	1.508 − 03	1.763 − 03	1.304 − 03
	1.693 − 03	1.290 − 03	1.948 − 03	1.474 − 03	1.620 − 03	1.234 − 03

Table A.7 continued

Photon energy (eV)	Lucite ($C_5H_8O_2$) $\bar{Z} = 6.56$ $\rho = 1180$ kg/m³ 3.248×10^{26} e/kg		Lithium fluoride (LiF) $\bar{Z} = 8.31$ $\rho = 2635$ kg/m³ 2.786×10^{26} e/kg		Carbon $\bar{Z} = 6$ $\rho = 2265$ kg/m³ 3.008×10^{26} e/kg	
	μ/ρ	μ_{en}/ρ	μ/ρ	μ_{en}/ρ	μ/ρ	μ_{en}/ρ
1.0 + 03	2.803 + 02	2.802 + 02	4.096 + 02	4.095 + 02	2.218 + 02	2.217 + 02
1.5 + 03	9.051 + 01	9.039 + 01	1.432 + 02	1.431 + 02	6.748 + 01	6.739 + 01
2.0 + 03	3.977 + 01	3.967 + 01	6.540 + 01	6.529 + 01	2.917 + 01	2.908 + 01
3.0 + 03	1.211 + 01	1.203 + 01	2.086 + 01	2.076 + 01	8.711 + 00	8.644 + 00
4.0 + 03	5.129 + 00	5.066 + 00	9.072 + 00	8.991 + 00	3.643 + 00	3.589 + 00
5.0 + 03	2.618 + 00	2.565 + 00	4.705 + 00	4.639 + 00	1.844 + 00	1.798 + 00
6.0 + 03	1.507 + 00	1.460 + 00	2.739 + 00	2.682 + 00	1.057 + 00	1.016 + 00
8.0 + 03	6.331 − 01	5.953 + 01	1.161 + 00	1.117 + 00	4.422 − 01	4.089 − 01
1.0 + 04	3.273 − 01	2.944 − 01	5.970 − 01	5.607 − 01	2.298 − 01	2.003 − 01
1.5 + 04	1.077 − 01	8.083 − 02	1.847 − 01	1.576 − 01	7.869 − 02	5.425 − 02
2.0 + 04	5.616 − 02	3.232 − 02	8.646 − 02	6.352 − 02	4.340 − 02	2.159 − 02
3.0 + 04	3.006 − 02	9.391 − 03	3.687 − 02	1.788 − 02	2.541 − 02	6.411 − 03
4.0 + 04	2.340 − 02	4.500 − 03	2.471 − 02	7.742 − 03	2.069 − 02	3.265 − 03
5.0 + 04	2.069 − 02	3.020 − 03	2.012 − 02	4.470 − 03	1.867 − 02	2.360 − 03
6.0 + 04	1.921 − 02	2.504 − 03	1.787 − 02	3.184 − 03	1.751 − 02	2.078 − 03
8.0 + 04	1.750 − 02	2.292 − 03	1.562 − 02	2.370 − 03	1.609 − 02	2.029 − 03
1.0 + 05	1.640 − 02	2.363 − 03	1.440 − 02	2.222 − 03	1.513 − 02	2.144 − 03
1.5 + 05	1.456 − 02	2.656 − 03	1.260 − 02	2.330 − 03	1.347 − 02	2.448 − 03
2.0 + 05	1.328 − 02	2.872 − 03	1.145 − 02	2.483 − 03	1.229 − 02	2.655 − 03
3.0 + 05	1.152 − 02	3.099 − 03	9.898 − 03	2.663 − 03	1.066 − 02	2.869 − 03
4.0 + 05	1.031 − 02	3.185 − 03	8.852 − 03	2.734 − 03	9.545 − 03	2.949 − 03
5.0 + 05	9.408 − 03	3.204 − 03	8.076 − 03	2.749 − 03	8.712 − 03	2.967 − 03
6.0 + 05	8.701 − 03	3.191 − 03	7.468 − 03	2.736 − 03	8.058 − 03	2.955 − 03
8.0 + 05	7.642 − 03	3.115 − 03	6.557 − 03	2.670 − 03	7.077 − 03	2.885 − 03
1.0 + 06	6.869 − 03	3.014 − 03	5.893 − 03	2.583 − 03	6.362 − 03	2.791 − 03
1.5 + 06	5.590 − 03	2.751 − 03	4.797 − 03	2.358 − 03	5.177 − 03	2.548 − 03
2.0 + 06	4.796 − 03	2.530 − 03	4.122 − 03	2.170 − 03	4.443 − 03	2.343 − 03
3.0 + 06	3.844 − 03	2.207 − 03	3.320 − 03	1.904 − 03	3.562 − 03	2.045 − 03
4.0 + 06	3.286 − 03	1.992 − 03	2.856 − 03	1.731 − 03	3.047 − 03	1.847 − 03
5.0 + 06	2.919 − 03	1.840 − 03	2.554 − 03	1.612 − 03	2.708 − 03	1.707 − 03
6.0 + 06	2.659 − 03	1.729 − 03	2.343 − 03	1.527 − 03	2.469 − 03	1.605 − 03
8.0 + 06	2.317 − 03	1.578 − 03	2.069 − 03	1.414 − 03	2.154 − 03	1.467 − 03
1.0 + 07	2.105 − 03	1.481 − 03	1.903 − 03	1.345 − 03	1.960 − 03	1.379 − 03
1.5 + 07	1.819 − 03	1.348 − 03	1.687 − 03	1.254 − 03	1.698 − 03	1.259 − 03
2.0 + 07	1.684 − 03	1.285 − 03	1.592 − 03	1.217 − 03	1.575 − 03	1.203 − 03

Table A.7 continued

Aluminum $\bar{Z} = 13$ $\rho = 2699$ kg/m³ 2.902×10^{26} e/kg		Copper $\bar{Z} = 29$ $\rho = 8960$ kg/m³ 2.749×10^{26} e/kg		Lead $\bar{Z} = 82$ $\rho = 1135$ kg/m³ 2.383×10^{26} e/kg	
μ/ρ	μ_{en}/ρ	μ/ρ	μ_{en}/ρ	μ/ρ	μ_{en}/ρ
1.076 + 02	1.074 + 02	1.003 + 03	1.002 + 03	5.210 + 02	5.198 + 02
3.683 + 01	3.663 + 01	4.223 + 02	4.219 + 02	2.356 + 02	2.344 + 02
2.222 + 02	2.164 + 02	2.063 + 02	2.059 + 02	1.285 + 02	1.274 + 02
7.746 + 01	7.599 + 01	7.198 + 01	7.158 + 01	1.965 + 02	1.954 + 02
3.545 + 01	3.487 + 01	3.347 + 01	3.313 + 01	1.251 + 02	1.242 + 02
1.902 + 01	1.870 + 01	1.834 + 01	1.804 + 01	7.304 + 01	7.222 + 01
1.134 + 01	1.115 + 01	1.118 + 01	1.092 + 01	4.672 + 01	4.598 + 01
4.953 + 00	4.849 + 00	5.099 + 00	4.905 + 00	2.287 + 01	2.226 + 01
2.582 + 00	2.495 + 00	2.140 + 01	1.514 + 00	1.306 + 01	1.256 + 01
7.836 − 01	7.377 − 01	7.343 + 00	5.853 + 00	1.116 + 01	8.939 + 00
3.392 − 01	3.056 − 01	3.352 + 00	2.810 + 00	8.636 + 00	6.923 + 00
1.115 − 01	8.646 − 02	1.083 + 00	9.382 − 01	3.032 + 00	2.550 + 00
5.630 − 02	3.556 − 02	4.828 − 01	4.173 − 01	1.436 + 00	1.221 + 00
3.655 − 02	1.816 − 02	2.595 − 01	2.196 − 01	8.041 − 01	6.796 − 01
2.763 − 02	1.087 − 02	1.583 − 01	1.290 − 01	5.020 − 01	4.177 − 01
2.012 − 02	5.464 − 03	7.587 − 02	5.593 − 02	2.419 − 01	1.936 − 01
1.701 − 02	3.773 − 03	4.563 − 02	2.952 − 02	5.550 − 01	2.229 − 01
1.378 − 02	2.823 − 03	2.210 − 02	1.030 − 02	2.014 − 01	1.135 − 01
1.223 − 02	2.745 − 03	1.557 − 02	5.811 − 03	9.985 − 02	6.229 − 02
1.042 − 02	2.817 − 03	1.118 − 02	3.636 − 03	4.026 − 02	2.581 − 02
9.276 − 03	2.863 − 03	9.409 − 03	3.135 − 03	2.323 − 02	1.439 − 02
8.446 − 03	2.870 − 03	8.360 − 03	2.943 − 03	1.613 − 02	9.564 − 03
7.801 − 03	2.851 − 03	7.624 − 03	2.835 − 03	1.248 − 02	7.132 − 03
6.842 − 03	2.778 − 03	6.605 − 03	2.686 − 03	8.869 − 03	4.838 − 03
6.146 − 03	2.684 − 03	5.900 − 03	2.563 − 03	7.103 − 03	3.787 − 03
5.007 − 03	2.447 − 03	4.803 − 03	2.313 − 03	5.222 − 03	2.714 − 03
4.324 − 03	2.261 − 03	4.204 − 03	2.156 − 03	4.607 − 03	2.407 − 03
3.541 − 03	2.018 − 03	3.599 − 03	2.016 − 03	4.234 − 03	2.351 − 03
3.107 − 03	1.877 − 03	3.318 − 03	1.981 − 03	4.197 − 03	2.463 − 03
2.836 − 03	1.790 − 03	3.176 − 03	1.991 − 03	4.272 − 03	2.600 − 03
2.655 − 03	1.735 − 03	3.108 − 03	2.019 − 03	4.391 − 03	2.730 − 03
2.437 − 03	1.674 − 03	3.074 − 03	2.092 − 03	4.675 − 03	2.948 − 03
2.318 − 03	1.645 − 03	3.103 − 03	2.165 − 03	4.972 − 03	3.114 − 03
2.195 − 03	1.626 − 03	3.247 − 03	2.286 − 03	5.658 − 03	3.353 − 03
2.168 − 03	1.637 − 03	3.408 − 03	2.384 − 03	6.205 − 03	3.440 − 03

Table A.8.

Collision mass stopping powers, S/ρ, in MeV cm^2/g, for electrons in various materials. The numbers following the E + or E − refer to the power of 10. For example, first entry 2.014 E + 01 should be read as 2.014×10^1.

Electron energy (MeV)	Carbon	Air	Water	Muscle	Fat
0.0100	2.014E + 01	1.975E + 01	2.256E + 01	2.237E + 01	2.347E + 01
0.0125	1.694E + 01	1.663E + 01	1.897E + 01	1.881E + 01	1.971E + 01
0.0150	1.471E + 01	1.445E + 01	1.647E + 01	1.633E + 01	1.709E + 01
0.0175	1.305E + 01	1.283E + 01	1.461E + 01	1.449E + 01	1.515E + 01
0.0200	1.177E + 01	1.157E + 01	1.317E + 01	1.306E + 01	1.365E + 01
0.0250	9.911E + 00	9.753E + 00	1.109E + 01	1.100E + 01	1.148E + 01
0.0300	8.624E + 00	8.492E + 00	9.653E + 00	9.571E + 01	9.984E + 00
0.0350	7.677E + 00	7.563E + 00	8.592E + 00	8.519E + 00	8.881E + 00
0.0400	6.948E + 00	6.848E + 00	7.777E + 00	7.711E + 00	8.034E + 00
0.0450	6.370E + 00	6.281E + 00	7.130E + 00	7.069E + 00	7.362E + 00
0.0500	5.899E + 00	5.819E + 00	6.603E + 00	6.547E + 00	6.816E + 00
0.0550	5.508E + 00	5.435E + 00	6.166E + 00	6.113E + 00	6.362E + 00
0.0600	5.177E + 00	5.111E + 00	5.797E + 00	5.747E + 00	5.979E + 00
0.0700	4.650E + 00	4.593E + 00	5.207E + 00	5.163E + 00	5.369E + 00
0.0800	4.247E + 00	4.198E + 00	4.757E + 00	4.717E + 00	4.903E + 00
0.0900	3.929E + 00	3.886E + 00	4.402E + 00	4.365E + 00	4.535E + 00
0.1000	3.671E + 00	3.633E + 00	4.115E + 00	4.080E + 00	4.238E + 00
0.1250	3.201E + 00	3.172E + 00	3.591E + 00	3.561E + 00	3.696E + 00
0.1500	2.883E + 00	2.861E + 00	3.238E + 00	3.210E + 00	3.330E + 00
0.1750	2.654E + 00	2.637E + 00	2.984E + 00	2.958E + 00	3.068E + 00
0.2000	2.482E + 00	2.470E + 00	2.793E + 00	2.769E + 00	2.871E + 00
0.2500	2.241E + 00	2.236E + 00	2.528E + 00	2.506E + 00	2.597E + 00
0.3000	2.083E + 00	2.084E + 00	2.355E + 00	2.335E + 00	2.418E + 00
0.3500	1.972E + 00	1.978E + 00	2.233E + 00	2.215E + 00	2.294E + 00
0.4000	1.891E + 00	1.902E + 00	2.145E + 00	2.129E + 00	2.204E + 00
0.4500	1.830E + 00	1.845E + 00	2.079E + 00	2.065E + 00	2.135E + 00
0.5000	1.782E + 00	1.802E + 00	2.028E + 00	2.016E + 00	2.081E + 00
0.5500	1.745E + 00	1.769E + 00	1.988E + 00	1.976E + 00	2.039E + 00
0.6000	1.716E + 00	1.743E + 00	1.956E + 00	1.945E + 00	2.005E + 00
0.7000	1.672E + 00	1.706E + 00	1.910E + 00	1.898E + 00	1.954E + 00
0.8000	1.643E + 00	1.683E + 00	1.879E + 00	1.866E + 00	1.921E + 00
0.9000	1.623E + 00	1.669E + 00	1.858E + 00	1.845E + 00	1.897E + 00
1.0000	1.609E + 00	1.661E + 00	1.844E + 00	1.830E + 00	1.880E + 00
1.2500	1.590E + 00	1.655E + 00	1.825E + 00	1.809E + 00	1.858E + 00
1.5000	1.584E + 00	1.661E + 00	1.820E + 00	1.802E + 00	1.849E + 00
1.7500	1.584E + 00	1.672E + 00	1.821E + 00	1.801E + 00	1.848E + 00
2.0000	1.587E + 00	1.684E + 00	1.825E + 00	1.804E + 00	1.850E + 00
2.5000	1.598E + 00	1.712E + 00	1.837E + 00	1.814E + 00	1.860E + 00
3.0000	1.611E + 00	1.740E + 00	1.850E + 00	1.826E + 00	1.872E + 00
3.5000	1.623E + 00	1.766E + 00	1.864E + 00	1.839E + 00	1.885E + 00
4.0000	1.636E + 00	1.790E + 00	1.877E + 00	1.851E + 00	1.897E + 00
4.5000	1.647E + 00	1.812E + 00	1.889E + 00	1.862E + 00	1.909E + 00
5.0000	1.658E + 00	1.833E + 00	1.900E + 00	1.873E + 00	1.920E + 00
5.5000	1.667E + 00	1.852E + 00	1.910E + 00	1.883E + 00	1.930E + 00
6.0000	1.676E + 00	1.870E + 00	1.919E + 00	1.892E + 00	1.939E + 00
7.0000	1.693E + 00	1.902E + 00	1.936E + 00	1.909E + 00	1.956E + 00
8.0000	1.707E + 00	1.931E + 00	1.951E + 00	1.924E + 00	1.972E + 00
9.0000	1.719E + 00	1.956E + 00	1.964E + 00	1.937E + 00	1.985E + 00
10.0000	1.730E + 00	1.979E + 00	1.976E + 00	1.949E + 00	1.997E + 00
12.5000	1.753E + 00	2.029E + 00	2.000E + 00	1.974E + 00	2.022E + 00
15.0000	1.770E + 00	2.069E + 00	2.020E + 00	1.995E + 00	2.042E + 00
17.5000	1.785E + 00	2.104E + 00	2.037E + 00	2.012E + 00	2.059E + 00
20.0000	1.797E + 00	2.134E + 00	2.051E + 00	2.026E + 00	2.073E + 00
25.0000	1.816E + 00	2.185E + 00	2.074E + 00	2.050E + 00	2.095E + 00
30.0000	1.832E + 00	2.226E + 00	2.092E + 00	2.068E + 00	2.113E + 00
35.0000	1.845E + 00	2.257E + 00	2.107E + 00	2.084E + 00	2.128E + 00
40.0000	1.856E + 00	2.282E + 00	2.120E + 00	2.097E + 00	2.141E + 00
45.0000	1.865E + 00	2.302E + 00	2.131E + 00	2.108E + 00	2.152E + 00
50.0000	1.874E + 00	2.319E + 00	2.141E + 00	2.118E + 00	2.161E + 00
55.0000	1.881E + 00	2.334E + 00	2.149E + 00	2.126E + 00	2.170E + 00
60.0000	1.888E + 00	2.347E + 00	2.157E + 00	2.134E + 00	2.178E + 00
70.0000	1.900E + 00	2.369E + 00	2.171E + 00	2.148E + 00	2.192E + 00
80.0000	1.911E + 00	2.387E + 00	2.183E + 00	2.160E + 00	2.203E + 00
90.0000	1.920E + 00	2.403E + 00	2.194E + 00	2.171E + 00	2.214E + 00

From Berger and Seltzer (4).

Table A.8 continued

Bone	Polystyrene	Lucite	Aluminum	Lead
2.068E + 01	2.223E + 01	2.198E + 01	1.649E + 01	8.428E + 00
1.742E + 01	1.868E + 01	1.848E + 01	1.398E + 01	7.357E + 00
1.514E + 01	1.621E + 01	1.604E + 01	1.220E + 01	6.561E + 00
1.344E + 01	1.437E + 01	1.423E + 01	1.088E + 01	5.946E + 00
1.213E + 01	1.296E + 01	1.283E + 01	9.845E + 00	5.453E + 00
1.023E + 01	1.091E + 01	1.080E + 01	8.339E + 00	4.714E + 00
8.912E + 00	9.485E + 00	9.400E + 00	7.288E + 00	4.182E + 00
7.939E + 00	8.440E + 00	8.367E + 00	6.510E + 00	3.779E + 00
7.190E + 00	7.637E + 00	7.573E + 00	5.909E + 00	3.463E + 00
6.596E + 00	7.000E + 00	6.942E + 00	5.431E + 00	3.208E + 00
6.112E + 00	6.481E + 00	6.429E + 00	5.040E + 00	2.997E + 00
5.709E + 00	6.051E + 00	6.003E + 00	4.715E + 00	2.821E + 00
5.370E + 00	5.688E + 00	5.644E + 00	4.439E + 00	2.670E + 00
4.827E + 00	5.108E + 00	5.070E + 00	3.999E + 00	2.426E + 00
4.412E + 00	4.666E + 00	4.631E + 00	3.661E + 00	2.237E + 00
4.085E + 00	4.317E + 00	4.286E + 00	3.394E + 00	2.087E + 00
3.820E + 00	4.034E + 00	4.006E + 00	3.178E + 00	1.964E + 00
3.336E + 00	3.520E + 00	3.496E + 00	2.782E + 00	1.738E + 00
3.010E + 00	3.172E + 00	3.152E + 00	2.514E + 00	1.583E + 00
2.775E + 00	2.923E + 00	2.904E + 00	2.320E + 00	1.471E + 00
2.599E + 00	2.735E + 00	2.719E + 00	2.175E + 00	1.387E + 00
2.354E + 00	2.475E + 00	2.461E + 00	1.973E + 00	1.269E + 00
2.194E + 00	2.305E + 00	2.292E + 00	1.840E + 00	1.193E + 00
2.079E + 00	2.187E + 00	2.175E + 00	1.748E + 00	1.140E + 00
1.996E + 00	2.101E + 00	2.090E + 00	1.681E + 00	1.102E + 00
1.932E + 00	2.035E + 00	2.026E + 00	1.631E + 00	1.074E + 00
1.883E + 00	1.984E + 00	1.975E + 00	1.594E + 00	1.053E + 00
1.845E + 00	1.943E + 00	1.935E + 00	1.564E + 00	1.037E + 00
1.815E + 00	1.911E + 00	1.903E + 00	1.541E + 00	1.026E + 00
1.770E + 00	1.864E + 00	1.856E + 00	1.508E + 00	1.009E + 00
1.740E + 00	1.832E + 00	1.825E + 00	1.487E + 00	1.000E + 00
1.719E + 00	1.810E + 00	1.803E + 00	1.474E + 00	9.957E − 01
1.705E + 00	1.794E + 00	1.788E + 00	1.466E + 00	9.939E − 01
1.686E + 00	1.773E + 00	1.767E + 00	1.458E + 00	9.966E − 01
1.680E + 00	1.766E + 00	1.760E + 00	1.460E + 00	1.004E + 00
1.681E + 00	1.765E + 00	1.759E + 00	1.467E + 00	1.014E + 00
1.684E + 00	1.768E + 00	1.762E + 00	1.475E + 00	1.024E + 00
1.696E + 00	1.778E + 00	1.772E + 00	1.492E + 00	1.044E + 00
1.709E + 00	1.791E + 00	1.784E + 00	1.509E + 00	1.063E + 00
1.722E + 00	1.804E + 00	1.797E + 00	1.525E + 00	1.080E + 00
1.735E + 00	1.816E + 00	1.809E + 00	1.539E + 00	1.095E + 00
1.747E + 00	1.828E + 00	1.821E + 00	1.552E + 00	1.108E + 00
1.758E + 00	1.839E + 00	1.832E + 00	1.563E + 00	1.120E + 00
1.768E + 00	1.849E + 00	1.842E + 00	1.574E + 00	1.132E + 00
1.778E + 00	1.859E + 00	1.851E + 00	1.583E + 00	1.142E + 00
1.795E + 00	1.876E + 00	1.868E + 00	1.600E + 00	1.160E + 00
1.810E + 00	1.891E + 00	1.883E + 00	1.614E + 00	1.175E + 00
1.823E + 00	1.904E + 00	1.896E + 00	1.627E + 00	1.189E + 00
1.835E + 00	1.916E + 00	1.908E + 00	1.638E + 00	1.201E + 00
1.860E + 00	1.940E + 00	1.932E + 00	1.661E + 00	1.226E + 00
1.879E + 00	1.960E + 00	1.952E + 00	1.679E + 00	1.246E + 00
1.896E + 00	1.975E + 00	1.968E + 00	1.694E + 00	1.262E + 00
1.909E + 00	1.989E + 00	1.982E + 00	1.707E + 00	1.277E + 00
1.931E + 00	2.010E + 00	2.004E + 00	1.728E + 00	1.299E + 00
1.949E + 00	2.027E + 00	2.022E + 00	1.744E + 00	1.318E + 00
1.963E + 00	2.041E + 00	2.036E + 00	1.758E + 00	1.332E + 00
1.976E + 00	2.053E + 00	2.049E + 00	1.770E + 00	1.345E + 00
1.986E + 00	2.064E + 00	2.059E + 00	1.780E + 00	1.356E + 00
1.996E + 00	2.073E + 00	2.069E + 00	1.789E + 00	1.365E + 00
2.004E + 00	2.081E + 00	2.077E + 00	1.797E + 00	1.374E + 00
2.012E + 00	2.089E + 00	2.085E + 00	1.804E + 00	1.381E + 00
2.025E + 00	2.102E + 00	2.098E + 00	1.816E + 00	1.395E + 00
2.037E + 00	2.113E + 00	2.109E + 00	1.827E + 00	1.406E + 00
2.047E + 00	2.123E + 00	2.120E + 00	1.837E + 00	1.415E + 00

Table A.9.1.
Cobalt-60 percent depth doses: 80 cm SSD*

Depth (cm)	Field size (cm) and backscatter factor (BSF)†									
	0 1.00	4 × 4 1.01$_4$	5 × 5 1.01$_7$	6 × 6 1.02$_1$	7 × 7 1.02$_5$	8 × 8 1.02$_9$	10 × 10 1.03$_6$	12 × 12 1.04$_3$	15 × 15 1.05$_2$	20 × 20 1.06$_1$
0.5	100.0	100.0	100.0	100.0	100.0	100.0	100.0	100.0	100.0	100.0
1	95.4	96.8	97.0	97.4	97.6	97.8	98.2	98.3	98.4	98.4
2	87.1	90.6	91.3	91.9	92.3	92.7	93.3	93.6	93.9	94.0
3	79.5	84.7	85.6	86.5	87.1	87.6	88.3	88.8	89.3	89.6
4	72.7	79.0	80.2	81.1	81.9	82.5	83.4	84.0	84.7	85.2
5	66.5	73.5	74.8	75.9	76.7	77.4	78.5	79.3	80.1	80.8
6	60.8	68.1	69.6	70.7	71.6	72.4	73.6	74.4	75.4	76.4
7	55.6	62.9	64.4	65.7	66.7	67.5	68.8	69.8	70.8	72.1
8	50.9	58.0	59.4	60.8	61.9	62.7	64.1	65.3	66.5	68.0
9	46.6	53.5	55.0	56.2	57.3	58.2	59.7	60.8	62.3	64.0
10	42.7	49.3	50.7	52.0	53.0	54.0	55.6	56.9	58.4	60.2
11	39.2	45.5	46.9	48.1	49.2	50.1	51.7	53.0	54.7	56.6
12	35.9	41.9	43.2	44.5	45.5	46.5	48.1	49.5	51.2	53.2
13	32.9	38.6	39.9	41.1	42.1	43.2	44.8	46.1	47.9	50.0
14	30.2	35.6	36.8	38.0	39.2	40.1	41.8	43.2	44.9	47.0
15	27.7	32.9	34.2	35.2	36.2	37.2	38.9	40.3	42.0	44.2
16	25.4	30.4	31.5	32.6	33.6	34.5	36.2	37.6	39.3	41.5
17	23.3	28.1	29.2	30.2	31.2	32.1	33.7	35.1	36.8	39.0
18	21.4	26.0	27.1	28.0	29.0	29.8	31.4	32.8	34.5	36.7
19	19.6	24.0	25.0	26.0	26.8	27.7	29.2	30.6	32.3	34.6
20	18.0	22.1	23.1	24.0	24.9	25.7	27.2	28.5	30.3	32.6
22	(15.3)	(18.9)	(19.8)	(20.6)	(21.4)	(22.1)	(23.7)	(24.9)	(26.5)	(28.8)
24	(12.9)	(16.1)	(16.9)	(17.7)	(18.4)	(19.1)	(20.5)	(21.8)	(23.2)	(25.4)
26	(10.8)	(13.7)	(14.4)	(15.1)	(15.8)	(16.5)	(17.8)	(18.9)	(20.4)	(22.5)
28	(9.1)	(11.7)	(12.3)	(12.9)	(13.6)	(14.2)	(15.5)	(16.5)	(17.9)	(19.9)
30	(7.7)	(10.0)	(10.6)	(11.1)	(11.7)	(12.3)	(13.5)	(14.4)	(15.7)	(17.5)

* Data are from the British Journal of Radiology (5).
† Values in parentheses represent extrapolated data.

Table A.9.2.
Cobalt-60 tissue-maximum ratios

	Field (cm) and S_p									
Depth (cm)	0 × 0 0.965	4 × 4 0.979	5 × 5 0.982	6 × 6 0.986	7 × 7 0.989	8 × 8 0.993	10 × 10 1.000	12 × 12 1.007	15 × 15 1.015	20 × 20 1.024
0.5	1.000	1.000	1.000	1.000	1.000	1.000	1.000	1.000	1.000	1.000
1.0	0.966	0.980	0.982	0.986	0.988	0.990	0.994	0.995	0.996	0.996
2.0	0.904	0.939	0.946	0.952	0.957	0.961	0.967	0.970	0.973	0.975
3.0	0.845	0.898	0.908	0.917	0.924	0.929	0.937	0.942	0947	0.951
4.0	0.792	0.857	0.870	0.880	0.808	0.895	0.905	0.911	0.919	0.925
5.0	0.741	0.815	0.829	0.841	0.851	0.858	0.870	0.879	0.889	0.898
6.0	0.694	0.771	0.788	0.801	0.811	0.820	0.834	0.843	0.855	0.867
7.0	0.649	0.728	0.745	0.759	0.771	0.781	0.796	0.808	0820	0.835
8.0	0.608	0.685	0.702	0.717	0.730	0.741	0.757	0.770	0.786	0.804
9.0	0.570	0.645	0.663	0.677	0.690	0.701	0.719	0.733	0.750	0.772
10.0	0.534	0.607	0.624	0.638	0.651	0.662	0.682	0.690	0.717	0.740
11.0	0.501	0.571	0.588	0.602	0.615	0.627	0.646	0.663	0.683	0.709
12.0	0.469	0.537	0.553	0.567	0.581	0.592	0.613	0.630	0.651	0.679
13.0	0.439	0.504	0.520	0.534	0.547	0.559	0.581	0.598	0.620	0.649
14.0	0.412	0.474	0.489	0.502	0.516	0.530	0.551	0.569	0.592	0.621
15.0	0.386	0.446	0.461	0.476	0.487	0.499	0.521	0.540	0.563	0.594
16.0	0.361	0.420	0.434	0.447	0.460	0.471	0.493	0.512	0.536	0.567
17.0	0.338	0.395	0.409	0.422	0.434	0.445	0.467	0.485	0.510	0.541
18.0	0.317	0.372	0.386	0.399	0.410	0.421	0.442	0.460	0.485	0.517
19.0	0.296	0.350	0.363	0.375	0.387	0.397	0.418	0.436	0.461	0.494
20.0	0.278	0.328	0.340	0.352	0.363	0.374	0.395	0.413	0.437	0.472
22.0	0.246	0.290	0.302	0.313	0.323	0.333	0.351	0.371	0.395	0.428
24.0	0.215	0.256	0.266	0.276	0.286	0.296	0.313	0.331	0.356	0.388
26.0	0.187	0.225	0.234	0.243	0.252	0.261	0.279	0.296	0.310	0.352
28.0	0.164	0.198	0.207	0.215	0.222	0.230	0.247	0.264	0.286	0.319
30.0	0.144	0.175	0.182	0.190	0.198	0.204	0.220	0.236	0.257	0.287

Calculated from percent depth dose data from Reference 5, using Equation 10.5. S_p is the phantom scatter factor, calculated by Equation 10.1.

Table A.9.3.
Cobalt-60 scatter-maximum ratios for circular fields

Depth d (cm)	Field radius (cm)											
	1	2	3	4	5	6	7	8	9	10	11	12
0.5	0.007	0.014	0.019	0.026	0.032	0.037	0.043	0.048	0.054	0.058	0.063	0.067
1	0.013	0.025	0.037	0.048	0.058	0.066	0.073	0.078	0.084	0.089	0.094	0.098
2	0.023	0.045	0.064	0.080	0.091	0.102	0.110	0.116	0.122	0.127	0.133	0.139
3	0.032	0.061	0.084	0.103	0.118	0.130	0.139	0.147	0.154	0.161	0.166	0.172
4	0.038	0.071	0.099	0.121	0.137	0.151	0.162	0.170	0.179	0.186	0.191	0.197
5	0.041	0.076	0.107	0.134	0.152	0.166	0.178	0.189	0.198	0.206	0.212	0.218
6	0.042	0.080	0.114	0.141	0.160	0.176	0.190	0.201	0.211	0.219	0.226	0.234
7	0.042	0.081	0.115	0.143	0.164	0.181	0.196	0.209	0.220	0.229	0.239	0.246
8	0.041	0.080	0.114	0.142	0.165	0.185	0.199	0.214	0.225	0.236	0.246	0.254
9	0.040	0.078	0.112	0.140	0.164	0.183	0.200	0.216	0.228	0.240	0.251	0.260
10	0.038	0.075	0.109	0.136	0.161	0.181	0.199	0.215	0.229	0.242	0.252	0.262
11	0.036	0.071	0.104	0.132	0.157	0.178	0.197	0.213	0.227	0.241	0.252	0.262
12	0.035	0.069	0.099	0.128	0.153	0.174	0.194	0.210	0.225	0.239	0.251	0.261
13	0.034	0.066	0.095	0.124	0.149	0.170	0.190	0.207	0.223	0.237	0.249	0.260
14	0.032	0.063	0.092	0.120	0.145	0.168	0.186	0.204	0.220	0.235	0.247	0.258
15	0.031	0.060	0.089	0.116	0.140	0.162	0.182	0.200	0.216	0.231	0.244	0.255
16	0.030	0.058	0.086	0.112	0.136	0.157	0.177	0.196	0.212	0.227	0.240	0.252
17	0.029	0.056	0.083	0.108	0.132	0.153	0.172	0.191	0.207	0.223	0.236	0.248
18	0.027	0.054	0.080	0.104	0.128	0.148	0.167	0.186	0.202	0.218	0.232	0.244
19	0.026	0.052	0.077	0.101	0.124	0.144	0.162	0.181	0.197	0.213	0.226	0.239
20	0.024	0.049	0.074	0.097	0.119	0.139	0.157	0.176	0.192	0.207	0.221	0234
22	0.022	0.044	0.067	0.088	0.109	0.128	0.146	0.163	0.180	0.194	0.208	0.222
24	0.020	0.040	0.060	0.080	0.099	0.118	0.136	0.152	0.168	0.182	0.196	0.208
26	0.018	0.036	0.054	0.073	0.091	0.108	0.125	0.142	0.156	0.170	0.184	0.196
28	0.016	0.032	0.049	0.067	0.083	0.098	0.115	0.132	0.156	0.159	0.172	0.184
30	0.015	0.030	0.045	0.061	0.076	0.089	0.105	0.121	0.134	0.146	0.159	0.170

	13	14	15	16	17	18	19	20	21	22	23	24	25
0.5	0.070	0.073	0.076	0.078	0.080	0.082	0.084	0.085	0.086	0.087	0.088	0.088	0.089
1	0.101	0.104	0.107	0.109	0.112	0.114	0.116	0.118	0.119	0.120	0.121	0.122	0.123
2	0.142	0.146	0.149	0.152	0.154	0.156	0.158	0.160	0.161	0.162	0.164	0.166	0.167
3	0.176	0.180	0.184	0.187	0.190	0.193	0.195	0.198	0.200	0.202	0.203	0.204	0.205
4	0.201	0.205	0.210	0.215	0.218	0.222	0.225	0.228	0.231	0.233	0.235	0.237	0.239
5	0.224	0.229	0.235	0.240	0.245	0.248	0.252	0.255	0.258	0.261	0.263	0.264	0.266
6	0.241	0.246	0.252	0.257	0.262	0.265	0.269	0.272	0.275	0.278	0.280	0.282	0.284
7	0.254	0.260	0.267	0.273	0.278	0.282	0.287	0.290	0.294	0.296	0.299	0.302	0.304
8	0.263	0.271	0.278	0.285	0.289	0.294	0.298	0.301	0.305	0.309	0.311	0.313	0.315
9	0.269	0.277	0.284	0.292	0.298	0.303	0.308	0.312	0.316	0.319	0.322	0.324	0.327
10	0.271	0.279	0.288	0.295	0.302	0.308	0.314	0.318	0.324	0.327	0.331	0.333	0.336
11	0.272	0.280	0.289	0.296	0.304	0.311	0.316	0.322	0.328	0.331	0.334	0.337	0.339
12	0.272	0.281	0.290	0.297	0.305	0.312	0.318	0.324	0.330	0.333	0.337	0.340	0.342
13	0.270	0.280	0.290	0.298	0.306	0.313	0.319	0.325	0.332	0.335	0.340	0.342	0.345
14	0.268	0.279	0.288	0.297	0.305	0.313	0.320	0.326	0.333	0.337	0.341	0.344	0.347
15	0.266	0.277	0.286	0.295	0.303	0.311	0.318	0.325	0.331	0.336	0.340	0.344	0.347
16	0.263	0.274	0.283	0.292	0.300	0.308	0.315	0.322	0.328	0.333	0.337	0.342	0.346
17	0.259	0.271	0.279	0.288	0.296	0.304	0.311	0.318	0.324	0.329	0.334	0.339	0.343
18	0.255	0.266	0.275	0.284	0.292	0.300	0.307	0.313	0.320	0.325	0.330	0.335	0.339
19	0.251	0.261	0.270	0.280	0.288	0.295	0.303	0.309	0.315	0.321	0.326	0.331	0.335
20	0.246	0.257	0.265	0.275	0.284	0.291	0.299	0.305	0.311	0.316	0.321	0.326	0.329
22	0.233	0.246	0.255	0.264	0.273	0.280	0.288	0.295	0.301	0.306	0.311	0.316	0.319
24	0.220	0.235	0.243	0.252	0.259	0.267	0.275	0.281	0.288	0.294	0.299	0.304	0.309
26	0.207	0.219	0.229	0.236	0.245	0.253	0.260	0.266	0.272	0.279	0.284	0.289	0.295
28	0.194	0.205	0.214	0.222	0.230	0.238	0.245	0.251	0.258	0.264	0.269	0.274	0.279
30	0.181	0.191	0.200	0.208	0.215	0.223	0.230	0.236	0.242	0.249	0.255	0.260	0.265

As discussed in Section 10.1D, SMRs are equal to SARs for cobalt-60. For higher energies, SARs cannot be as accurately measured. The SAR data in the above table are taken from Johns and Cunningham (2).

Table A.10.1.
4-MV x-ray percent depth doses: 100 cm SSD*

Depth (cm)	0.0 × 0.0 0.97	4.0 × 4.0 0.98	6.0 × 6.0 0.99	8.0 × 8.0 0.99	10.0 × 10.0 1.00	12.0 × 12.0 1.00	15.0 × 15.0 1.01	20.0 × 20.0 1.01	25.0 × 25.0 1.02	30.0 × 30.0 1.02
1.0	100.0	100.0	100.0	100.0	100.0	100.0	100.0	100.0	100.0	100.0
2.0	93.2	96.5	97.0	97.2	97.4	97.4	97.4	97.7	97.9	97.9
3.0	86.9	91.3	92.3	92.7	92.9	93.2	93.6	94.0	94.4	94.3
4.0	81.1	85.4	87.3	88.0	88.5	89.1	89.4	90.2	90.5	90.3
5.0	75.6	81.1	83.1	84.3	84.8	85.2	85.4	86.4	87.0	86.9
6.0	70.5	76.0	78.4	79.6	80.3	80.9	81.6	82.6	82.9	83.1
7.0	65.9	71.1	73.8	75.4	76.4	77.0	77.8	78.8	79.3	79.7
8.0	61.4	66.4	69.4	71.3	72.5	73.3	74.1	75.2	75.9	76.5
9.0	57.4	62.1	65.1	67.1	68.6	69.5	70.3	71.6	72.4	73.2
10.0	53.5	58.0	61.0	63.1	64.8	65.8	66.7	68.2	69.1	70.0
11.0	50.1	54.6	57.4	59.6	61.3	62.3	63.3	64.8	65.9	66.8
12.0	46.9	51.3	54.0	56.2	57.9	58.9	59.9	61.5	62.7	63.8
13.0	43.7	48.1	50.8	53.0	54.6	55.7	56.7	58.3	59.7	60.9
14.0	40.7	45.0	47.6	49.8	51.5	52.5	53.6	55.2	56.7	58.1
15.0	38.2	42.1	44.7	46.8	48.5	49.6	50.7	52.5	54.0	55.4
16.0	35.7	39.2	41.8	43.9	45.6	46.7	48.0	49.9	51.4	52.7
17.0	33.3	36.4	39.1	41.1	42.7	43.9	45.3	47.3	48.8	50.1
18.0	31.0	33.8	36.5	38.4	40.0	41.3	42.8	44.9	46.3	47.5
19.0	29.1	31.8	34.3	36.2	37.8	39.0	40.5	42.6	44.1	45.5
20.0	27.2	29.9	32.2	34.0	35.6	36.8	38.2	40.4	42.0	43.5
21.0	25.4	28.0	30.2	31.9	33.5	34.6	36.0	38.2	40.0	41.6
22.0	23.7	26.2	28.2	29.9	31.4	32.5	33.9	36.2	38.0	39.7
23.0	22.3	24.6	26.6	28.2	29.6	30.7	32.1	34.3	36.1	37.7
24.0	20.9	23.1	25.1	26.6	27.9	28.9	30.2	32.4	34.1	35.7
25.0	19.5	21.7	23.6	25.0	26.2	27.1	28.5	30.7	32.3	33.7
26.0	18.2	20.3	22.1	23.4	24.6	25.4	26.8	28.9	30.4	31.8
27.0	17.1	19.1	20.8	22.1	23.2	24.1	25.3	27.4	28.9	30.4
28.0	16.0	17.9	19.6	20.8	21.9	22.7	23.9	25.9	27.5	29.0
29.0	15.0	16.7	18.3	19.5	20.6	21.4	22.5	24.4	26.1	27.7
30.0	14.0	15.6	17.2	18.3	19.3	20.1	21.2	23.0	24.8	26.4

Field size (cm)† and S_p

* Source-surface distance.
† Data are from the University of Minnesota, EMI-4 Linac. S_p is the phantom scatter correction factor (Equation 10.2).

Table A.10.2.
4-MV x-ray tissue-maximum ratios

Depth (cm)	Field size (cm)									
	0.0 × 0.0	4.0 × 4.0	6.0 × 6.0	8.0 × 8.0	10.0 × 10.0	12.0 × 12.0	15.0 × 15.0	20.0 × 20.0	25.0 × 25.0	30.0 × 30.0
1.0	1.000	1.000	1.000	1.000	1.000	1.000	1.000	1.000	1.000	1.000
2.0	0.951	0.984	0.989	0.991	0.993	0.993	0.994	0.996	0.999	0.998
3.0	0.904	0.948	0.959	0.963	0.966	0.968	0.973	0.977	0.981	0.981
4.0	0.860	0.903	0.924	0.931	0.937	0.943	0.947	0.955	0.958	0.957
5.0	0.817	0.874	0.894	0.909	0.914	0.919	0.922	0.931	0.938	0.939
6.0	0.777	0.833	0.858	0.875	0.882	0.889	0.896	0.907	0.912	0.913
7.0	0.739	0.793	0.822	0.842	0.853	0.861	0.870	0.881	0.887	0.892
8.0	0.702	0.753	0.785	0.809	0.823	0.834	0.843	0.856	0.863	0.870
9.0	0.668	0.716	0.749	0.774	0.791	0.803	0.814	0.829	0.838	0.846
10.0	0.635	0.679	0.713	0.739	0.759	0.773	0.785	0.802	0.813	0.823
11.0	0.606	0.651	0.683	0.709	0.730	0.745	0.757	0.774	0.787	0.798
12.0	0.577	0.622	0.653	0.679	0.701	0.716	0.729	0.747	0.761	0.774
13.0	0.548	0.594	0.623	0.649	0.671	0.687	0.701	0.720	0.735	0.749
14.0	0.519	0.565	0.593	0.620	0.642	0.659	0.673	0.692	0.709	0.725
15.0	0.495	0.535	0.565	0.591	0.614	0.631	0.647	0.668	0.686	0.701
16.0	0.471	0.505	0.537	0.563	0.585	0.603	0.620	0.643	0.662	0.678
17.0	0.447	0.475	0.509	0.535	0.557	0.575	0.594	0.619	0.639	0.654
18.0	0.423	0.445	0.481	0.507	0.528	0.547	0.567	0.594	0.615	0.631
19.0	0.404	0.426	0.459	0.485	0.505	0.524	0.544	0.571	0.594	0.611
20.0	0.384	0.407	0.438	0.462	0.482	0.501	0.521	0.549	0.572	0.590
21.0	0.365	0.388	0.416	0.439	0.460	0.478	0.498	0.526	0.550	0.570
22.0	0.346	0.369	0.395	0.417	0.437	0.455	0.475	0.503	0.528	0.550
23.0	0.330	0.352	0.378	0.399	0.418	0.436	0.455	0.482	0.508	0.529
24.0	0.315	0.335	0.360	0.381	0.400	0.416	0.435	0.462	0.488	0.508
25.0	0.299	0.318	0.343	0.364	0.381	0.397	0.414	0.442	0.467	0.487
26.0	0.283	0.301	0.326	0.346	0.362	0.377	0.394	0.421	0.447	0.466
27.0	0.270	0.286	0.311	0.330	0.346	0.361	0.378	0.404	0.429	0.449
28.0	0.258	0.272	0.296	0.315	0.330	0.345	0.362	0.386	0.411	0.431
29.0	0.245	0.257	0.281	0.300	0.314	0.329	0.346	0.369	0.393	0.414
30.0	0.232	0.242	0.266	0.284	0.298	0.312	0.330	0.352	0.375	0.397

* Calculated from data in Table A.10.1, using Equation 10.4.

Table A.10.3.

4-MV x-ray scatter-maximum ratios for circular fields

Depth (cm)	Radius (cm)												
	2.0	4.0	6.0	8.0	10.0	12.0	14.0	16.0	18.0	20.0	22.0	24.0	26.0
1.0	0.000	0.000	0.000	0.000	0.000	0.000	0.000	0.000	0.000	0.000	0.000	0.000	0.000
2.0	0.035	0.039	0.042	0.042	0.041	0.043	0.052	0.049	0.045	0.040	0.036	0.032	0.027
3.0	0.039	0.059	0.062	0.068	0.071	0.074	0.079	0.077	0.076	0.074	0.073	0.071	0.069
4.0	0.045	0.070	0.080	0.086	0.092	0.098	0.100	0.099	0.097	0.095	0.093	0.092	0.090
5.0	0.048	0.093	0.099	0.102	0.109	0.117	0.124	0.122	0.120	0.118	0.116	0.114	0.112
6.0	0.048	0.095	0.108	0.118	0.126	0.133	0.135	0.136	0.137	0.138	0.139	0.140	0.141
7.0	0.049	0.098	0.111	0.125	0.137	0.147	0.154	0.155	0.156	0.157	0.159	0.160	0.161
8.0	0.046	0.101	0.126	0.139	0.148	0.156	0.161	0.166	0.170	0.174	0.179	0.183	0.187
9.0	0.042	0.098	0.131	0.145	0.154	0.163	0.171	0.175	0.178	0.182	0.186	0.190	0.193
10.0	0.048	0.096	0.131	0.148	0.160	0.171	0.179	0.185	0.192	0.198	0.204	0.210	0.216
11.0	0.048	0.097	0.131	0.150	0.163	0.175	0.185	0.191	0.198	0.204	0.210	0.217	0.223
12.0	0.041	0.092	0.127	0.150	0.163	0.176	0.188	0.195	0.202	0.209	0.215	0.222	0.229
13.0	0.043	0.093	0.129	0.153	0.167	0.179	0.191	0.200	0.209	0.218	0.227	0.236	0.244
14.0	0.043	0.091	0.131	0.152	0.165	0.178	0.191	0.201	0.211	0.221	0.231	0.241	0.251
15.0	0.036	0.084	0.122	0.147	0.165	0.180	0.193	0.200	0.206	0.212	0.218	0.224	0.230
16.0	0.031	0.080	0.119	0.145	0.164	0.180	0.195	0.203	0.211	0.220	0.228	0.236	0.244
17.0	0.036	0.080	0.119	0.143	0.160	0.178	0.196	0.208	0.219	0.229	0.240	0.251	0.262
18.0	0.033	0.075	0.112	0.140	0.159	0.177	0.193	0.203	0.213	0.222	0.232	0.241	0.250
19.0	0.033	0.074	0.113	0.140	0.158	0.175	0.193	0.202	0.211	0.220	0.229	0.238	0.247
20.0	0.029	0.072	0.109	0.138	0.156	0.175	0.193	0.203	0.213	0.222	0.232	0.242	0.251
21.0	0.030	0.068	0.104	0.131	0.151	0.171	0.189	0.203	0.216	0.229	0.242	0.255	0.268
22.0	0.025	0.063	0.098	0.126	0.145	0.164	0.184	0.198	0.212	0.226	0.241	0.255	0.269
23.0	0.031	0.061	0.093	0.123	0.142	0.159	0.178	0.191	0.202	0.214	0.226	0.237	0.249
24.0	0.029	0.061	0.092	0.122	0.138	0.153	0.172	0.187	0.202	0.216	0.230	0.245	0.259
25.0	0.026	0.055	0.086	0.115	0.135	0.152	0.169	0.182	0.195	0.207	0.220	0.233	0.246
26.0	0.028	0.057	0.085	0.108	0.126	0.145	0.167	0.178	0.190	0.201	0.212	0.223	0.234
27.0	0.026	0.051	0.080	0.108	0.128	0.146	0.162	0.174	0.185	0.196	0.208	0.219	0.231
28.0	0.025	0.052	0.079	0.104	0.120	0.137	0.159	0.171	0.183	0.194	0.205	0.216	0.228
29.0	0.021	0.049	0.075	0.098	0.115	0.133	0.152	0.165	0.177	0.189	0.201	0.214	0.226
30.0	0.023	0.048	0.072	0.096	0.111	0.126	0.145	0.160	0.174	0.189	0.204	0.219	0.234

Calculated from Table A.10.1, using Equation 10.6.

Table A.11.1
10-MV x-ray percent depth doses

Depth (cm)	0 × 0	A/P and field size (cm)								
		1.00 4 × 4	1.50 6 × 6	2.00 8 × 8	2.50 10 × 10	3.00 12 × 12	3.75 15 × 15	5.00 20 × 20	6.25 25 × 25	7.50 30 × 30
0	5.0	6.5	8.5	10.7	12.5	14.5	17.0	21.0	24.5	28.0
0.2	37.0	40.0	43.0	45.0	46.5	48.0	50.0	52.5	54.0	56.0
0.5	65.0	67.0	69.0	70.5	72.0	73.0	74.0	76.0	77.0	79.0
1.0	86.0	88.0	89.0	90.0	91.0	91.5	92.0	93.0	94.0	95.0
1.5	94.5	95.5	96.0	96.5	97.0	97.0	97.5	98.0	98.0	98.5
2.0	96.5	97.5	98.0	98.0	98.0	98.5	99.0	99.0	99.5	99.5
2.5	100.0	100.0	100.0	100.0	100.0	100.0	100.0	100.0	100.0	100.0
3.0	97.4	99.0	99.0	99.0	99.0	99.0	99.0	99.0	99.0	99.0
4.0	92.3	96.4	96.4	96.4	96.4	96.5	96.5	96.5	96.5	96.5
5.0	87.5	91.6	91.8	91.9	92.1	92.2	92.3	92.5	92.6	92.7
6.0	83.0	87.0	87.4	87.7	87.9	88.1	88.3	88.6	88.8	89.0
7.0	78.7	82.6	83.2	83.6	83.9	84.2	84.5	84.9	85.2	85.5
8.0	74.7	78.5	79.2	79.7	80.1	80.4	80.8	81.4	81.8	82.1
9.0	70.8	74.6	75.4	76.0	76.5	76.9	77.3	78.0	78.4	78.8
10.0	67.2	70.8	71.8	72.5	73.0	73.5	74.0	74.7	75.3	75.7
11.0	63.8	67.3	68.4	69.1	69.7	70.2	70.8	71.6	72.2	72.7
12.0	60.6	63.9	65.1	65.9	66.6	67.1	67.7	68.6	69.3	69.8
13.0	57.5	60.7	62.0	62.8	63.5	64.1	64.8	65.7	66.5	67.1
14.0	54.6	57.7	59.0	59.9	60.7	61.3	62.0	63.0	63.8	64.4
15.0	51.9	54.8	56.2	57.1	57.9	58.5	59.3	60.4	61.2	61.8
16.0	49.3	52.1	53.5	54.5	55.3	55.9	56.8	57.8	58.7	59.4
17.0	46.8	49.5	50.9	52.0	52.8	53.5	54.3	55.4	56.3	57.0
18.0	44.5	47.0	48.5	49.5	50.4	51.1	52.0	53.1	54.0	54.8
19.0	42.3	44.7	46.1	47.2	48.1	48.8	49.7	50.9	51.8	52.6
20.0	40.2	42.4	43.9	45.0	45.9	46.7	47.6	48.8	49.7	50.5
22.0	36.3	38.3	39.8	41.0	41.9	42.6	43.5	44.8	45.8	46.6
24.0	32.8	34.6	36.1	37.2	38.2	38.9	39.9	41.1	42.1	43.0
26.0	29.7	31.2	32.7	33.9	34.8	35.5	36.5	37.8	38.8	39.6
28.0	26.9	28.1	29.7	30.8	31.7	32.5	33.4	34.7	35.7	36.5
30.0	24.3	25.4	26.9	28.0	28.9	29.6	30.6	31.8	32.9	33.7

Data are from Khan *et al.* (6) for the Toshiba LMR-13 Linac. $S_p \simeq 1.0$ for this energy.

Table A.11.2
10-MV x-ray tissue-maximum ratios*

Depth d (cm)	A/P and field size (cm)†									
	0 × 0	1.00 4 × 4	1.50 6 × 6	2.00 8 × 8	2.50 10 × 10	3.00 12 × 12	3.75 15 × 15	5.00 20 × 20	6.25 25 × 25	7.50 30 × 30
0	0.048	0.062	0.081	0.102	0.119	0.138	0.162	0.200	0.233	0.267
0.2	0.354	0.382	0.411	0.430	0.444	0.459	0.478	0.502	0.516	0.535
0.5	0.625	0.644	0.663	0.678	0.692	0.702	0.711	0.731	0.740	0.759
1.0	0.835	0.854	0.864	0.874	0.884	0.888	0.893	0.903	0.913	0.922
1.5	0.927	0.936	0.941	0.946	0.951	0.951	0.956	0.961	0.961	0.966
2.0	0.956	0.966	0.970	0.970	0.970	0.975	0.980	0.980	0.985	0.985
2.5	1.000	1.000	1.000	1.000	1.000	1.000	1.000	1.000	1.000	1.000
3.0	0.983	1.000	1.000	1.000	1.000	1.000	1.000	1.000	1.000	1.000
4.0	0.950	0.992	0.992	0.993	0.993	0.993	0.993	0.993	0.993	0.994
5.0	0.918	0.960	0.963	0.965	0.966	0.967	0.968	0.970	0.971	0.972
6.0	0.887	0.930	0.934	0.937	0.939	0.941	0.944	0.947	0.949	0.951
7.0	0.858	0.899	0.906	0.910	0.913	0.916	0.920	0.924	0.928	0.931
8.0	0.829	0.870	0.878	0.884	0.888	0.892	0.896	0.902	0.906	0.910
9.0	0.801	0.841	0.851	0.858	0.863	0.867	0.873	0.880	0.885	0.889
10.0	0.774	0.813	0.824	0.832	0.838	0.843	0.850	0.858	0.864	0.869
11.0	0.748	0.786	0.798	0.807	0.814	0.820	0.827	0.836	0.843	0.849
12.0	0.723	0.760	0.773	0.783	0.791	0.797	0.805	0.815	0.823	0.830
13.0	0.699	0.734	0.749	0.759	0.768	0.774	0.783	0.794	0.803	0.810
14.0	0.676	0.709	0.725	0.736	0.745	0.752	0.762	0.774	0.783	0.791
15.0	0.653	0.684	0.701	0.713	0.723	0.731	0.741	0.753	0.764	0.772
16.0	0.631	0.661	0.678	0.691	0.701	0.710	0.720	0.734	0.744	0.753
17.0	0.610	0.638	0.656	0.669	0.680	0.689	0.700	0.714	0.726	0.735
18.0	0.589	0.615	0.634	0.648	0.659	0.669	0.680	0.695	0.707	0.717
19.0	0.570	0.593	0.613	0.628	0.639	0.649	0.661	0.676	0.689	0.699
20.0	0.551	0.572	0.593	0.608	0.620	0.629	0.642	0.658	0.671	0.681
22.0	0.514	0.532	0.553	0.569	0.582	0.592	0.605	0.622	0.636	0.647
24.0	0.480	0.494	0.516	0.533	0.546	0.556	0.570	0.588	0.602	0.614
26.0	0.449	0.458	0.481	0.498	0.511	0.522	0.536	0.555	0.570	0.583
28.0	0.419	0.425	0.448	0.465	0.479	0.490	0.505	0.524	0.539	0.552
30.0	0.392	0.394	0.417	0.434	0.448	0.459	0.474	0.494	0.509	0.523

* Data are calculated from Table A.11.1 and are from Reference 7.
† Projected at depth d.

Table A.11.3.
10-MV x-ray scatter-maximum ratios

Depth d (cm)	Field radius (cm) at depth d												
	2	4	6	8	10	12	14	16	18	20	22	24	26
2.5	0	0	0	0	0	0	0	0	0	0	0	0	0
3.0	0.017	0.017	0.017	0.017	0.017	0.017	0.017	0.017	0.017	0.017	0.017	0.017	0.017
4.0	0.042	0.042	0.043	0.043	0.043	0.043	0.043	0.043	0.044	0.044	0.044	0.044	0.044
6.0	0.043	0.048	0.053	0.056	0.058	0.060	0.062	0.063	0.065	0.066	0.067	0.068	0.069
8.0	0.041	0.052	0.060	0.066	0.070	0.074	0.077	0.080	0.082	0.084	0.086	0.088	0.090
10.0	0.039	0.055	0.066	0.074	0.080	0.085	0.089	0.093	0.097	0.100	0.102	0.105	0.107
12.0	0.037	0.056	0.070	0.080	0.087	0.094	0.099	0.104	0.109	0.112	0.116	0.119	0.122
14.0	0.033	0.056	0.072	0.084	0.093	0.101	0.107	0.113	0.118	0.123	0.127	0.130	0.134
16.0	0.030	0.055	0.073	0.086	0.097	0.106	0.113	0.119	0.125	0.130	0.135	0.140	0.144
18.0	0.026	0.053	0.073	0.088	0.099	0.109	0.117	0.124	0.131	0.137	0.142	0.147	0.151
20.0	0.021	0.051	0.072	0.088	0.101	0.111	0.120	0.128	0.135	0.141	0.147	0.152	0.157
22.0	0.018	0.048	0.071	0.087	0.101	0.112	0.121	0.129	0.137	0.144	0.150	0.155	0.161
24.0	0.014	0.045	0.069	0.086	0.100	0.112	0.121	0.130	0.138	0.145	0.152	0.158	0.163
26.0	0.009	0.042	0.066	0.084	0.098	0.110	0.121	0.130	0.138	0.145	0.152	0.158	0.164
28.0	0.006	0.039	0.063	0.082	0.096	0.109	0.119	0.129	0.137	0.145	0.152	0.158	0.164
30.0	0.002	0.035	0.060	0.079	0.094	0.106	0.117	0.127	0.136	0.143	0.151	0.157	0.163

Data are calculated from Table A.11.1 and are from Reference 7.

References

1. Task Group 21, Radiation Therapy Committee, American Association of Physicists in Medicine: A protocol for the determination of absorbed dose from high energy photon and electron beams. *Med Phys* 10:741, 1983.
2. Johns HE, Cunningham JR: *The Physics of Radiology*, 4th ed. Springfield, IL, Charles C Thomas, 1983.
3. Hubbell JH: Photon mass attenuation and energy-absorption coefficients from 1 keV to 20 MeV. *Int J Appl Radiat Isotopes* 33:1269, 1982.
4. Berger MJ, Seltzer SM: *Stopping Powers and Ranges of Electrons and Positrons*, 2nd ed. Washington, DC, US Department of Commerce, National Bureau of Standards, 1983.
5. Hospital Physicists' Association: Central axis depth dose data for use in radiotherapy. *Br J Radiol* (Suppl. 11) 1978.
6. Khan FM, Moore VC, Sato S: Depth dose and scatter analysis of 10 MV x-rays. *Radiology* 102:165, 1972.
7. Khan FM: Depth dose and scatter analysis of 10 MV x-rays (letter to the editor). *Radiology* 106:662, 1973.

Index

Page numbers in *italics* denote figures; those followed by "t" or "f" denote tables or footnotes, respectively.